Oxford

Diagnosis and management of dementia: a manual for memory disorders teams

Diagnosis and management of dementia

A manual for memory disorders teams

Edited by
Gordon K. Wilcock
Department of Care of the Elderly, University of Bristol, Frenchay Day Hospital, Bristol, UK

Romola S. Bucks
Department of Care of the Elderly, University of Bristol, The BRACE Centre, Blackberry Hill Hospital, Bristol, UK

Kenneth Rockwood
Division of Geriatric Medicine, Dalhousie University, Queen Elizabeth II Health Sciences Centre, Halifax, Canada

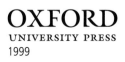

OXFORD
UNIVERSITY PRESS
1999

OXFORD
UNIVERSITY PRESS

Great Clarendon Street, Oxford OX2 6DP

Oxford University Press is a department of the University of Oxford
and furthers the University's aim of excellence in research, scholarship,
and education by publishing worldwide in

Oxford New York

Athens Auckland Bangkok Bogotá Buenos Aires Calcutta
Cape Town Chennai Dar es Salaam Delhi Florence Hong Kong Istanbul
Karachi Kuala Lumpur Madrid Melbourne Mexico City Mumbai
Nairobi Paris São Paulo Singapore Taipei Tokyo Toronto Warsaw

and associated companies in Berlin Ibadan

Oxford is a registered trade mark of Oxford University Press

Published in the United States
by Oxford University Press Inc., New York

British Library Cataloguing in Publication Data
(Data available)

Library of Congress Cataloging in Publication Data
(Data applied for)

ISBN 0 19 262815 1 (Hbk)
ISBN 0 19 262822 4 (Pbk)

Typeset by Footnote Graphics, Warminster, Wilts
Printed in Great Britain by Biddles Ltd., Guildford, Surrey

Contents

Preface

Gordon K. Wilcock, Romola S. Bucks, and Kenneth Rockwood

Organized services for people with memory disorders are growing. This growth is variously spurred by an increase in the numbers of people with memory problems (largely a reflection of the prevalence of dementia in an ageing population) and by an increased appreciation of the complexity of needs of such patients (witness simply the new diagnostic categories for vascular dementia, dementia with Lewy bodies, and frontotemporal dementia). Further growth is likely, especially now that we appear to have crossed the threshold of effective treatment for many patients with dementia.

With this increased appreciation of the needs of patients with dementia, and of the ability to meet them, has come recognition of the necessity for an interdisciplinary approach to management. On the medical side alone a person with dementia will usually require, in addition to the services of the medical dementia specialist (usually a geriatrician, psychiatrist, or neurologist), the skills of a family physician, neuroradiologist, nuclear medicine physician, neuropsychologist, or even neurosurgeon. Nurses, counselling and clinical psychologists, social workers, occupational therapists, speech therapists, pharmacists, and clergy also have important roles to play in caring for individuals and their families. And this is not to forget those important voluntary services and social services which provide essential support to sufferers and their family members.

The effective organization of such disparate resources does not just happen, but requires an understanding both of the patients' needs and the skills of the various professions, as well as realistic expectations about what can be achieved. We have brought this book together to help achieve effective care through memory disorders teams, whether they work in a specialized memory disorders clinic or in the community.

The contributors are experts in their areas and, as can be seen from many of the chapters, they enjoy and are challenged by their work—and are often not shy about challenging others to do better. In editing, we have chiefly attempted to arrive at clarity of expression and to avoid duplication (although we have been mindful that some repetition is necessary to give individual chapters coherence). We have not, however, attempted to minimize controversy, nor have we sought to impose uniformity of tone or approach.

The book is organized along the following lines. Section 1 covers *'Establishing and organizing a clinic'*, including the administrative and information needs of a memory disorders team as well as the possible staff members and what they can offer to the assessment process. Section 2 covers the *'Diagnostic process'* and includes a discussion about when normal ageing changes become abnormal as well as chapters on differentiating common and uncommon dementing conditions. Section 3 looks at *'Management'* issues in dementia from the hospital through to primary care, from the perspective of both the carer and the patient. In the *Appendix* we report the results of a survey of the memory disorders services run by the authors of this book at the time it was being prepared. We believe the results of this survey demonstrate both the common core features and the fascinating variability in practice across the world. We hope that readers will find this section helpful in deciding how their own services will be run.

Perhaps the greatest challenge in providing diagnostic services and care in dementia is the heterogeneity of patients and their needs. This heterogeneity poses both theoretical and practical difficulties. We welcome attempts to embrace this individuality of patients. In particular, we support the growing awareness of the experience of the individual with dementia—often a neglected dimension in service provision. Notwithstanding this heterogeneity, the use of staging approaches to dementia (particularly Alzheimer's disease) has been advocated by some of the authors as a way of matching services with needs. Thus, the book makes reference to presymptomatic, mild, moderate, and severe dementia as useful organizing principles. We do not, however, advocate the use of algorithms or care maps. We are aware of the need for flexibility in the application of the principles involved in assessing and managing people with dementia, depending also on the context in which the reader is working. The key must be in individualizing care.

Care of patients with dementia is complex however, and must include the carers and the environments in which we operate. From this readily flows the rationale of multidimensional care. We believe, nevertheless, that such care must be grounded in accurate diagnosis coupled with first-rate clinical treatment, hence our inclusion of chapters from a wide variety of backgrounds.

We are grateful to our parent institutions (the Universities of Bristol and Dalhousie) for the ongoing support of our work, and to our colleagues who have supported this endeavour. We especially acknowledge our patients and their carers for all they have taught us.

Contributors

M. Agg Information Officer, Department of Care of the Elderly, The BRACE Centre, University of Bristol, Blackberry Hill Hospital, Bristol, UK

C. Ballard Clinical Scientist/Honorary Consultant Psychiatrist, MRC Neuro-chemical Pathology Unit, Newcastle General Hospital, Newcastle, UK

B. Lynn Beattie Professor, Division of Geriatric Medicine, Vancouver Hospital and Health Sciences Centre, University of British Columbia, Vancouver, Canada

M. Bird NH & MRC Social Psychiatry Research Unit, The Australian National University, Canberra, Australia

J. Byrne Senior Lecturer in Psychiatry of Old Age, University of Manchester, Withington Hospital, Manchester, UK

L.M.T. Byrne Research Psychologist, Department of Care of the Elderly, The BRACE Centre, University of Bristol, Blackberry Hill Hospital, Bristol, UK

R.S. Bucks Clinical Neuropsychologist, Department of Care of the Elderly, The BRACE Centre, University of Bristol, Blackberry Hill Hospital, Bristol, UK

A. Burns Professor, School of Psychiatry and Behavioural Sciences, Withington Hospital, Manchester, UK

D. Carr Assistant Professor of Internal Medicine, Division of Geriatrics and Gerontology, Washington University in St Louis, School of Medicine, Older Adult Health Center, St Louis, USA

A. Carswell Associate Professor, Director, School of Rehabilitation Sciences, University of British Columbia, Vancouver, Canada

R. Eastwood Professor, St Louis University Health Sciences Center, Department of Psychiatry, St Louis, USA

H. Feldman Clinical Associate Professor, Division of Neurology, Vancouver & Health Sciences Centre, University of British Columbia, Vancouver, Canada

S.H. Ferris Professor, Department of Psychiatry, New York University School of Medicine, New York, USA

F. Forette Professor, Hospital Broca, Fondation National de Gerontologie, Paris, France

S. Gauthier Director, Alzheimer's Disease Research Unit, McGill Centre for Studies in Ageing, Verdun, Canada

J. Gilliard Director, Dementia Voice, Blackberry Hill Hospital, Bristol, UK

J.E. Graham Department of Anthropology and Sociology, University of British Columbia, Vancouver, Canada

K. Hildebrand Manager, Scientific Affairs, CroMedica Global Inc, Victoria, Canada

K.A. Jobst University Department of Medicine and Therapeutics, Gardiner Institute, Western Infirmary, Glasgow, UK

R.W. Jones Director, The Research Institute for the Care of the Elderly, St Martin's Hospital, Bath, UK

J. Lindesay Professor, Department of Psychiatry, University of Leicester, UK

D.A. Loewenstein Mount Sinai Medical Center, Department of Psychiatry, Miami Beach, USA

L.H. Mallery Division of Geriatric Medicine, Dalhousie University, Queen Elizabeth II Health Sciences Centre, Halifax, Canada

J. Marcusson Professor, Department of Geriatric Medicine, University Hospital of Linkoping, Linkoping, Sweden

J. Matthews Administrator, Bristol Memory Disorders Clinic, The BRACE Centre, University of Bristol, Blackberry Hill Hospital, Bristol, UK

B.L. Miller Professor, Department of Neurology, University of California, San Francisco, Mount Zion Hospital, San Francisco, USA

E. Mohr Professor, Chairman and Chief Executive Officer, CroMedica Global Inc, Victoria Canada

J.C. Morris Director, Memory and Aging Project, Washington University School of Medicine, St Louis, USA

J.T. O'Brien Brighton Clinic, Newcastle General Hospital, Newcastle, UK

D. O'Neill Consultant Physician, Age-Related Health Care, Meath Hospital, Dublin, Ireland

S. Page Senior Clinical Nurse, Memory Assessment Service, School of Psychiatry and Behavioural Sciences, Withington Hospital, Manchester, UK

W. Pryse-Phillips   Professor, Division of Neurology, Memorial University of Newfoundland, Health Sciences Centre, St John's, Canada

P.V. Rabins   Professor, Department of Psychiatry, Behavioural Sciences, The Johns Hopkins University, Baltimore, USA

D.N. Ripich   Associate Dean, Department of Communication Sciences, Case Western Reserve University, Cleveland, USA

K. Rockwood   Division of Geriatric Medicine, Dalhousie University, Queen Elizabeth II Health Sciences Centre, Halifax, Canada

I. Skoog   Associate Professor, Department of Psychiatry, Sahlgrenska Hospital, University of Gothenburg, Gothenburg, Sweden

J.P. Sloan   Clinical Associate Professor, Department of Family Practice, The University of British Columbia, Vancouver Hospital and Health Sciences Centre, Vancouver, Canada

R. Spiegel   Professor, Sandoz Pharmaceuticals Ltd, Basle, Switzerland

S. Stevens   Speech and Language Therapy Department, Hammersmith Hospital, London, UK

R. Suarez   Research Fellow, School of Medicine, Harbour-UCLA Medical Center, Torrance, USA

L.-O. Wahlund   Karolinska Institute, Department of Clinical Neuroscience, Division of Geriatric Medicine, Huddinge University Hospital, Huddinge, Sweden

K. Wesnes   Director, Cognitive Drug Research Ltd, Reading, UK

G.K. Wilcock   Professor, Department of Care of the Elderly, University of Bristol, Frenchay Day Hospital, Bristol, UK

R. Woods   Professor, School of Psychology, University of Wales, Bangor, UK

Commonly used abbreviations

AAMI	age-associated memory impairment
AD	Alzheimer's disease
ADL	activities of daily living
AIDS	acquired immune deficiency syndrome
BADLS	Bristol Activities of Daily Living Scale
BEHAVE-AD	Behavioural Pathology in Alzheimer's Disease Rating Scale
CAMCOG	Cambridge Cognitive Examination
CAMDEX	Cambridge Mental Disorders in the Elderly Examination
CANTAB	Cambridge Neurophysical Test Automated Battery
CDR	Clinical Dementia Rating
CERAD	Consortium to Establish a Registry for Alzheimer's Disease
C5R	Consortium of Canadian Centers for Clinical Cognitive Research
CT	computed tomography
DAFS	Direct Assessment of Functional Status
DAT	dementia of Alzheimer type
DLB	dementia with Lewy bodies
DSM	Diagnostic and Statistical Manual of Mental Disorders (various editions)
EEG	electroencephalography
FLD	frontal lobe dementia
GDS	Global Deterioration Scale
GP	general practitioner
ICD-10	International Classification of Diseases, 10th revision
MMSE	Mini-Mental State Examination
MRI	magnetic resonance imaging

NART	National Adult Reading Test
NINCDS-ADRDA	National Institiute of Neurological and Communicative Disorders and Stroke – the Alzheimer's Disease and Related Disorders Association
NINDS-AIREN	National Institiute for Neurological Disorders and Stroke with support from the Association Internationale pour la recherche et l'Enseignement en Neurosciences
NPH	normal pressure hydrocephalus
NPI	Neuropsychiatric Inventory
NSAID	non-steroidal anti-inflammatory drug
OBRA	Omnibus Budget Reconciliation Act
PET	positron emission tomography
RAVLT	Rey Auditory Verbal Learning Test
SPECT	single photon emission computed tomography
SSRI	serotonin selective re-uptake inhibitor
TSH	thyroid stimulating hormone
WAIS(-R)	Wechsler Intelligence Scale – (revised)
WMS(-R)	Wechsler Memory Scale – (revised)

1 Introduction

J. Lindesay and J.C. Morris

Specialist services for patients with memory disorders have a relatively short history and have tended to develop separately from other provision for people with dementia, such as psychogeriatric services. One increasingly popular service model, the memory clinic, has its origins in the United States, where they were first established in the mid-1970s with the aim of providing an outpatient diagnostic, treatment, and advice service for individuals with milder forms of dementia. Their genesis was to a great extent a response to the unmet needs of families of dementing individuals, who were frustrated by the apparent reluctance of many physicians to diagnose dementia in patients who lacked insight into their cognitive difficulties and who appeared superficially normal by virtue of preserved social skills and competence for basic activities of daily living. Despite this interest in dementia, they were called 'memory clinics' in order to focus attention on memory impairment as an important early sign of the disorder, and to get around the problem that dementia was often not recognized by the patients' doctors. It was also thought that the idea of a 'dementia clinic' would be unattractive and stigmatizing, and might discourage referrals (Fraser 1992). These clinics enabled interested and experienced specialists from various disciplines to collaborate in the diagnosis, management, and research into what, at that time, was an under-appreciated group of disorders. In the two decades since the first clinics were set up, their numbers have steadily grown in the United States and elsewhere; a survey carried out in 1993 in the British Isles identified 20 memory clinics active at that time (Wright and Lindesay 1995). The experience of these specialist memory disorders services has contributed significantly to the greater awareness of the problems associated with mild dementia, and so to the development of community-based services for patients and caregivers. These services have also been important in combating therapeutic nihilism and in promoting the concept of dementia (notably Alzheimer's disease) as a treatable disorder.

What exactly are memory clinics? For the most part, they have developed as local initiatives by interested individuals with particular objectives, and there is no explicitly or universally agreed operational model. However, published descriptions indicate that they are broadly similar and follow the original United States model of a hospital-based, outpatient, multidisciplinary service providing a range of detailed assessment, management, and advisory services, and acting as a focus for research and teaching activities (Reding *et al.* 1985; Knopman *et al.* 1985; Van der Cammen *et al.* 1987; Bayer *et al.* 1987; Philpot and Levy 1987; Rai and Phonsathorn 1990; Harrison and Jones 1993; McMurdo *et al.* 1993; Kelly *et al.* 1995). They tend to be based in departments of old age psychiatry, neurology, and geriatrics, but clinics are also run by neuropsychiatrists and clinical psychologists with an interest in this area. The last 20 years have also seen a considerable development of mainstream, community-based psychogeriatric services, particularly in the United Kingdom, and in comparison with these services memory clinics have been criticized on a number of counts: in particular, that their activities are restricted to small, non-representative patient populations; they are too research-focused; they are hospital-based, and have only a limited role in long-term care and support; and that their activities are marginal to and poorly co-ordinated with those of other services. The cost-effectiveness of memory clinics has also been called into question. As a result, services such as these can have difficulty in justifying their existence and in funding their activities. It is therefore necessary to identify why they are important and precisely how they add value to existing service provision for this patient group.

What, then, is the role of specialist services for patients with memory disorders, such as memory clinics, in the future development of health services? As good mainstream primary care and psychogeriatric services develop, they will have less of a part to play in the routine clinical assessment and long-term management of elderly patients with dementia, but there will still be a need for tertiary referral services for diagnostically difficult cases. Where psychogeriatric services are less well developed, and where most care for demented patients is provided at the primary care level, memory clinics are still a valuable, multidisciplinary source of expertise for those seeking help with management problems, particularly those that are more commonly encountered in patients with mild dementia, such as unsafe driving, inappropriate use of medication, financial imprudence, and family denial of the disorder.

Patient advocacy will also continue to be an important activity. Even in areas with good specialist psychogeriatric services, there is still a need for a high-profile service to act as a focus for particular groups of patients, for example those with presenile dementia, who often present significant diagnostic problems and whose needs for care and support are still inadequately met both by general adult psychiatric services and those specializing in older people. These patients are a valuable and often willing research population and memory disorders services might undertake to be responsible for their assessment and follow-up, and to co-ordinate inputs from the various statutory and voluntary services as they are needed. By this means, these services could also be the advocate for this group and encourage service developments. Taking on such a role may also be useful in securing long-term, core funding from the purchasers of health services.

One of the most important continuing functions for specialist memory disorders services, at least in some centres, will be to provide well-characterized and motivated patient samples for research. In particular, the evaluation of new pharmacological treatments for Alzheimer's disease and other dementias will require carefully selected cohorts of subjects for prelicensing Phase II and III trials, and for longer-term naturalistic studies of any drugs that are eventually licensed for these disorders (Skerritt *et al.* 1996). The inclusion and exclusion criteria for these trials are such that most patients with dementia referred to geriatric and psychogeriatric services do not meet them, and there is still a need for a distinct and separate initiative to attract and recruit eligible subjects. Longer-term studies will also need to evaluate the impact of treatments on non-cognitive features of Alzheimer's disease, such as agitation, delusions, and hallucinations, which occur more commonly in the later stages of the disorder. Non-pharmacological treatment strategies, such as memory training, prosthetic cognitive aids, exercise programmes, reality orientation, and reminiscence also need equally rigorous evaluation, and well-defined clinical samples will be crucial for the development and validation of the specific diagnostic markers and tests that will be needed if future treatments are to be targeted effectively. The cost-effectiveness of any future diagnostic markers and specific treatments will also need to be established. Post-mortem studies are still necessary to provide the neuro-pathological validation of clinical diagnosis and for neurochemical research but these are increasingly difficult to carry out in patient populations cared for by dispersed community services. Specialist memory disorders services are well placed to recruit and follow up patients (and carers) willing to co-operate in this particular area of research activity.

Memory clinics currently make a useful contribution to the undergraduate and postgraduate education of doctors, psychologists, and other health professionals. They enable trainees to develop an expertise in the use of intensive procedures for assessing cognitive function that is difficult to obtain anywhere else, and the multidisciplinary approach of the memory clinic to assessment and diagnosis helps them to experience and appreciate the contribution of professions other than their own to this process. In the survey of memory clinics by Wright and Lindesay (1995), 65 per cent reported that education was one of their major activities; ideally, this should be an explicit (and funded) function of all such services.

The scope of this book

To date, most of the publications from memory clinics have been research-oriented. The purpose of this book is to provide a practical guide to the setting up and organization of services, both clinic and community oriented, for patients with memory disorders, and to review the various diagnostic and management issues that such services raise. Memory clinics are an increasingly common model of service for this patient group but alternative approaches, such as specialist outreach teams, will also be discussed and are equally important. The first section deals with organizing and establishing a memory disorders service, and addresses administrative aspects, information management, patient assessment, and research functions. It is important that these services have policies with regard to patient referral and follow-up that accord with their intended functions; for example if the primary aim of the service is to identify subjects with Alzheimer's disease for research purposes, then it would not be a good idea to have an open referral policy, as this would probably significantly reduce the case yield. Similarly, services which routinely follow up all patients will have less capacity to assess new referrals than those which limit follow-up to those cases where there is continuing diagnostic uncertainty.

The multidisciplinary approach to assessment in both memory clinics and general psychogeriatric services is well established. However, a number of important issues in this respect remain to be clarified, which the reader interested in developing or reviewing a memory clinic may need to keep in mind. For example to what extent do the various professional assessments overlap? Does the clinician's formal assessment of cognitive function contribute anything to the diagnostic process which is not provided by neuro-psychological testing? If not, would the clinician's time be better spent in more detailed examination of non-cognitive psychopathology? What contribution does expert clinical judgement make to the diagnostic process, particularly in early and difficult cases? Increased specialization of professional input might improve the service's cost-effectiveness but would it reduce its educational value? A related issue is the question of skill mix. Memory clinics in particular vary considerably in the number and range of professions involved in the assessment process; is there a combination of professions/ skills which provides an optimal trade-off between diagnostic accuracy and cost?

The second section of this book deals with the diagnostic process and this also raises a number of issues that memory disorders services need to consider. For diagnosis of the dementias, it is important that assessment and data collection procedures keep pace with scientific developments. Our knowledge of clinical subtypes and underlying causes and risk factors is increasing rapidly, and this new understanding is already having an impact both on research and on clinical practice. For example drug trials in Alzheimer's disease increasingly require apolipoprotein E genotyping and the identification of patients meeting diagnostic criteria for Lewy body dementia in order to evaluate the impact of treatments on particular patient groups. In the future, memory disorders services may also have to take into account the emergence of new disorders, such as the new variant of Creutzfeldt-Jakob disease which has been linked with bovine spongiform encephalopathy in the United Kingdom (Will *et al.* 1996).

Memory clinics also see a significant number of patients whose subjective memory complaints are not associated with objective evidence of the cognitive deficits necessary for a diagnosis of dementia. In some cases, the memory impairment is related to an episode of depression or anxiety, and resolves when this is treated. In others, the presence of an isolated memory deficit in the absence of any functional psychiatric disorder to account for it may result in the diagnosis of 'age-associated memory impairment' or 'age-related cognitive decline'. Although this is recognized and coded by DSM-IV as 'a condition that may be a focus of clinical attention' (American Psychiatric Association 1994), it remains a controversial concept (see Chapter 13). Long-term follow-up studies are needed to establish whether it is in fact homogeneous or made up of a diverse group of individuals, some experiencing normal ageing and others in the earliest stages of a dementing process.

Although this book is concerned with the diagnosis and management of dementia, it should be noted that not all memory disorders services have dementia as their main area of interest or activity. For example the memory clinic described by Kopelman and Crawford (1996) deals principally with amnesic syndromes and memory impairments associated with non-progressive brain damage. As these authors point out, although the concept of the memory clinic has been dominated by the dementias, these other groups of patients with organic memory impairments also have assessment and management needs which are poorly met by mainstream services and they require the expertise and focus that a specialist clinic provides. Should the activities of existing memory disorders services be expanded to include this group of patients or would their needs be better served by a separate, dedicated service?

The third section of this book discusses the role of memory disorders services in relation to the management of patients with dementia. The specific research interests of services will inevitably involve them in the treatment and follow-up of selected groups of patients. However, to what extent should they be involved in the routine management of their patients? This will depend on the availability of alternative service provision; in an area with a comprehensive infrastructure of both primary care and specialist psychogeriatric services, a memory clinic will be able to confine itself to a tertiary, advisory role and dedicate its limited resources to assessment and diagnosis. In localities less well served by other services for demented patients and their carers, it may have to assume a greater responsibility for longer-term management. In general, memory disorders services should aim to complement other services and not duplicate them, and there should be clear and agreed referral procedures in both directions.

The future

It is likely that specialist services for patients with memory disorders will be among the first to encounter the important practical and ethical issues that will be raised by developments in our understanding of the dementias and our ability to treat them. The first generation of drugs with a symptomatic effect in mild to moderate Alzheimer's disease has been under development and evaluation for a number of years now, and three of these (tacrine, rivastigmine, and donepezil) have already received licences in the United States, United Kingdom, Canada, and other countries. This is raising important questions about how suitable patients should be identified and managed. There is also the so-called problem of the 'unspecified model' of successful treatment (Rockwood and Morris 1996); given that very few patients with dementia are likely to have a reversal of all their symptoms, or to be entirely protected from the development of new ones, memory disorders services are likely to play an important role in describing and defining the effects of pharmacological treatments. In the absence of a specific diagnostic marker for Alzheimer's disease, the availability of a treatment will considerably increase the demand on services such as memory clinics that are in a position to make a clinical diagnosis with a high degree of accuracy. Indeed, given recent estimates of a substantial age-associated annual incidence of Alzheimer's disease over the age of 65 years (Herbert *et al.* 1995), it is likely that demand could considerably outstrip the ability of existing memory disorders services to meet it. Any programme of public screening for dementia using a brief test, such as the Mini-Mental State Examination, would generate significant numbers of false-positives (Wilcock *et al.* 1994), and they would burden still further the diagnostic assessment services. A more practical solution to this problem would be to improve the diagnostic skills of mainstream primary care and psycho-geriatric services, and memory disorders services could make an important contribution to this by educating health professionals and by validating structured assessment tools for use in other settings.

The availability of treatment, including potential treatments in the context of drug trials, also highlights the important and unresolved issue of consent in relation to dementia. To be meaningful, consent requires competence and whether or not an individual is competent depends upon the nature and complexity of the particular decision involved—that is, it is decision specific.

Mildly demented patients may well be competent to consent to treatment or to participation in a drug trial but there is as yet no legal framework for providing such treatments to incompetent patients. Proxy consent by relatives has no legal validity, although this is usually sought in the case of subjects being recruited into trials. The doctor's common law duty of care is another consideration, although this may be of limited applicability in relation to new treatments with limited impact on the course of the disease. In the future, provision may be made for such decisions to be taken by professional advocates/ guardians/ care managers charged with acting in the overall best interests of the patient, but for now the law has yet to catch up with scientific advance in this area of medicine. Similar issues will also be raised in connection with decisions to withhold or stop treatments—hence the need for studies to determine how long patients will continue to receive benefit from antidementia drugs. Another related issue is the extent to which dementing patients can and should be involved in other decisions regarding their care, welfare, and safety, and this is turn raises questions about how, when, and if they should be told their diagnosis (Gilliard and Gwilliam 1996).

As our understanding of the molecular genetics of Alzheimer's disease advances, memory disorders services will also need to be aware of the ethical and practical issues with regard to presymptomatic testing for this disorder (Lovestone and Harper 1994). Apart from a few families with a specific mutation causing their Alzheimer's disease, no such test is yet available; the apolipoprotein allele E4 is associated with increased risk of developing the disorder but it is by no means diagnostic or predictive. However, the eventual development of such a test, particularly one which accurately identifies patients at future risk, would require services to offer pretest counselling to help patients and their families appreciate the implications of a positive result, and post-test support and follow-up to help them adjust to it. The experience of Huntington's disease services will be useful in developing policies and protocols for any future testing for Alzheimer's disease (Burns and Harris 1996).

Another issue raised by the prospect of genetic testing and other forms of presymptomatic screening for the dementias is that of confidentiality. Who will have legitimate access to this information—the patient only, their family, their health insurance company? As the example of HIV testing has shown, the answers to these questions are not straightforward, and are determined as much by public attitudes and financial considerations as by medical ethics and clinical judgement. Clinicians looking after patients with dementia in memory clinics, community mental health services, and elsewhere already face dilemmas about confidentiality in relation to driving and other potential hazards, such as gun ownership. Whilst severe dementia is clearly incompat-ible with driving, in milder cases it can be very difficult to judge when public safety takes precedence over individuals' wishes, particularly if they depend on their car to maintain an independent and fulfilling life. Although licensing authorities issue guidelines as to who is and is not fit to drive, these can be difficult to interpret in the borderline case, particularly in the absence of any objective and reliable means of measuring driving safety. These tricky ethical and medico-legal issues are among the various management problems discussed in Chapter 19.

Scientific advances in the diagnosis and treatment of Alzheimer's disease and other dementias have the potential to transform services for this group of patients in the years to come. It may be that in a perfect world there would be no need for such services (Fraser 1992), but for the foreseeable future memory clinics will have an important role, not only in contributing to basic research but also in monitoring its impact on practice and in developing protocols and procedures which will enable as many individuals as possible to benefit from significant developments.

References

Key references recommended by the authors are marked with an *.

American Psychiatric Association (1994) *Diagnostic and statistical manual of mental disorders* (4th edition). American Psychiatric Association, Washington.

Bayer, A., Pathy, J. and Twining, C. (1987) The memory clinic: A new approach to the detection of early dementia. *Drugs*, **33** (Suppl.), 84–9.

Burns, A. and Harris, J. (1996) Ethical issues in dementia. *Psychiatric Bulletin*, **20**, 107–8.

*Fraser, M. (1992) Memory clinics and memory training. In: *Recent advances in psychogeriatrics*, Vol. 2 (ed. T. Arie), pp. 105–15. Churchill Livingstone, London.

Gilliard, J. and Gwilliam, C. (1996) Sharing the diagnosis: A survey of memory disorders clinics, their policies on informing people with dementia and their families, and the support they offer. *International Journal of Geriatric Psychiatry*, **11**, 1001–3.

Harrison, M. and Jones, R.W. (1993) Don't forget memory clinics. *Geriatric Medicine*, **23**, 39–42.

Herbert, L.E., Scherr, P.A., Beckett, L.A., Albert, M.S., Pilgrim, D.M., Chown, M.J., *et al.* (1995) Age-specific incidence of Alzheimer's disease in a community population. *Journal of the American Medical Association*, **273**, 1354–9.

Kelly, C.A., Harvey, R.J., Stevens, S.J., *et al.* (1995) Specialist memory clinic:

The experience at the Hammersmith Hospital. *Facts and Research in Gerontology*, **1**, 21–30.

Knopman, D.S., Deinard, S., Kitto, J., Hartman, M. and MacKenzie, T. (1985) A clinic for dementia. Two years experience. *Minnesota Medicine*, **68**, 687–92.

*Kopelman, M. and Crawford, S. (1996) Not all memory clinics are dementia clinics. *Neuropsychological Rehabilitation*, **6**, 187–202.

Lovestone, S. and Harper, P. (1994) A genetic test for Alzheimer's disease? *Psychiatric Bulletin*, **8**, 645.

McMurdo, M.E.T., Grant, D.J., Gilchrist, J., Findlay, D., McLennan, J. and Lawrence, B. (1993) The Dundee Memory Clinic: the first 50 patients. *Health Bulletin*, **51**, 203–7.

*Philpot, M. and Levy, R. (1987) A memory clinic for the early diagnosis of dementia. *International Journal of Geriatric Psychiatry*, **2**, 195–200.

Rai, G. and Phonsathorn, V. (1990) Depression in patients with early dementia of Alzheimer type. *Care of the Elderly*, **2**, 371–2.

*Reding, M., Haycox, J. and Blass, J. (1985) Depression in patients referred to a memory clinic. *Archives of Neurology*, **42**, 894–6.

Rockwood, K. and Morris, J.C. (1996) Global staging measures in dementia. In: *Clinical diagnosis and management of Alzheimer's disease* (Ed. S. Gauthier). Martin Dunitz, London.

Skerritt, U., Pitt, B., Armstrong, S. and O'Brien, A. (1996) Recruiting patients for drug trials: a difficult task. *Psychiatric Bulletin*, **20**, 708–10.

Van der Cammen, T.J.M., Simpson, J.M., Fraser, R.M., Preker, A.S. and Exton-Smith, A.N. (1987) The memory clinic: A new approach to the detection of dementia. *British Journal of Psychiatry*, **150**, 359–64.

Wilcock, G.K., Ashworth, D.L., Langfield, J.A. and Smith, P.M. (1994) Detecting patients with Alzheimer's disease suitable for drug treatment: comparison of three methods of assessment. *British Journal of General Practice*, **44**, 30–3.

Will, R.G., Ironside, J.W., Zeidler, M., Cousens, S.N., Estibeiro, K., Alperovitch, A., *et al.* (1996) A new variant of Creutzfeldt-Jakob disease in the UK. *Lancet*, **347**, 921–5.

*Wright, N. and Lindesay, J. (1995) A survey of memory clinics in the British Isles. *International Journal of Geriatric Psychiatry*, **10**, 379–85.

1 Establishing and organizing a clinic

2 Administrative and organizational aspects

B.L. Beattie, R.S. Bucks, and J. Matthews

As the number of elderly people increases, so does the demand for services aimed at diagnosing and managing cognitive impairment, especially dementia. There is a stronger imperative than ever to study changing cognitive and functional ability in order to improve understanding, treatment, and quality of life. Though a small number of memory teams see patients who do not have dementing disorders (e.g. epilepsy, head injury, or amnesia; see Kopelman and Crawford 1996), most concentrate on older patients. For convenience this chapter focuses on patients with dementia, although the general principles apply whichever group is being served.

The multidisciplinary nature of memory teams makes them ideally suited to addressing the complexities of dementia diagnosis and care. Though there are other ways of organizing services and assessment procedures, memory disorders teams are one solution to the problem of efficiently co-ordinating the many investigations and the quantity of information which are required for an early diagnosis and intervention. This chapter will address some of the practical issues in developing a memory disorders team. Elements of the organization and rationale behind setting up a team may be useful to others who do not work in such a team.

Getting started

The critical first step in setting up a memory disorders team is to write a protocol containing the team's objectives, in clear and unambiguous terms. This will help in determining the staffing structure of the team, the referral criteria, the types of problems the team wishes to address, the length of patient follow-ups, and the means of recording information. These factors have important implications for resources, including staffing and space. For example a team providing primary care would have different needs and priorities than a secondary or tertiary referral clinic. Over time, the requirements for the team may change and thus need reviewing. Opportunity to do so should be built into the objectives.

Each of the following sections is preceded by a list of questions. As part of the process of developing the team, the members could consider these questions. By doing so, a draft protocol will emerge, although some questions will not be suitable to every clinical service and the list of questions is by no means exhaustive. Where the question is self explanatory it is not addressed in the text.

Relationship to local services

♦ How does the proposed service differ from existing services?
♦ How will the team liaise with other services?
♦ What provision will be made for the team to refer to other services?
♦ What voluntary services are there and how will the team work with them?
♦ What catchment area is the team serving?
♦ How will the service be publicized?

It is essential to establish how the new team will fit in with existing services. The new team may choose to concentrate on assessment and diagnosis but make limited interventions, preferring instead to refer for follow-up to the local or community health care system. Alternatively, the team may be part of a continuum of geriatric or psychiatric services in a district or region, or part of a health maintenance organization or community-based health service. It is necessary to clarify the types of referral the team will accept. The team will also need to clarify how referrals on to other agencies will be funded.

Referral criteria

♦ What age limits will be imposed?
♦ Which patients will be appropriate to refer to the service?
♦ Will self referral be accepted?
♦ Will referrals be accepted from any health care professional?
♦ Will the team see people with brain injury, depression/anxiety, or suspected dementia only?
♦ Will patients be seen from within or outside the catchment area?
♦ Will the general practitioner/ primary care physician need to have completed a basic screen?

The role the new team plays will be defined by the catchment area it serves and the other services available. It is unlikely, however, that the expectation

Table 2.1 Results from a survey of university memory clinics involved in the Consortium of Canadian Centres for Clinical Cognitive Research (C5R)

Number of patients	Site 1 Dalhousie	Site 3 Laval	Site 4 McGill	Site 5 Ottawa	Site 6 Toronto	Site 7 Western Ontario	Site 9 Calgary	Site 10 UBC	Total
New referrals	150	125	312	156	100	80	111	131	1165
Follow-ups	75	51	624	70	200	40	87	49	1196

of most teams will be to see all the persons in the vicinity with suspected dementia. The team could choose to see persons with unusual syndromes, difficult behaviour, psychosocial crises, early diagnosis, or those interested in taking part in research protocols or therapeutic programmes.

If family members or other care workers initiate the referral, then, obtaining doctor (usually the primary care physician) approval is important. The protocol should specify whether self referral is acceptable. Failure adequately to define the referral criteria may lead to inappropriate referrals. It may also lead to the expectations of either the referring agent or the patient not being met.

Given that memory impairment affects large numbers of the population of elderly persons, the potential numbers of patients referred to a new team may be substantial. The number of persons seen at follow-up directly affects the number who can be seen for a first appointment. Follow-up visits increase incrementally. A survey, carried out with the teams involved in the Consortium of Canadian Centres for Clinical Cognitive Research (C5R) demonstrates the large variation in the numbers of new referrals seen per year and in the numbers who were seen for follow-up (Table 2.1). Some of the variation can be explained by availability of personnel, by type of research being undertaken, and by variations in patterns of practice in local services. The issue of follow-up is discussed in more detail later in the chapter.

Some of the disciplines which may be represented in the team

- Physician/Geriatrician/Neurologist   Chapter 4;
- Psychiatrist   Chapter 5;
- Psychologist/Neuropsychologist   Chapters 7 and 18;
- Social worker   Chapter 16;
- Nurse   Chapter 11;
- Occupational therapist   Chapter 10;
- Speech and language therapist   Chapter 9;

- ◆ Geneticist   Chapter 19;
- ◆ Counsellor   Chapters 16 and 18;
- ◆ Psychology technicians/Assistants   Chapter 7.

Memory disorders teams are examples of multi- or interdisciplinary groups. They have the advantage of bringing together skilled health care professionals to provide a multidimensional assessment. There are core roles and responsibilities which need to be accounted for within the team, though there will be a degree of overlap in which team members can provide those skills. In an era of limited funding, some teams choose to employ 'cross-trained' individuals; for example a nurse who also acts as a psychometric technician and offers some counselling. Each team will need to decide the skills required, after which decisions can be made about who provides those skills. It will be apparent in the subsequent paragraphs which aspects of the multidimensional assessment may be undertaken by a number of different professionals. The chapters identified in the list above explore the roles of these teams members in more detail.

Many memory disorders teams begin with those staff already in post. Indeed, the creation of a team is an opportunity to develop links across departmental boundaries. Funding for other staff may sometimes be obtained through research grants, allowing expansion of the clinical services.

Doctors/physicians

Doctors with expertise in evaluating people with dementia or other cognitive decline may be drawn from geriatric medicine, psychiatry, neurology, and primary care. These individuals must have training, patience, good people skills, and an interest in chronic cognitive disease. They must also be sensitive to the dilemmas of patients and their caregivers.

Neuropsychologist (plus technician or assistant)

The expertise of a neuropsychologist or behavioural neurologist is extremely helpful, especially if the team has chosen to identify very early cases of dementia. If psychology assistants or technicians are available, then the role of the neuropsychologist can also be extended to develop and undertake research activities. The technician/assistant conducts neuropsychological testing and scoring whilst the neuropsychologist is responsible for their supervision, interpretation, and reports. The neuropsychologist may also offer advice to patients and caregivers on techniques and devices to aid in the management of cognitive disorders (see Chapter 18 for a discussion of non-pharmacological approaches to treatment).

Social worker, counsellor, community psychiatric nurse, and/or clinical psychologist

The activities of these team members are to provide assessment of the social situation, to explore relationship issues, and to facilitate the counselling and development of coping strategies for the caregivers and the patients, as appropriate. Team members will need a good knowledge of community services, both formal systems and informal, such as Alzheimer Disease societies. Any of these personnel may also facilitate development of support groups to meet the special needs of family members of patients or of the patients themselves, especially those who are mildly impaired and have insight. Support for caregivers is discussed in more detail in Chapter 16 and strategies for helping sufferers are covered in Chapter 19.

Nurse

Nurses are able to assist the patient when they are to be examined and can take samples for laboratory testing. In some memory disorders teams the nurse also undertakes cognitive assessment, interviews the patient and their relatives, and, in the case of community teams, may also conduct a home assessment (see Chapter 11, Assessment in the community). The nurse may also have a role in the functions described in the paragraph above.

Administration and other staff

◆ Who will act as co-ordinator/ administrator for the team?
◆ How much time will they need to do this?
◆ What secretarial support will the team need?
◆ What could volunteers do for the team?
◆ Will there be someone who arranges for autopsy consent?

Administration staff are invaluable members of the team. Good telephone skills are critical. Administration staff must have an understanding of how cognitive change affects sufferers and their caregivers in order to be able to communicate well with them. Empathy is essential, though skills in closing a conversation may also be useful.

Co-ordinator/ administrator

The team needs a co-ordinator or administrator. This person may be a nurse or from another discipline, and must have excellent organizational skills as all other teams members will depend on them for information about the timetable and the patients. The administrator will be responsible for collating background information about the patient prior to assessment. Ideally, the team would also have a booking clerk and secretary. In reality, many smaller teams rely on medical secretaries or an administrator to fulfil all these roles. As the team grows this arrangement needs reviewing. The co-ordinator/ administrator may also be able to play a more direct role in patient care, perhaps taking part in support groups or conducting focus groups and patient satisfaction surveys.

Volunteers and other personnel

Volunteers can be invaluable. They may act as escorts, they may accompany patients while family members talk to staff members, they may offer refreshments and keep patients and their family company. Overall, they provide a friendly welcome to patients and families. This is important when the co-ordinator or nurse is tied up with other duties. Depending on the team's location there may also be students from medicine, psychiatry, nursing, social work, or psychology. These students may be involved with assessments, interventions, and research programmes but will need appropriate supervision, training, and indemnity.

Where and when

- ◆ Where will assessments be carried out?
- ◆ On which days will the team assess patients?
- ◆ Who will see the patients?
- ◆ How long will each part of the assessment take?

Where will the clinic be held?

This depends largely on the availability of local resources. Ideally, the team should meet in a setting which is private, comfortable, and free from distractions and where there is an interview room large enough to accommodate family members or others providing collateral information. The location needs to have a warm and welcoming atmosphere so that visitors feel comfortable despite their (or their family member's) apprehensions about their appointment. Possible locations include a hospital outpatient clinic, general practice surgery, mental health resource centre, social services building, or other community centre. Community settings may be less stigmatizing than hospitals, especially if the service is psychiatry based. Some teams will choose to assess individuals in their own home (but see Chapter 11).

On which days will the clinic be held?

Many teams, if operating on a clinic basis, start with one half day per week and grow. Given the frailty of some patients, however, it may be more appropriate to spread the assessment over two separate appointments. Each team will organize the assessment days differently. In British Columbia, patients are seen on two separate days. In Bristol, the assessments are divided so that the clinical assessments are performed on one day, and the CT scan on another. Testing can be tiring and breaks are advisable. In addition, dividing the assessment over 2 days may allow the patient or their family to ask questions they may have forgotten on the first day.

Referral process

◆ Will telephone, fax, or only written referrals be accepted?
◆ What information is to be gathered before assessment?
◆ What is the maximum interval between referral and assessment?
◆ How will urgent referrals be dealt with?
◆ What documentation will be kept?
◆ How will patients be notified of their appointment and how long before the date?
◆ Will patients/carers be sent information about the appointment and, if so, in what format?

Documentation

It is important to obtain documentation of previous consultations. This may include medical consultations, previous CT scans, laboratory results, and community or other assessments (for example psychology, psychiatry, occupational therapy, or community nursing). This recorded information assists where individuals or their family members may not recall events clearly.

Wait(ing) lists and urgent referrals

The use of a waiting list is important. There are circumstances when a critical change in behaviour or other factor affecting the family may require an urgent appointment. However, some teams may choose not to provide an acute evaluation service but to refer to other services such as geriatric medicine or psychiatry, which may be better able to respond to urgent situations.

Clinic information

Information about the clinic should be sent to the family prior to the appointment. If the patient lives alone, it may be necessary to send duplicate information to the relative or friend who will come with them. This should include; information about the clinic format, instructions for parking, and a map of the clinic location. If the team serves ethnic minority groups then, ideally, this information should be available in their first language.

The assessment process

♦ Will the patient always see a doctor first?

♦ Will a triage system be used?

♦ Will a structured programme or flexible approach be adopted?

♦ Will there be time for breaks?

The timetable will need to allow for new patient assessments, follow-up appointments, and should have a degree of flexibility to deal with additional assessments identified during interviews or testing (these may be conducted on the day or additional appointments may be made to see the patient in their own home or on site). Patients and family members should be contacted 2 or 3 weeks in advance of their appointment time. Some teams make a reminder telephone call the morning or the day before the appointment in order to make sure that a friend or family member is available.

If the patient and/ or family member are to see a number of team members for assessment, inclusion of break times will be important. Each patient may be seen by key team members; alternatively, a triage assessment conducted by a nurse could determine subsequent assessments, though systems of this type are by no means without controversy.

At a clinic

If the patients are to be seen in a clinic, then the following points should be considered:

♦ Will there be a facility to arrange transport to the clinic?

♦ Who will greet the patients and their families/ carers on arrival?

♦ Will they sign a consent form? If they do not, how will you determine consent has been given?

♦ Will a carer/ friend be present during all aspects of the assessment?

♦ Will there be an opportunity for the carer/ friend to speak to someone alone?

♦ Will there be an opportunity for the patient to speak to someone alone?

Signing in

In some North American services, there is a formal signing in process. In many United Kingdom services, consent is assumed from the patient's agreement to stay for assessment. Whatever approach is taken, verbal consent to assessment should probably be checked before each new assessment. In the case of clinical or academic research, informed consent must be obtained in writing and will include a signature from the patient and their relative.

Who is present during the interview/ assessment?

Patients may be interviewed with trusted family members or friends present and/ or on their own. Indeed, when gathering factual data such as a review of symptoms and past medical history, collateral information is invaluable. The doctor may explain that she or he is interested in hearing both points of view (from the patient and relative) even though the answers may differ. Most patients and families are satisfied with this approach. There are times however, when family members are uncomfortable with contradicting their relatives, or patients become irate when they are contradicted. An opportunity for the family member to give information separately may be found while the patient is preparing for the physical examination (though doing so without the patient's consent may present legal difficulties). An opportunity to speak to the patient separately, either before or after the physical examination, may also prove useful. Despite choosing to have a family member present during the interview, the patient may still have concerns which they do not wish to raise in the presence of that family member.

Whilst it is generally considered better to conduct neuropsychological or cognitive assessments without the relative present, there will be times when the patient is less anxious if their relative stays with them. An individual approach should be taken to deciding who should be present at each stage of the assessment process.

Assessing the carers

Opportunity should be given to family members to talk of their own difficulties in caring for a person with dementia. This interview may be undertaken by a social worker, counsellor, or nurse. Chapter 16 on Carer support looks at the difficulties carers may experience in more detail.

Health records/ patient notes

◆ How will data from the team be recorded?
◆ Which data does the team need to code?
◆ Who will be responsible for coding and collating the data?
◆ Where will the records be stored and will all team members have access?

Traditionally, many centres have had paper records although there are increasing opportunities for computerization. For a detailed discussion of systems and data see Chapter 3, Information management. Whilst computerized systems are powerful, it may also be helpful to have a card index system which all team members can access (see Helpful hints, below).

Recording of information must be formalized. This means training all new team members in standardized methods of assessment, clinical interpretation, and record keeping. It also means monitoring the standards of practice of current team members on a regular basis. However, not all information obtained during assessment may be necessary or appropriate for coding onto a database.

Helpful hints

A few suggestions from established and successful teams have been included.

Card index system

This provides detailed information about the patient, their general practitioner, and the family. It is easily accessible to all staff, without having to access either the computerized system or the patient's notes/ chart.

Sample:

HOSPITAL NUMBER	SURNAME
FULL NAME	D.O.B.
ADDRESS	
TELEPHONE NUMBER	
NEXT OF KIN	
GENERAL PRACTITIONER	

On the reverse side, record a history of the patient's attendances (dates of visits), relevant medical history, and family details, especially contact details for the next of kin or primary caregiver if different, plus other details such as hospital admissions, medical consultations, previous CT scans, and calls from the family physician or community team.

Alphabetical, chronological, and demographic record of referrals

Recording all referrals in this way gives an overview of trends (for example which areas refer more than others, age groups of referrals, and how many received within a certain period). All of which assist in administering the work load and in targeting publicity to potential referring agents.

Forward diary

Recording follow-up appointments in a forward diary provides immediate information on outstanding appointments. Extra clinics can be booked to accommodate the numbers of people for follow-up.

Patient notes

A single set of patients notes (the health record) should be kept, containing assessments from all team members. As well as clinic assessment sheets and dementia screen results (blood, urine, radiographs etc.), this will include any copies of relevant correspondence. If the notes may be required for research, they should be marked 'not for destruction', since many hospital medical records departments will have a rolling programme of destroying notes of deceased or discharged patients after a certain time span.

Policy manual

This should contain a set of all clinic assessment sheets and standards of practice for all team members, for use as a training tool for new staff members and for audit purposes.

Feeding back the results

- To the team:
  - Will there be a post assessment meeting and when/ where will it be held?
  - Who will attend?
- To the referring agent:
  - Who will feedback to the referring agent?
  - What form will the feedback take?
  - How long after the appointment(s) will the referring agent hear from the team?
- To the patient and their family:
  - When will feedback be given?
  - Who will be present?
  - Will the patient be told their diagnosis?
  - Will they be given written or taped information to take away regarding the team's findings?
  - Will follow-up be offered once this diagnosis is given?

Feedback to the team

Many teams find it essential to have a forum to share information and come to consensus. Usually 1 to 2 hours once a week will allow review of new assessments and follow-ups. Having a formal process with documentation to be completed facilitates consistency. Team discussion is helpful and team members learn from each other, becoming increasingly sophisticated in their approach to evaluation. If students are involved, they can take part in the presentations and discussion. The team co-ordinator would be responsible for assembling a list of current patients for discussion and ensuring the health records and relevant documentation are available.

Feedback to the referring agent

Some teams may choose for each team member to write separate feedback, others may pool their information and appoint a team member to feedback on their behalf. The team will need to decide what format this feedback should take, in particular whether it will include actual test results or summaries of the relevant findings. A survey of referring physicians or agencies to determine their needs is often helpful, as it is sometimes the case that the information needed by the person referring is different from the documentation needed by the team.

Feedback to the patient and their family

The family conference or meeting with the patient and significant others is an important part of the clinic process. It is helpful to provide an opportunity for the patient and family members to sit down and review the assessment and recommendations. The team will need to decide which staff will be present when feedback is given (for example doctor, counsellor, nurse, psychologist, or a combination). In addition, the team must establish a policy about disclosing the diagnosis to patients (see e.g. Gilliard and Gwilliam 1996). This policy might include decisions about the following: will the patient be alone, with their carer or other family members; who will be told first; what will they be told and how? Personalized information sheets or tapes to take away help reinforce what has been discussed during the meeting. These may also include general information about support groups and local agencies as well as advice about benefits and legal information. A telephone call, a few weeks after the meeting, could give families the opportunity to ask questions they did not think of at the time.

Subsequent visits

- Will a further appointment be required following extra investigations or treatment?
- Will there be follow-up visit(s)? After what interval?
- How long before patients are discharged?

Developing coping strategies may need reinforcement and encouragement. Follow-up can be extremely beneficial to families, providing support and time to overcome reluctance to utilize community services. Though, as has been indicated, follow-up visits also limit the availability of new patient assessments.

After what interval and how often?

Follow-up can be variable depending on the needs of the patient and the family, the objectives of the team, and the available resources. If the team is responsible for a primary care role, higher frequency may be needed (e.g. every 3–6 months). If treatment has been recommended (such as B_{12} replacement or antidepressant medication) the team may wish to see the patient for reassessment within 3 months or less. If diagnosis is unclear, follow-up over 6 to 9 months may be indicated. Otherwise, if there is a need to measure change over time and the team offers a consultation service, visits every 12 to 18 months may suffice.

How long?

In a study by O'Neill *et al.* (1992), longitudinal assessment of patients attending a memory clinic specializing in early diagnosis demonstrated that the majority of patients had achieved a stable diagnosis by the time they had been seen four times over a period of 2 years (initial visit, 6 month follow-up, 12-month follow-up, 24-month follow-up). A decision was therefore made to stop following up patients (unless otherwise clinically indicated) after the fourth visit.

Patients with dementia can live many years and, theoretically, dementia services could continue to see them on a regular basis for this time. Whilst maintaining contact may play an important role in supporting the caregiver and might have the added benefit of improving the take up rate of autopsy confirmation of diagnosis, unless clinically indicated, repeated assessment would not be appropriate. One solution may be to institute annual telephone contact as a substitute for clinical follow-up, as has been undertaken by some cancer institutes.

Other strategies for dealing with the problem of handling follow-ups may include: increasing base line staffing; increasing the follow-up interval (this may be helpful for only a limited time although there will be deaths); or defining the types of patients to be seen for follow-up, such as only those with mild to moderate impairment.

Neuropathological confirmation of diagnosis

Neuropathological diagnosis still remains the lynchpin for the diagnosis of the dementias. Long-term relationships with patients and families are vital if they are to take part in such a programme. Teams which wish to adopt an autopsy programme will need a policy to deal with this which includes the following:

♦ information for patients and families about the value of neuropathological examination;

♦ information about the process of autopsy;

♦ information about consent;

♦ information about local legislation for tissue donation for diagnostic purposes;

♦ information about personal advance directives (living wills).

The policy should also include what to do in the event of a death at the weekend or night time and how to accommodate persons seen in the clinic who die at a distance.

Research

♦ Will the team engage in research?

♦ How and by whom will the data be recorded for research purposes?

♦ Will the team become involved in treatment trials?

♦ Who will be responsible for each research project?

♦ How will the team control access to patients and their families for research?

♦ Will the research programme require the involvement of other specialties?

Memory disorders teams provide opportunities for research, especially collaborative projects. These opportunities are discussed in more detail in Chapter 12. In addition, connections with formal training programmes and with colleges or universities may provide students wishing to undertake research projects or theses. For example some teams carry out genetic research requiring the skills of a geneticist to interpret family trees, history, and background information and to analyse blood samples. As understanding about the genetics of dementia increases, it is likely that teams will need to think about genetic counselling in the not too distant future.

Research activities however, have legal implications, implications for the management of information (discussed in Chapter 3), and for the use of resources. In addition, successful teams may be exhausted by their successes. For example obtaining research grants imposes an increasing level of stress on perhaps an already busy team. In addition, research activities must be known to all the staff in order not to overburden patients' families and team members. It is essential to identify one individual who will be responsible for overseeing each project. This individual must liaise with the co-ordinator.

Other issues

♦ How will the team be financed?

♦ Will the team be associated with any other institutions or organizations?

♦ Will the team accept students and what will their role be?

♦ Will the team make time to discuss administrative issues?

Financing the team

Many new teams are financed from within existing budgets. Financing from charitable organizations or from the pharmaceutical industry may limit the team's autonomy, by shifting the focus of the team towards trials of medications, when the team may wish to concentrate on education, social support, and memory management (Bender 1996). Likewise research grants encourage the team to focus on the patients as subjects rather than as individuals with needs. These are not reasons to avoid these sources of funding altogether, but they do highlight the necessity of being clear about the team's objectives.

Administration and team building

Building and maintaining the team requires regular meetings. All team members including administrative staff should attend these meetings, contributing items for the agenda. Encouraging the participation of all team members is important. Rotating the chair for this meeting may help.

Looking forward

Memory disorders teams are still a relatively new concept. As understanding of the dementias grows, as diagnostic accuracy increases, and as new treatments (both pharmacological and psychological) become available, so the concept of a 'memory disorders team' will also develop. Any new service has both positive and negative attributes. The development of memory disorders teams, however, has become a focus for increasing interest in cognitive impairment, in behavioural change, in psychiatric disorders in dementia, in new technologies, and in therapies. By structuring a clinic or team well (clearly defining its objectives), by reviewing progress on a regular basis, and by being responsive to criticism and feedback from users, these teams will provide examples of innovative and quality services. Setting up a team is a time consuming process. However, an organized service, with clear objectives, is in a better position to argue for much needed resources.

References

Key references recommended by the authors are marked with an *.

* Bender, M. (1996). Memory Clinics: Locked doors on the gravy train. *PSIGE Newsletter*, September.

* Gilliard, J. and Gwilliam, C. (1996). Sharing the diagnosis: a survey of memory disorders clinics, their policies on informing people with dementia and their families, and the support they offer. *International Journal of Geriatric Psychiatry*, **11**, 1001–3.

Kopelman, M. and Crawford, S. (1996). Not all memory clinics are dementia clinics. *Neuropsychological Rehabilitation*, **6,** 187–202.

O'Neill, D., Surmon, D. J., and Wilcock, G. K. (1992). Longitudinal diagnosis of memory disorders. *Age Ageing*, **21**, 393–7.

3   Information management

Janice E. Graham and Maggie Agg

The increase over the past two decades in international epidemiological surveys of the aged, dementia disease case registries, and the computerization of clinical practices, has resulted in a multiplicity of databases whose reliability and validity vary dramatically. Their value to those who access patient and population information for clinical and research purposes depends on systematic organization and quality control. In order for information systems to meet quality assurance requirements, these databases should include individual case-specific data, apply standardized criteria and outcomes, and be rigorous in data accuracy and completion. If these databases are also to be used for clinical research then they should include 'all *known* characteristics that affect outcome' (Black 1997). Details omitted, or more often unknown when the database was set up, may be needed later. Acquiring this missing information may require considerable labour, and/ or it may not be available. When designing an information system, these considerations should be taken into account and the system needs to be able to respond to new demands on the information it contains.

This chapter considers the implications for the design and management of information systems which record the work of memory disorders teams operating in a climate of rapid change in the understanding of dementia. We shall discuss the practical details of team organization as well as the complexities of building databases which can contribute to further understandings and, we hope, may lead to better identification, care, treatment, and ultimately prevention for those encountering cognitive decline. The organization of information systems for a memory disorders team should reflect the needs of the people being referred and their primary caregivers, as well as the research and medical–scientific interests of the staff. It is our belief that a successful information system arises only when there is dialogue and exchange among all these players.

Defining the team

Memory disorders services have been in existence since the late 1970s in the United Kingdom (personal communication, Gordon Wilcock). In the United

States they originated in the mid-seventies (Lindesay 1995). Their priorities and structures have many common features which suggest general principles for organizing the collection, storage, and manipulation of information.

Successful information management is fundamental to the operation of such services. The best way to proceed is: to identify the strengths of that organization and its personnel; to recognize the patterns of, and potential bottlenecks to communication; and to decide which tools are best suited to the information needs of the service. Understandably, many memory teams come into existence without the intensive planning suggested here. They may inherit existing data storage systems or may not have the perfect complement of staff available at all times. Whether it is possible to computerize at the outset or to organize the optimal number of clinic sessions for the projected population, for example, the issues discussed here may suggest alternatives for information systems in clinics already in existence as well as facilitate the planning for a new clinic.

Memory disorders teams which have published their early experiences, included, in many cases, their aims and objectives and these have been collected below. All had at least one and most had several objectives in common (Knopman *et al.* 1985; Philpot and Levy 1987; Bayer *et al.* 1990; Van der Cammen *et al.* 1987; McMurdo *et al.* 1993; Almeida *et al.* 1993).

- ♦ a centre for the assessment and possible treatment of memory disorder;
- ♦ a centre for the ongoing monitoring of those diagnosed with a memory disorder;
- ♦ a research centre to refine methods of detection of memory impairment and dementia;
- ♦ a research centre into the causes of memory disorder;
- ♦ a resource for advice and counselling to those who are referred for assessment;
- ♦ a centre for collaboration of services for dementia sufferers and their families;
- ♦ a teaching centre for health professionals;
- ♦ a centre of excellence for the wider dissemination of memory issues;
- ♦ a centre for the recruitment of volunteers for therapeutic trials.

No single label adequately identifies the multiple roles performed at any given institution but most will include several of the above objectives in their mandate. The first stage, therefore, is to make explicit the reasons for the team's projected or actual existence. Chapter 2 discusses this in detail. What will it achieve? Which tasks are essential for its success? What possible changes to the service or its working environment are likely to determine its effectiveness in the future? Having identified the *modus operandi* of the memory disorders team it then becomes possible to define its information needs. It is a good idea for the key personnel to identify which tasks, individually, they want the system to perform. Then they can engage in a group consultation, drawing from as many existing and future potential interests as possible, in order to arrive at a consensus on how to proceed. This consultation process allows for important insights and input from the administrative, clinical, and research interests, all of whom will be accessing the information system in future.

Organizing the clinic

Once the priorities have been established, the uses of a computerized information system will be seen to fall into four broad categories:

♦ administration
♦ audit
♦ clinical and diagnostic
♦ research.

Some data may fall into more than one of these categories. Careful design at the outset will ensure that the relational flow between the relevant discrete items is readily accessible (or protected) as necessary. Figure 3.1 offers a simplified diagram of information movement.

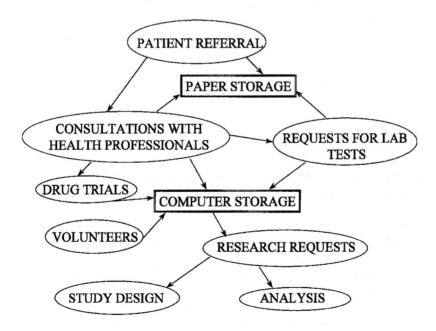

Fig. 3.1 Clinically-generated information flow within a memory disorders team.

Collecting the information

The specifics of the clinic routines determine the order in which data are collected. These tasks are (1) administrative, (2) clinical, and (3) research based:

1. **Administrative data** are generated from:

 ◆ referrals—these originate in different ways; some clinics accept only from general practitioners and hospital departments, others allow self-referrals;

 ◆ appointments;

 ◆ clinics—ensuring staff complement, transport for patients, schedules;

 ◆ clinic meetings—collating information about follow-up and further tests;

 ◆ letters generated by the consultations—to other professionals, to the patient.

 Patients may have pre-existing case notes if they are already known to the hospital or a set may be generated once they have been added to the waiting list. At the same time, a record will be added to the hospital database. Any data collected after this point will be particular to the memory disorders team and the design of the system can reflect its priorities.

2. **Clinical data** are generated from:

 ◆ patient's medical, social, and family history;

 ◆ physical examination;

 ◆ record of neuropsychological and other assessments;

 ◆ results of laboratory, radiological, and neurophysiological investigations;

 ◆ diagnostic outcome;

 ◆ treatment recommendations;

 ◆ future contact with the team for that patient.

 Once the record for a patient is coded there is the possibility that he or she will be invited to participate in research projects. Data may also be collected from healthy volunteers (often spouses or a cohort of caregivers), who agree to undergo some of the same procedures as the patients in order to provide control data.

3. **Research data** are generated from:

 ◆ both the administrative and clinical data above;

 ◆ demographic characteristics and details of patients and volunteers;

 ◆ details of research projects;

♦ personnel involved in research;

♦ details of approaches to participants in projects and their responses.

All these information-generating events are consolidated in the design of the database.

Recording information

Different means for efficient recording of information arise from the source and the nature of the information, see Table 3.1.

Where the same data are required for clinical and research purposes decisions should be made concerning the most efficient and effective approach to collection. The database software can be designed to generate the case note and assessment forms, which can then be completed by the clinicians during assessment. These can be coded directly into the relational database, allowing cross-referencing for all the demands of the computerized information system (administrative, clinical, and research). Since the examination must be conducted in a way that is appropriate both for the clinician and for the patient, however, a user-friendly form must be designed. The patient and clinician's requirements for a calm, thorough, and efficient clinic visit remain a priority, and can be assisted by designing the form to aid the consultation (rather than a consultation to complement the form).

The collection of data will evolve as new technology arrives, but probably

Table 3.1 Data sources

Data source	Data capture	Destination
Clinic appointment	Appointment card, telephone message	Patient
Consultation	Paper form	Database, case notes
Patient demographic characteristics	Paper form, computer keyboard	Database, case notes
Neuropsychological testing	Paper form, computer keyboard	Database, case notes
Physical, neurological, and medical examination	Paper form, computer keyboard	Database, case notes
Telephone data collection	Paper form	Database
Laboratory results	Paper form, computer	Database, case notes
Letter to GP	Dictaphone then word processor	Patient's GP
Telephone message	Notepad beside phone	Staff member
Staff activity	Research diary	Staff members

still relies to some extent on paper-based routines, which suit both patient and staff. This need not compromise the efficiency of the computerized system. Elucidating the information flows will yield the best design for the databases and forms. The story to be recorded begins from the time of the patient referral and continues through the appointment, the clinical consultation and assessments, the laboratory testing and neuroimaging, the diagnosis, and the follow-up. If measurement outcomes include, as they often do, institutionalization and ultimately death, then these too should be carefully tracked, dated, and recorded.

Storing information

The heart of the computerized data storage system will be a database or spreadsheet application. It may be part of a hospital or university network or it may be accessible through a local area network which serves the clinic's computing needs. It may be on a single computer. The standard software commercially available is sufficiently flexible to allow the customizing of a system without recourse to specialist computer help other than that offered as part of network support. The expertise which staff members bring may determine whether outside help is sought at this stage. There will be a requirement for regular reports and alerting messages if important contradictions are detected and some programming experience will be needed. Any system chosen must be able to read data held on software that is more primitive and these data must be easily exportable to statistical software.

Three methods of storing computerized information are outlined below:

1. A **spreadsheet** stores information as a series of lists on separate sheets. It is very useful for numerical data where summary information is often required, for example daily totals, means, etc. and is therefore a good auditing tool.

2. A **database** is used where the information to be stored is more varied in type. It allows sizeable text entries as well as all the numerical types (see Table 3.2) and is designed to make retrieval of the data easy so that a subset can be viewed on the screen rather than the whole file. Like the spreadsheet, the data can be distributed over any number of files and summary statistics can be performed on them. The entry of data is made easier by the use of forms, which can be customized to show only fields relevant to a particular entry procedure.

3. A **relational database** is one in which the files can be linked by sharing a common field so that subsets of data may be retrieved from more than one file if they relate to, for example, a subject who has the same patient ID number in both files.

Table 3.2 Database terms

Database term	Description
Field	The column containing the information on a particular subject for every entry e.g. SURNAME, VISIT NUMBER, VISIT DATE are all fields.
Record	Corresponds to a row of the table. A record in the DIAGNOSES table would contain the diagnosis details for a single person on a particular visit.
One-to-many relationship	Two tables are connected according to a logic which allows only one entry for a patient in the first table and any number of entries for that patient in the second table. The symbols used in Fig. 3.2 are 1----- ∞. In a 1-----1 relationship only one entry per patient (or patient visit) is possible in either table.
Referential integrity	An entry in one table for a patient can be required before a related table will be permitted to add an entry for that patient. For example, in Fig. 3.2 there needs to be an entry in the PATIENT'S HISTORY table above before one can be put into the DIAGNOSES table for that patient.
SQL	Structured query language—a programming language for creating and using databases which underpins the operation of relational databases.
Validation rule	The values specified during the design of the table for a particular field. If data entered falls outside these values they will not be accepted.
Default value	The value inserted during the creation of a new record in a particular field, usually the missing data code for that field. It can be overwritten with the required value where available. The ambiguity of a blank field is avoided.
Retrieval	The selection of a subset of data which corresponds to a chosen cohort. The criteria for choosing are specified in a query and can range from the simple (all female patients) to the fiendishly convoluted (e.g. all patients over age 70 with no family history of dementia but with diagnosis X whose B12 value is within certain limits, who live at home in a particular geographical area, and have indicated that they are willing to participate in research).

Relational databases have a particular advantage for the storage of data collected over time from patients who make repeated visits. The initial visit will yield demographic data, which need only be updated at subsequent visits. There are also data that are coded for each visit from psychological assessments, diagnoses, etc. Tables can be constructed with the once-only data in a form that is separate from the repeated data. These are linked by a common field (patient ID) and thus no duplication of patient data at each visit is required. This relational system can be used to ensure that there is consistency for each patient if it is set up with referential integrity between the tables. Referential integrity makes it impossible to enter details of a visit if the

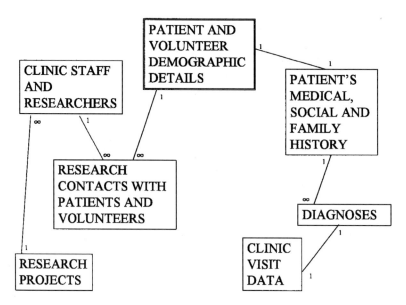

Fig. 3.2 The relationships within a database designed for a team with a strong research element. Separate tables for each category are linked according to the relational logic which minimizes the need for duplication of information coded and reduces the coding errors (relationships 1—1, and 1—∞ as defined in Table 3.2).

basic data is not already present in the demographics table. The relational design is particularly useful in a team setting where one system is needed to correlate all the research project details with the personnel, patient volunteers, outside volunteers, and the approaches made to individuals when studies are being set up. Figure 3.2 shows the relationships of the tables in a database used for clinical and research purposes.

Choosing database software

The rapid evolution of database software makes powerful packages easily affordable. If personal computers, perhaps linked by a local area network, are in use, the package of choice is usually windows-based relational database software. This will be user-friendly for those unfamiliar with programming and yet allowing the retrieval procedures to be couched in structured query language (SQL). Some of the database terms are defined more fully in Table 3.3. The power of personal computer software does not match that of ORACLE, the relational database software used on mainframes. ORACLE can support databases of the size that may be required for disease case registries. ORACLE requires familiarity with SQL and does not have an intuitive user interface. It is possible to import and export data between these systems and others. However, the choice will most likely be guided by

Table 3.3 Data types

Data type	Description
Text	Single character
	Words
	Paragraphs
Number	Integer
	Floating point decimal, large or small
Date/time	Various formats
Counter	Updates with each entry
Currency	Monetary values
Yes/no	Boolean (only 2 possibilities)

practical factors such as which system is recommended by the computer support available to the clinic.

Coding information

The structure of the data, the form in which it is stored, depends to some extent on the system chosen. Database and spreadsheet software offers a wide range of formats within one file, enabling the designer to choose the data type. Table 3.2 details the most commonly used formats.

The more closely one can specify the data type, the greater the chances that the data will be entered correctly. Database software has advantages over most spreadsheets in that validation rules and default values may be specified in order further to reduce coding errors.

The most important requirement of the data coder(s) is consistency of approach so that the same data are collected from all personnel. To ensure reliability of data, a standard operating procedure (SOP) must be established in handbook form and made easily available to all who might be involved in data coding and entry. The SOP is a step-by-step manual specifying the tasks to be carried out and the order in which to do them. It is independent of personnel and intelligible to a newcomer.

There will always be judgements to be made by the coder, especially when free text has to be condensed or translated to a code. Guidelines, however, are invaluable for streamlining the process. Similarly, where clinicians have several options for recording a specific value into a variable field it is important that they are made aware of the codes for all these options. A coding manual must be readily available, and may even be designed to appear on-line when entering the information on the computer, or appear as an end note to the page when using paper. These guidelines are best devised in consultation with those who actually use the system. A comprehensive SOP will enable the data entry to be carried out by a non-specialist in computers or medicine.

Using information

Relational databases enable the retrieval of information to be refined to a high art as long as the design of the tables is fully understood by the retriever, who must have ready access to the manuals used by the coders. The quality of the information retrieved will be related directly to the quality of the understanding between the designer, the coder, and the retriever.

Most user-friendly spreadsheets or databases allow for only a limited amount of statistical work. These tend to be associated with the immediate administrative needs of the clinic. Additional, specialized statistical packages will be required for most research demands and whether analysis is carried out in-house or not, much labour may be saved if the data types used in the database are chosen to correspond to the requirements of the analysis. For instance, if gender is coded as a number rather than a text character it will not need transposing once imported to the statistical package.

The data collected directly for research purposes will vary according to the nature of the project.

• A **prospective study** will require the identification of a cohort of suitable and willing participants with the data collection being organized by the researchers. In such cases, the clinical data will be a starting point (a particular diagnosis, age range, etc.) For prospective studies there needs to be a register of all patients' involvement in previous projects (including trials of therapeutic agents) and any information relevant to their eligibility as well as their suitability for being approached for participation. In clinics that recruit healthy volunteers to act as controls in research projects, similar data will be collected. Even the most willing volunteers may falter if they are called on too often.

• A **database-driven** study will require the data to be in a form suitable for statistical analysis. It is this requirement which can cause much discussion and recrimination, for there is nothing so powerful as 20/20 hindsight for deciding on the priorities by which the data storage is chosen and in what detail. Each research project comes up with new reasons for adding a field or changing the coding of a field. As identified at the outset of this chapter, the most useful strategy is to consult as widely as possible among colleagues and other teams, visiting them to observe clinic routines and information systems in action, for they are usually more than willing to share their trials and tribulations, thereby safeguarding one from re-inventing the wheel.

Research considerations

The number and size of databases used in medicine have multiplied, as the technology becomes more accessible and cheaper. They range from the small spreadsheet used for administration in a clinic to large disease registries designed to contain all relevant cases from a geographical catchment area. The analysis of the team's *raison d'être* will have established whether the information collected will contribute to a wider data pool or be tailored for team use only. Issues surrounding standardization remain pivotal in quality assurance. The reliability, validity, and generalizability of the information collected will determine its usefulness and how accurately the data can be analysed.

Standardization and diagnostic criteria

The advantages of standardizing and systematizing clinical data are clear, but the real-life situations met by memory disorders teams do not lend themselves to the collection of clear-cut 'facts' and 'illness categories'. In an elderly population, especially, there are likely to be comorbidities (Mitnitski *et al.* 1997) and atypical presentations (Jarrett *et al.* 1995). The temptation to pigeon-hole uncommon presentations into previously recognized categories may result in the loss of new information.

Criteria for the diagnosis of dementia and cognitive impairment are still evolving (Graham *et al.* 1996a, b, c; Graham *et al.* 1997). To define data fields in this fluid situation is challenging. A new generation of operationalized and criteria-related classification systems for dementia is found in publications from the American Psychiatric Association (1987, 1994) and World Health Organization (1993) and differential diagnostic criteria for Alzheimer's disease in McKhann (1984), vascular dementia in Chui *et al.* (1992), Roman *et al.* (1993), Hachinski (1994), Erkinjuntti *et al.* (1994), frontotemporal dementia in Lund and Manchester Group (1994), and dementia of the Lewy-body type in McKeith *et al.* (1992, 1994, 1996). Diagnoses derived through use of such systems are viewed as more objective and reliable. They allow comparisons between different data sets as the subjects fulfil the same criteria. The conclusions derived from the analysis of these data can be generalized to a defined population. However, they are not free of criticism (Lopez *et al.* 1990, 1994; Kukull *et al.* 1990; Romanoski *et al.* 1988; Leach and Levy 1994).

Frailty, a term widely used for ageing people, remains ill-defined (Campbell and Buchner 1997), despite being the subject of considerable theoretical and methodological analysis (Kaufman 1994; Rockwood *et al.* 1994; Campbell 1997). Should we abandon collecting the 'bits and pieces' that are the essential components of geriatric medicine because we have not identified the category, the data field, in which it can fit? The key, in both data collection and information retrieval, remains to balance the need for relevance (Mumford 1991) with the need for conciseness and efficiency. Feinstein (1994) discusses the dangers of limiting the meaning and sense of data collected now to existing and future users.

To address concerns about accuracy and reliability, a minimal data set (MDS) was implemented by all long-term care facilities in the United States (Morris *et al*. 1990, 1995). Although research applications may be limited (Teresi and Holmes 1992), this standardized assessment documents the resident's functional, medical, psychosocial, and cognitive status, with evidence gaining for the validity of its cognition scale (Hartmaier *et al*. 1994, 1995). In the United Kingdom, the Medical Research Council published a recommended minimum data set for use in memory clinics (Wilcock *et al.* 1989). The applicability of such research instruments is challenged by the following conceptual and methodological considerations:

♦ most diagnostic criteria are expressed in general constructs which require further translation into a set of specific behavioural and psychometric tests;

♦ concise, accurate clinical evaluations are needed;

♦ well-established normative data for cognitive performance in later life is incomplete;

♦ some dementias are characterized by changes in motivation, judgement, and behaviour, whereas those cognitive areas being assessed by standard batteries may remain intact;

♦ it remains difficult to develop tests of memory loss and other deficits that are not biased against persons of lower education or those from minority linguistic and cultural groups (floor and ceiling effects);

♦ inter-rater agreement in applying many diagnostic criteria remain modest;

♦ the clinical diagnosis of many dementia subtypes require autopsy to confirm and there is some debate about the validity of post-mortem findings;

♦ comorbidity is common; differentiation between vascular dementia and possible Alzheimer's with vascular components, for example, remains problematic. Variation between individual cases and symptom overlap complicates diagnosis.

♦ concepts about and knowledge of dementia are rapidly evolving.

Notwithstanding these constraints, large databases allow the prevalence and incidence of diseases to be determined. They can be interrogated to establish symptomotologies for populations and individuals. Characteristics (genetic, environmental, social, cultural, functional, and demographic) can be assessed for possible determinants of health and illness and the success of therapies can be monitored and assessed. Diagnostic and prognostic strategies and conclusions can be drawn.

Paradoxically, constant evolution in diagnostic criteria and in clinical practice mean that a database may be threatened with obsoleteness just as it attains the appropriate sample size to provide statistical power. Wyatt (1994) argues for, and we would concur with, the necessity of regular upgrading discussions by developers and clinicians after the computerized clinical data system is implemented.

Looking to the future

There are a number of different ways in which databases can be developed in the future. Future analyses of existing databases should offer insights into more sensitive and valid systems for classifying cases. Future developments of database systems should allow clinicians to use them as 'expert systems' supporting diagnosis and/ or service provision. And finally, data systems will be able to record more information about the subjective experience of people with dementia in ways which should make the first two developments more valid.

Using databases which allow improvement in diagnostic criteria

A number of commentators have pointed out problems with the standard approaches for case identification (Copeland 1981,1990; Brayne and Calloway 1990). While standardization of clinical approaches is necessary and can result in highly reliable diagnoses of individual cases (Graham 1996a), patients often do not fit neatly into clear-cut diagnostic categories. In short, reliability may be achieved only at the expense of validity. It has been proposed that a more useful approach might be to gather data on as many relevant symptoms and signs as is practicable, and then, in addition to recording the clinical diagnoses, estimate, by way of algorithms, how they fit given patterns in an individual patient (Graham 1996b, 1996c; Mitnitski *et al*. 1997). Thus, one may have a patient who has a 90 per cent fit with Alzheimer's disease, a 5 per cent fit with vascular dementia, and a 5 per cent fit with depression. Another may have a 50 per cent fit with dementia of the Lewy body type, 30 per cent fit with vascular dementia, 10 per cent with Alzheimer's disease and 10 per cent unspecified. Such an approach seeks to define patients precisely as they exist clinically, with untidy details that do not fit *a priori* definitions, while simultaneously not ignoring the patterns by which clinicians work. However, Feinstein cautions against measurements that lack 'common sense', or those that are appropriate to specific clinical settings only. If algorithms are to become more common, then the traditional search for summary and parsimony in the items recorded within the database will have to be reconsidered.

Medical diagnosis is an interpretation constructed by piecing together information provided by the patient as a series of symptoms (by a patient narrative or interview) and signs (by physical examination and tests). These symptoms and signs, along with other coded information, are increasingly being collected and inscribed in clinical and epidemiological databases in order to address important medical and research questions as well as to inform and direct health care policy and planning. There are many different routes to the interpretation of a diagnosis. Graham *et al.* (1996b) suggest that there are many paths to diagnosis, each of which can be internally consistent and justified. The task is to establish the most probable, the most reliable and valid path given the present body of knowledge. As a cultural product, data are produced rather than simply collected. The individual items, the data gathered in a medical examination for example, are targeted constructs which represent a dialogue between what the patient is experiencing and what the physician uncovers in the examination.

Using databases to support clinical practice

Expert tools or neural networks which may support the work of clinicians in the future rely on databases for their development (Szolovits 1979). Where we are not sure how the patterns may play out, we need to gather information that might inductively lead us to solutions later. Furthermore, there is merit in research on the database itself. The development of more powerful software means that information systems need not only be regarded as 'simple' systems which collect, store, and display data, but may also act as 'advisory' systems, providing interactive feedback and, for example, clinical reminders prompting the clinician to perform an annual assessment which can be printed out on the day sheets of a memory disorders team (see Wyatt 1991).

Expanding on the range of information collected

Feinstein (1994) has taken aim at the impoverishment of traditional systems of classification. Emphasis on objective measurements or 'hard data' neglects the 'soft data' and taxonomies that would describe clinical phenomenon. These clinical taxonomies ignore

> patterns of symptoms, severity of illness, effects of comorbid conditions, timing of phenomena, rate of progression of illness, functional capacity, and other clinical distinctions which distinguish groups of patients who otherwise seem deceptively similar because they have the same diagnosis, laboratory results, and demographic status (pp. 800).

Most importantly, the patients themselves are seldom asked to rate their own health and quality of life, their beliefs and values, or the weight they apply to their own conditions and to potential interventions. These clinical distinctions, the subjective experiences of individuals with dementia, are seldom contained in databases, which thereby lack the ability to be relevant or applicable to individual patients (Feinstein 1994).

However such databases develop in the future, attention to classification *processes* (e.g. disability) instead of *entities* (e.g. disease) will free the clinician and researcher from existing constraints of inappropriate and outdated taxonomic categories.

Conclusions

The discussion up to this point may have persuaded the putative clinic organizer that the effort of creating a satisfactory information system will not repay the work involved. The reality is far more encouraging. With the co-operation of those who will work there and attention to the following pointers, the process will be very rewarding:

♦ involve at the outset as many as possible of the potential players who will be using the data;

♦ agree on the intentions and objectives;

♦ choose easily reducible criteria for measuring important variables, e.g. diagnoses, assessment scales, research ambitions, costs;

♦ decide how much of the information will be stored on computer, and for what purposes, in light of the above;

♦ consult with computer support in choosing the system and while the databases are being built. If a more sophisticated management information system is required and the expertise of the staff is stretched, some specialist input at this stage may pay dividends;

♦ select a computerized system that will be user-friendly to all staff, both for storage and for retrieval;

♦ ensure that the software chosen is compatible with all others with which it is likely to communicate, including more powerful statistical packages;

♦ establish standard operating procedures (SOPs) using as much consultation with staff as possible;

♦ design thorough induction routines for new staff members and make the SOP manuals readily available and user-friendly, keeping in mind new members and staff changes;

♦ build in regular reviews of the usefulness and relevance of the information stored.

A successful memory disorders team is one where the patients, clinicians, researchers, and administrative staff can elicit, access, and provide information accurately, efficiently, and effectively. The recent advances in early identification of cognitive impairment and in identifying potentially modifiable risk factors for dementia subtypes provide us with hope where little existed only a few years ago. Improved understanding of the patient's perspective is contributing to better care for sufferers of dementia and their carers. A good information system, available to service providers and researchers, is a cornerstone of these advances.

References

Key references recommended by the authors are marked with an *.

Almeida OP, Hill K, Howard R, O'Brien J, and Levy R. Demographic and clinical features of patients attending a memory clinic. *International Journal of Geriatric Psychiatry* 1993; **8**: 497–501.

American Psychiatric Association. *Diagnostic and Statistical Manual of Mental Disorders*, third edition—revised, Washington D.C.: American Psychiatric Association 1987.

American Psychiatric Association. *Diagnostic and Statistical Manual of Mental Disorders*, fourth edition, Washington, D.C.: American Psychiatric Association 1994.

Bayer AL. Richards V, and Phillips G. The Community Memory Project—a multidisciplinary approach to patients with forgetfulness and early dementia. *Care of the Elderly*, 1990; **2**, 236–238.

Black N. Developing high quality clinical databases. *British Medical Journal* 1997; **315**: 381–2.

Brayne C, Calloway P. The case identification of dementia in the community: a comparison of methods. *International Journal Geriatric Psychiatry* 1990; **5**: 309–16.

Campbell AJ and Buchner DM. (1997). Unstable disability and the fluctuations of frailty. *Age & Ageing* 1997; **26**: 315–8.

Chui HC, Victoroff JI, Margolin D, Jagust W, Shankle R, Katzman R. Criteria for the diagnosis of ischemic vascular dementia proposed by the State of California Alzheimer's Disease Diagnostic and Treatment Centers. *Neurology* 1992; **42**: 473–80.

Copeland JRM. What is a case, a case for what? In, *What is a case? The problems of definition in psychiatric community surveys* (JK Wing, P Bebbington, LN Robbins, ed.). London: Grant McIntyre, 1981:7–11.

Copeland JRM. Suitable instruments for detecting dementia in community samples. *Age & Ageing* 1990; **19**: 81–3.

Erkinjuntti T, Hachinski VC, Sulkava R. Alzheimer disease and vascular dementia. In: *Dementia: presentations, differential diagnosis, and nosology* (VOB Emery and TE Oxman, ed.). Baltimore: Johns Hopkins University Press, 1994: 208–31.

Feinstein AR. Clinical judgement revisited: the distraction of quantitative models. *Annals Internal Medicine* 1994; **120**: 799–805.

Graham JE, Rockwood K, Beattie BL, McDowell I, Eastwood, MR, Gauthier S. (a) Standardization of the diagnosis of dementia in the Canadian Study of Health and Aging. *Neuroepidemiology* 1996; **15**: 246–56.

Graham JE, Mitnitski AB, Mogilner AJ, Gauvreau D, Rockwood K. (b) Symptoms and signs in dementia: synergy and antagonism. *Dementia* 1996; **7**: 331–5.

Graham JE, Mitnitski AB, Mogilner AJ, Gauvreau D, Rockwood K. (c) An algorithmic approach to the differential diagnosis of dementia. *Dementia* 1996; **7**: 324–30.

Graham JE, Rockwood K, Beattie BL, Eastwood R, Gauthier S, Tuokko H, McDowell I. Prevalence and severity of cognitive impairment with and without dementia in an elderly population. *Lancet* 1997; **349**: 1793–6.

Hachinksi V. Vascular dementia: a radical redefinition. *Dementia* 1994; **5**: 130–2.

Hartmaier SL, Sloane PD, Guess HA, Koch GG. The MDS cognition scale: a valid instrument for identifying and staging nursing home residents with dementia using the minimum data set. *Journal of the American Geriatrics Society* 1994; **42**: 1173–9.

Hartmaier SL, Sloane PD, Guess HA, Koch GG, Mitchell CM, Phillips CD. Validation of the minimum data set cognitive performance scale: agreement with the mini-mental state examination. *Journal of Gerontology* 1995; **50A**: M128–33.

Jarrett PG, Rockwood K, Carver D, Stolee P, Cosway S. Illness presentation in elderly patients. *Archive of Internal Medicine* 1995; **155**: 1060–4.

Kaufman SR. The social construction of frailty: an anthropological perspective. *Journal of Aging Studies* 1994; **8**:45–58.

Knopman DS, Deinard S, Kitto J, Hartman M, Mackenzie T. A clinic for dementia. Two years experience. *Minnesota Medicine* 1985; **68**: 687–92.

Kukull WA, Larson EB, Reifler BV, Lampe TH, Yerby MS, Hughes JP. Interrater reliability of Alzheimer's disease diagnosis. *Neurology* 1990; **40**: 257–60.

Leach J, Levy R. Reflections on the NINCDS/ADRDA criteria for the diagnosis of Alzheimer's disease. *International Journal of Geriatric Psychiatry* 1994; **9**: 173–9.

Lindesay J. Memory clinics: past, present and future. *Alzheimer's Review* 1995; **5**: 97–100.

Lopez OL, Larumbe MR, Becker JT, Rezek D, Rosen J, Klunk W, DeKosky

ST. Reliability of NINDS-AIREN clinical criteria for the diagnosis of vascular dementia. *Neurology* 1994; **44**: 1240–5.

Lopez OL, Swihart AA, Becker JT, Reinmuth OM, Reynolds CF, Rezek DL, *et al*. Reliability of NINCDS-ADRDA clinical criteria for the diagnosis of Alzheimer's disease. *Neurology* 1990; **40**: 1517–22.

Lund and Manchester Groups Clinical and neuropathological criteria for frontotemporal dementia: consensus statement. *Journal of Neurology Neurosurgery and Psychiatry* 1994; **57**: 416–18.

McKeith I, Perry RH, Fairbairn AF, Jabeen S, Perry EK. Operational criteria for senile dementia of Lewy body type. *Psychological Medicine* 1992; **22**: 911–22.

McKeith IG, Fairbairn AF, Perry RH, Thompson P. The clinical diagnosis and misdiagnosis of senile dementia of Lewy body type (SDLT). *British Journal of Psychiatry* 1994; **165**: 324–32.

McKeith IG, Galasko D, Kosaka K, Perry EK, Dickson DW, Hansen LA, *et al*., for the Consortium on Dementia with Lewy Bodies. Consensus guidelines for the clinical and pathologic diagnosis of dementia with Lewy bodies (DLB). *Neurology* 1996; **47**: 1113–24.

McKhann G, Drachman D, Folstein M, Katzman R, Price D, Stadlan EM. Clinical diagnosis of Alzheimer's disease: report of the NINCDS-ADRDA Work Group under the auspices of Department of Health and Human Services Task Force on Alzheimer's Disease. *Neurology* 1984; **34**: 939–44.

McMurdo MET, Grant DJ, Gilchrist J, Findlay D, McLennan J, Lawrence B. The Dundee Memory Clinic: the first 50 patients. *Health Bulletin* 1993; July: 203–7.

Mitnitski AB, Graham JE, Mogilner AJ, Rockwood K. Vector diagnostics in dementia derived from Bayes' theorem. *American Journal of Epidemiology* 1997; **146**: 665–71.

Morris JN, Hawes C, Fries BE, *et al*. Designing the national resident assessment instrument for nursing facilities. *Gerontologist* 1990; **30**: 293–307.

Morris JN, Murphy K, Nonemaker S. *Long term care facility resident assessment instrument (RAI) user's manual*. Baltimore, Maryland: Briggs Health Care Products, 1995.

Mumford E. Need for relevance in management information systems: what the NHS can learn from industry. *British Medical Journal* 1991; **302**: 79–83.

Philpot MP, Levy R. A memory clinic for the early diagnosis of dementia. *International Journal of Geriatric Psychiatry* 1987; **2**: 195–200.

Rockwood K, Fox RA, Stolee P, Robertson D, Beattie BL. Frailty in elderly people: an evolving concept. *Canadian Medical Association Journal* 1994; **150**: 489–495.

Roman GC, Tatemichi TK, Erkinjuntii T, Cummings JL, *et al*. Vascular dementia: diagnostic criteria for research studies. *Neurology* 1993; **43**: 250–60.

Romanoski AJ, Nestadt G, Chahal R, *et al.* Interobserver reliability of a 'Standardized Psychiatric Examination' (SPE) for case ascertainment (DSM-III). *Journal of Nervous and Mental Disease* 1988; **176**: 63–71.

Szolovits P, ed. *Artificial intelligence in medicine.* Washington, D.C.: American Association for the Advancement of Science, 1979.

Teresi JA, Holmes D. Should MDS data be used for research? *Gerontologist* 1992; **32**: 148–51.

Van der Cammen TJM, Simpson JM, Fraser RM, Preker AS, Exton-Smith AN. The memory clinic: a new approach to the detection of dementia. *British Journal of Psychiatry* 1987; **150**: 359–64.

Wilcock GK, Hope RA, Brooks DN, Lantos PL, Oppenheimer C, Reynolds GP, Rossor MN, Davies MB. Recommended minimum data sets to be collected in research studies on Alzheimer's disease. *Journal of Neurology Neurosurgery and Psychiatry* 1989; **52**: 693–700.

World Health Organization. *The ICD-10 classification of mental and behavioural disorders: diagnostic criteria for research.* Geneva: World Health Organization, 1993.

Wyatt J. Computer-based knowledge systems. *Lancet* 1991; **338**: 1431–6.

Wyatt JC. Clinical data systems, part 3: development and evaluation. *Lancet* 1994; **344**: 1682–8.

4 Medical assessment

G.K. Wilcock and I. Skoog

Introduction

Although more than 70 diseases can cause dementia, three are probably responsible for 70 to 80 per cent of all cases: Alzheimer's disease; vascular dementia; and dementia associated with Lewy bodies. Most other causes are by themselves uncommon, but together they may constitute 10 to 25 per cent of patients referred for a dementia evaluation, and they are important to recognize as several of them are potentially treatable or involve a process which may be retarded by appropriate treatment. Furthermore, several potentially treatable physical and mental disorders may be superimposed on a primary dementia and thus aggravate this condition. In patients with a primary dementia, these conditions are often neglected. In people under 65, up to 20 per cent may have a treatable or remediable aggravating factor, although the proportion decreases with age to less than 5 per cent in those aged 65 and over (Smith and Kiloh 1981). All comorbid conditions, which may aggravate the dementia, become more common with age.

It is important that all patients with a suspected diagnosis of dementia, and demented patients with a sudden deterioration in their condition, receive a careful medical examination and further investigation as a basis for planning medical, psychological, and social care. This should be undertaken even if one of the major dementias has been diagnosed, as treatable factors may be neglected unless the patient is carefully evaluated. These other factors may also affect the prognosis and pattern of progression of the disorder. In addition, treatment for Alzheimer's disease is already becoming available in some countries (e.g. rivastigmine). This type of dementia must therefore be distinguished from other causes, including those where alternative treatment strategies will be appropriate, such as for some of the vascular dementias. It has to be emphasized that mixed types of dementias are common, which further complicates the clinical evaluation.

Examination of the patient will often provide clues that are important to the differential diagnosis of a person's cognitive impairment. The findings may help differentiate between an acute confusional state (delirium) and a dementing illness, or indicate that the patient is suffering with a combination of an acute confusional state on top of an underlying dementia, for example by revealing evidence of the potential causes of any of these conditions. There may also be evidence of potential underlying causes for dementia, of risk factors which might contribute to or aggravate the patient's condition, or of comorbidity that may be important in anticipating the prognosis for an individual and planning his or her future care.

The advent of new treatments, for example for Alzheimer's disease, should also be borne in mind during the examination of a patient since one may find evidence indicating that certain types of medication (e.g. cholinergic agonists) may be contraindicated, e.g. it is important not to forget that some abnormalities of the cardiovascular system imply the need for caution in prescribing cholinergically-active drugs. There are many other examples that are potentially important in relation to treatment, including the possibility that extrapyramidal abnormalities in the nervous system may indicate the presence of a Lewy body-associated dementia with the need for considerable caution if the prescription of neuroleptics is deemed unavoidable. This is discussed further in Chapter 17.

This chapter is not meant to be an exhaustive list of the potential findings on examination in relation to all possible causes of confusion and dementia. It is meant to highlight some of the more important inter-relationships and to emphasize the need for careful assessment of the patient. We appreciate that what is described will not be possible, or perhaps even appropriate, in all settings, especially where community assessment is undertaken by non-medically qualified staff. Nevertheless, it should be apparent that a considerable amount of useful information can be obtained without the type of detailed medical assessment which is usually only undertaken by medically qualified staff.

Much of the information presented in the section which follows will usefully be supplemented by cross referral to other chapters where the reader feels this appropriate, for example in relation to pointers to less commonly encountered underlying causes of dementia identified during the assessment.

History

A person with dementia usually has difficulty providing a reliable history and it is therefore mandatory to obtain information from other sources, such as a reliable and close informant who knows the patient well (e.g. a relative, a neighbour, or a home carer). Other available information should also be collected, for example from case records.

Cognitive symptoms

The first step in the medical assessment is to obtain an impression of the pattern and severity of the cognitive dysfunction. Are the symptoms adequate for a diagnosis of dementia? Even if not, a thorough medical evaluation should be performed in a patient with a history of significant cognitive decline. Otherwise important clinical conditions may be missed. The current level of cognitive function should be assessed in the context of the patient's previous educational level and their professional and intellectual ability. Previous personality is also important as this may modify the presentation of the illness (see Chapters 5 and 7).

Onset, progression, and symptom pattern

The duration of the symptoms and the nature of the presenting complaint, together with the mode of onset and progression, may provide important clues. For example the typical picture of Alzheimer's disease is that of an insidious onset of memory problems followed by progressively worsening impairment of language and the development of apraxia or agnosia. Vascular dementia is more commonly associated with a sudden onset, perhaps with stepwise progression and the development of a fragmented pattern of symptoms of cognitive deficit (such as early language disturbance or agnosia). However, in up to 30 per cent of cases with vascular dementia the clinical course may be similar to that of typical Alzheimer's disease, and in a proportion of Alzheimer cases the onset may be atypical.

In evaluating the history, one has to be careful. A 'sudden onset' may mean a sudden realization of the condition by the relatives or others, such as when a husband or wife who took care of the patient dies or when the patient comes to medical attention because of another condition. A very fast progression is seen in some secondary dementias and in conditions such as Creutzfelt–Jakob's disease (CJD).

It is important to seek information about core symptoms that relate to impairment in memory, language, and praxis, as already mentioned, but in addition, to enquire about orientation in time and space, ability to concentrate or whether easily distractible, ability to plan and carry through activities, and visuospatial function (such as a history of misinterpreting distances or misjudging distance and location of objects).

Interviewing a close informant is often the best way to establish the presence of personality change, behavioural disturbances, and the presence of 'psychiatric' symptoms such as visual hallucinations (which, if present early in the course, may point to a Lewy body dementia), paranoid, and other delusions. The picture painted by the history will then start unravelling the differential diagnosis, allowing one to begin to differentiate between conditions such as Alzheimer's disease (mainly cortical symptoms with dysfunction of the temporal and parietal lobes giving rise to e.g. apraxia, aphasia, agnosia, and memory disturbance), vascular dementia, the Lewy body dementias (with hallucinations and subcortical symptoms such as psychomotor slowness and motoric symptoms), and those associated initially with predominantly frontal lobe symptoms (personality changes, loss of initiative, poverty of speech), such as in frontal lobe dementia, amyotrophic lateral sclerosis (ALS), and some vascular dementias.

The pattern in which the symptoms emerge is also important. The time course between dementia onset and certain disorders may point in the direction of a certain cause of the dementia, for example dementia evolving in connection with a stroke suggests a vascular dementia. Urinary incontinence and gait disturbance early in the course may point in the direction of normal pressure hydrocephalus or, in some cases, vascular dementia, and early extrapyramidal symptoms may suggest a dementia in relation to Lewy body disease or subcortical ischaemic white-matter lesions. The symptom pattern may also indicate some of those conditions that do not strictly speaking fulfil the criteria for a diagnosis of dementia, for example cognitive and behavioural changes associated with depression and more focal lobar syndromes such as primary progressive aphasia. It has to be emphasized again that there is an overlap in the symptomatology between different types of dementia and it is not uncommon that more than one condition is present in the same patient.

Past medical history

Conditions that have occurred in the past may play a part in the development of the patient's present state of cognitive impairment. Any link should always be assumed to be possible rather than definite unless there is clear evidence supporting an aetiological relationship.

Past history of **head injury** sufficient to render the patient unconscious may be relevant not only to the possibility of Alzheimer's disease, but also to normal pressure hydrocephalus. Head trauma may also result in the development of a subdural haematoma, although this is unusual as a cause of progressive intellectual impairment, but it can be associated with fluctuating neurological function which can sometimes have a cognitive component. The trauma required to produce a subdural haematoma may be almost negligible, and in any person whose condition waxes and wanes, especially if associated with fluctuating clouding of consciousness or focal signs, this possibility should be considered. If present, signs of increased intracranial pressure are a helpful pointer in this direction, although they may also indicate the possibility of a cerebral tumour. Both of these conditions may be potentially treatable and may be diagnosed with a CT or MRI scan.

Epilepsy is similarly important as it may lead to anoxic damage, direct damage from repeated or sustained fits, and some of the drugs taken to control epilepsy may also have an effect upon intellect. Similarly **thyrotoxicosis,** whether treated surgically or medically, may be associated with the development of **hypothryroidism** in later life, with a consequent impact upon intellectual ability.

Any past history that confirms the presence of **a disorder of any of the major body systems** may be relevant in a patient with dementia. Both cardiovascular disease, for example myocardial infarction, dysrhythmic episodes and cerebrovascular disease (e.g. with a history of transient episodes of focal symptoms or stroke) are equally important, as are metabolic disorders, especially diabetes mellitus, whether requiring insulin or oral treatment, and whether related to episodes of hyperglycaemia or hypoglycaemia. Renal disease is infrequently a contributory factor but should be considered where appropriate. Hepatic impairment is also well known to cause intellectual dysfunction, but it is rarely a cause of dementia, and is more usually associated with an acute confusional state. Generalized systemic disorders, such as systemic lupus erythematosus and rheumatoid arthritis, may lead to dementia-like symptoms through different mechanisms, and so may disorders with hyperviscosity of the blood, such as polycythaemia vera and different forms of hyperlipidaemia, and vasculitis, such as temporal arteritis.

Past history of a **carcinoma,** even if many years before the apparent onset of the dementia, and also in the absence of focal signs, could be relevant. In practice, however, with the exception of a few tumours such as carcinoma of the breast or lungs, secondary involvement of the brain is unusual if more than 2 or 3 years have elapsed since the primary carcinoma was diagnosed and treated.

Coexisting medical conditions

A significant abnormality in many of the major body systems, even if arising relatively recently, may be associated with the development of cognitive impairment. Although one usually seeks symptoms by using a systemic or functional inquiry when taking the history, one must not forget to enquire about disturbance of gait or the presence of incontinence which may be pointers to normal pressure hydrocephalus if they occur early on in the course of an apparent dementia. Similarly, symptoms suggestive of raised intracranial pressure (e.g. headache, vomiting) or cerebral tumour should be sought.

A careful assessment of medication is also essential, not just because of the possibility that some medicines, for example hypnotics, sedatives, anticholinergic drugs, digitalis, and others may impair intellect, but also because others, for example neuroleptics, should be used with great caution in patients with a suspected diagnosis of dementia associated with Lewy body disease.

Depression (evidence for a primary depression versus primary dementia)

If the patient is suffering with depression masquerading as dementia, there will often be clues in the history in addition to the presence of symptoms that suggest a diagnosis of depression. Differentiation is not always easy however, since depression and dementia frequently coexist and it is sometimes necessary to institute a trial of anti-depressant treatment before a final decision is made as to whether or not a genuine dementia is also present. This is discussed further in Chapter 5.

In a depressive illness, the symptoms suggesting cognitive impairment or dementia often have a relatively fast onset compared to the pattern in most primary dementias. The patient will often complain about his or her symptoms or exaggerate them. Concentration difficulties are often more marked in depression and there may be associated agitation. Other clues pointing to a diagnosis of depression include a history of the patient being worse in the morning, suicidal feelings, anxiety, or other affective symptoms. Cortical dysfunction such as aphasia, agnosia, or apraxia is rare in uncomplicated depression.

Many people with a depressive illness have a past history of similar episodes. Prior episodes of depression have also been suggested to occur more frequently in those developing dementia in later life although the evidence is contradictory. A family history of depression is more common in those with a depressive illness than in an uncomplicated dementia. If the patient has already been prescribed an anti-depressant, preferably an SSRI rather than an anticholinergic tricyclic anti-depressant, the way in which they have responded, if at all, may also be helpful in differentiating between the presence of pseudodementia of the depressive type, a primary dementia, or a combination of both. Depression superimposed on a primary dementia is most often evident in the early phase of dementia, but should be treated as a depression as it may cause suffering in the patient and it may worsen the patient's dementia.

Alcohol

Despite the fact that a history of heavy alcohol use or abuse is well known to be under-reported, and difficult to confirm, its relative importance as an aetiological or contributory factor to a person's cognitive impairment is nevertheless easily overlooked. In addition to the toxic effect of alcohol upon the brain, which may persist for some considerable time after the intake has been reduced, there is also the effect of the dietary and vitamin deficiencies, such as thiamine deficiency, that so often accompany alcohol abuse. Thiamine deficiency leading to Wernicke's encephalopathy (with eye signs, gait disturbance, and confusion) should be considered a medical emergency and appropriate treatment should be administered immediately. Alcohol abusers are also at increased risk for head trauma. If there is *any* suspicion of over indulgence in alcohol, further corroborative evidence should be sought from the history, and particular attention paid to eliciting supportive signs on physical examination. One should also request the relevant laboratory investigations, for example measurement of the level of γ-glutamyl trans-peptidase and an index of thiamine status such as the level of erythrocyte transketolase activity.

Family history

A family history is especially important for the diagnosis of certain specific causes of dementia, such as Huntingdon's disease and CJD, although both these conditions may occur sporadically. It is also important in the rare cases of familial Alzheimer's disease or familiar vascular dementias, such as CADASIL (cerebral autosomal dominant arteriopathy with subcortical infarcts and leukoencephalopathy). In addition, information about a familial history of Down's syndrome should be obtained.

In many cases one often finds that there is a rather vague description of a person with forgetfulness in the years before they died and it is not easy to decide whether or not this constituted a dementing illness. Unless there is a very clear family history of dementia, with an autopsy or otherwise confirmed underlying cause, the fact that another member or members of the family have had a similar illness is not very helpful in arriving at a diagnosis. This information may, however, be helpful when providing advice about the prognosis in the patient being evaluated, especially if there is a familial trend. In relation to family history, relatives often have concerns about their own risk of becoming demented.

Social assessment

Although this is likely to be of little diagnostic value, assessment of the social background to the patient is important when considering future management planning (see Chapters 16, 18, and 19). The issues covered should include the family situation and social support networks, financial background, living arrangements, existing needs for health and social support, and the impact on these of comorbidities such as impaired mobility and poor eyesight. There may also be a number of practical issues that have to be taken into account, such as driving a motor car, managing money, and hazard risks such as the use of a gas cooker. This aspect of the history indicates areas that need more careful consideration when the patient is undergoing neuro-psychological assessment.

Features which may help differentiate delirium from dementia

Delirium is usually the result of either an acute illness, often infective in nature, or an unwanted effect of medication, especially drugs with an anticholinergic effect, or psychotropic drugs, such as benzodiazepines or high dose neuroleptics, and sometimes even other drugs such as digitalis.

Infection constitutes the commonest acute illness, and respiratory and urinary tract infections probably account for more acute confusional states than any other single cause. Nevertheless infection anywhere may be relevant. Lower urinary tract obstruction with bladder distension is a common, and often overlooked, cause of confusion in the elderly male. In addition, as already mentioned, impairment of any major organ system may contribute to intellectual impairment and, although this can sometimes result in a dementia, delirium is more frequently the result. The onset is usually fairly rapid, that is over hours or days rather than months, and features of the history may point the physician in the direction of an underlying cause. However, delirium may sometimes develop more slowly in older adults. The symptoms often fluctuate over the day and are worse at night.

Confusion which results from drug treatment is often associated with the initiation of new therapy or a change in an existing regime, but can occur in a patient whose medication has not been altered for some while, for example if undiagnosed renal impairment has allowed a drug to accumulate to levels that are toxic.

The diagnosis of delirium or dementia is not necessarily a mutually exclusive process. Both frequently coexist and manifest or incipient dementia is probably the most common underlying cause of confusion. It is not unusual to be asked to assess a patient who appears to have become acutely confused. Although initially it is assumed that this is the result of a delirium, it is surprising how often the patient is left with cognitive impairment after the acute problem has resolved. This may result from brain damage caused by the acute episode, but it may also indicate that there was an unremarkable or unnoticed degree of intellectual impairment before the acute episode drew the carer's attention to the fact that something was amiss.

Examination of the patient

General appearance

Clinical examination is especially important in the patient with dementia as he or she will often have problems in expressing symptoms verbally. Before the advent of high technology medicine, an experienced medical attendant, whether physician, nurse or worker in a different discipline, gained much useful information by just observing their patient's general appearance.

Although we try and teach this skill even today, the pressure to demonstrate one's knowledge about the latest technology, and at the same time to process patients as quickly as possible, often results in less attention than is warranted being given to the patient's presentation. Exploring this does not take long, and much useful information can be gained in the first few seconds whilst the patient walks into a consulting room or the examiner into the patient's home and while the usual pleasantries are being exchanged.

Does the patient look ill or toxic? Is he or she short of breath or does he or she have a cough? Skin colour is important, for example the presence of cyanosis, jaundice, paleness (indicating possible anaemia), or plethoric appearance (suggesting polycythaemia). Are there signs of hypo- or hyperthyroidism? Does the patient look parkinsonian, for example with the typical emotionless facial appearance, or stooped posture, or both? Does their appearance and the way they respond suggest the presence of depression? Are there manifestations of malnutrition? Is the patient showing signs of pain?

Superficial assessment of gait may indicate that more formal assessment of this part of the neurological examination must be undertaken carefully, whilst evidence of dysarthria or dysphasia may have similar implications for the assessment of speech and language.

The smell of infected urine, in the house or from the clothing of a person who has been incontinent, indicates the need to exclude a toxic confusional state caused by a urinary tract infection. The smell of alcohol points one in the direction of an alcohol related dementia or delirium.

Although not part of assessing a patient's general appearance, it is important not to forget to use a thermometer if a delirium is suspected, and to examine the regional lymph nodes during more formal examination, if this is undertaken. Useful information can also be obtained from the manner in which a person reacts to being examined, for example the presence of obvious discomfort or distress during abdominal examination or the manipulation of a limb.

It is essential to obtain an impression as to whether communication is hampered by impaired vision or hearing, a receptive aphasia, bradyphrenia, or difficulty with expression.

Mental state examination

In the assessment, a short mental evaluation, including testing of cognitive function, should always be instituted to assess the patient's mental ability and reveal signs of global or focal impairment. Neuropsychological assessment, however, is described in detail in Chapter 7 and is beyond the scope of this chapter. Whilst we appreciate that in some settings, such as the patient's own home, all that may be possible is a relatively simple assessment such as the mini mental state examination, in others more extensive assessment may be both desirable and practical. A mental state examination should also include an informal observation of the patient during the examination, assessing language, reasoning, memory, and also specifically apraxia, aphasia, agnosia, and left–right orientation.

Psychiatric assessment

Although this is dealt with in detail in Chapter 5, important information can often be obtained during the course of normal history taking and physical examination, without formal psychiatric assessment. This includes general appearance and its relevance to underlying psychiatric disorder, alterations in mood, evidence of increased suspiciousness and paranoid ideas, delusions or hallucinations, disturbance of behaviour, personality change, attention to hygiene, alertness and orientation, and impairment of judgement and insight. If a formal psychiatric assessment is considered appropriate, this should be undertaken by a psychiatrist or an appropriate member of the nursing profession.

Central nervous system

Examination of the central nervous system is usually helpful in confirming the presence of one of the three commonest causes of dementia, even if only by excluding other potential underlying CNS disorders. Pointers to the presence of cerebrovascular disease or dementia associated with Lewy bodies are the least that should be sought, having excluded any obvious CNS cause of a delirium, such as encephalitis.

Wherever possible a formal neurological examination should be undertaken. Abnormal signs should be sought in the pyramidal and extrapyramidal motor system, especially asymmetry of reflexes, abnormalities of plantar response, facial or limb weakness, evidence of rigidity or bradykinesia, or tremor. These may help indicate the presence or absence of cerebrovascular disease, Parkinson's disease, dementia associated with Lewy bodies, or amyotrophic lateral sclerosis, etc. Myoclonus may indicate the possibility of CJD, especially in the presence of a rapidly progressing dementia with other neurological features, including abnormality of pyramidal or extrapyramidal motor function and cerebellar signs.

Posture and gait pattern may indicate extrapyramidal disorders, cerebrovascular disease, and other conditions such as normal pressure hydrocephalus and Wernicke's encephalopathy. The presence of involuntary movements, particularly when associated with other relevant symptoms or signs, may be indicators of Huntingdon's disease or, if myoclonic in nature, of CJD.

The presence of primitive reflexes is a feature of many dementias once they are well advanced. The earlier occurrence of primitive reflexes however is more frequently a feature of those disorders which are particularly associated with frontal lobe disease. Useful reflexes for testing in this regard include the grasp reflex, the snout reflex, and the palmomental reflex.

Cranial nerve examination includes evaluation of the presence of nystagmus, pupillary abnormalities or abnormal eye movements which may indicate underlying cerebellar or brainstem lesions. These include Wernicke's encephalopathy, the increasingly rare case nowadays of neurosyphilis, and, in conjunction with other abnormal findings in the CNS, of a whole range of neurological disorders associated with dementia (see Chapter 15). One-sided pupillary dilatation may indicate space-occupying lesions (such as tumour or subdural haematoma) and papilloedema is an indication of increased intracranial pressure. Examination of other aspects of cranial nerve and cerebellar function may also be helpful in this respect.

Assessment of sensation is often less helpful, especially of vibration and proprioception which are often impaired in the distal part of the lower limbs in elderly people. Nevertheless, sensory impairment may suggest the presence of cerebrovascular disease (especially one-sided such as in pure sensory stroke in relation to a lacunar infarct) or peripheral neuropathy associated with vitamin B12 deficiency, diabetes, or other neurological or systemic illnesses.

Cardiorespiratory examination

Examination of the chest may reveal signs suggesting the presence of infection or heart failure. More rarely it may reveal signs of a pleural effusion suggesting a more significant underlying lesion, for example a carcinoma of the bronchus which may cause dementia by cerebral metastases, or occasionally via a non-metastatic mechanism.

The presence of hypertension, or evidence of this from fundoscopy, the rate and rhythm of the pulse, and the presence of cardiac murmurs or bruits in the carotid vessels all point to a potential vascular cause for cognitive impairment. Similarly the presence of peripheral vascular disease, especially in association with a past history of myocardial infarction, may also point in this direction. A blood pressure measurement after 5 minutes resting with the patient in the sitting position should be performed. High blood pressure may indicate a vascular dementia and low blood pressure should alert the physician to be careful with drugs which may lower blood pressure. This should be complemented with measurement in the standing position. Orthostatic hypotension is common in many types of dementia and may lead to further brain damage caused by hypotensive episodes.

Finally, one should be alert for signs of vasculitis, for example a temporal arteritis with pain on palpation over the temporal region.

Abdominal examination

The findings on abdominal examination are more likely to indicate potential causes of delirium rather than help elucidate the underlying nature of a dementia. There are, however, a few notable exceptions such as dementia secondary to chronic alcohol intoxication. Obvious signs of hepatic or renal disease, the presence of abnormal masses or free fluid, may all be relevant. Constipation is sometimes considered to be a cause of confusion but more often it is the drugs that are responsible for, or are aggravating, the constipation that are really the culprit (e.g. opiate based analgesics, anticholinergic drugs such as tricyclic antidepressants, and some anti-parkinsonian agents). One should also look for bladder distension. It is important to observe the patient's reaction during palpation, as people with dementia often have difficulty indicating where their pain is.

Musculoskeletal system

Although less directly relevant, examination of the musculoskeletal system can be helpful. Joint infection may result in a delirium, and occasionally arthritis is part of a more systemic condition that may also be affecting cerebral function such as an arthritis associated with a collagen–vascular disorder. Similarly, the presence of arthritis may explain an abnormal gait pattern which otherwise might be misinterpreted, for example as part of the diagnostic triad of normal pressure hydrocephalus. Muscle atrophy may be a sign of malnutrition.

Summary

The state of our current knowledge about the conditions which cause delirium and dementia is such that the majority of the useful diagnostic information often comes from a carefully taken history and examination of the patient. Most of the investigations are helpful by way of excluding infrequently occurring problems and it is essential that these are sought and treated when discovered.

Our understanding of the basic pathological processes responsible for many of the commoner causes of dementia is increasing rapidly, and with it the move towards developing diagnostic indicators. At the time of writing however, there is no clear evidence to suggest that a particular diagnostic test is of value in the routine clinical context for any of the three most commonly occurring causes of dementia, that is Alzheimer's disease, vascular cognitive impairment, and dementia associated with Lewy bodies, although research is moving in that direction. Therefore, much of the diagnostic process has to be based on a careful bedside evaluation including a detailed clinical history and examination.

Bibliography

Key references recommended by the authors are marked with an *.

Bannister R. *Brain's Clinical Neurology*. Seventh Edition. Oxford: Oxford University Press, 1992.

Brun A, Englund E, Gustafson L, Passant U, Mann DMA, Neary D, Snowden JS. Clinical and neuropathological criteria for frontotemporal dementia. *Journal of Neurology, Neurosurgery, and Psychiatry* 1994; **57**: 416–18.

Erkinjuntti T, Sulkava R, Kovanen J, Palo J. Suspected dementia: evaluation of 323 consecutive referrals. *Acta Neurologica Scandinavia* 1987; **76**: 359–64.

Erkinjuntti T, Wikström J, Palo J, Autio L. Dementia among medical inpatients. Evaluation of 2000 consecutive admissions. *Archives of Internal Medicine* 1986; **146**: 1923–6.

*Geldmacher DS, Whitehouse PJ. Evaluation of dementia. *New England Journal of Medicine* 1996; **335**: 330–6.

Graham JE, Mitnitski AB, Mogilner AJ, Gauvreau D, Rockwood K. An algorithmic approach to the differential diagnosis of dementia. *Dementia* 1996; **7**: 324–30.

Larson EB, Reifler BV, Featherstone HJ, English DR. Dementia in elderly outpatients: A prospective study. *Annals of Internal Medicine* 1984; **100**: 417–23.

Larson EB, Reifler BV, Sumi SM, Canfield CG, Chinn NM. Diagnostic evaluation of 200 elderly outpatients with suspected dementia. *Journal of Gerontology* 1985; **40**: 536–43.

Larson EB, Reifler BV, Sumi SM, Canfield CG, Chinn NM. Diagnostic tests in the evaluation of dementia A prospective study of 200 elderly outpatients. *Archives of Internal Medicine* 1986; **146**: 1917–22.

McLean S. Assessing dementia. Part I: Difficulties, definitions and differential diagnosis. *Australia and New Zealand Journal of Psychiatry* 1987; **21**: 142–74.

McKeith IG, Galasko D, Wilcock GK, Byrne EJ. Lewy body dementia—diagnosis and treatment. *British Journal of Psychiatry* 1995; **167**: 709–17.

*McKeith IG, Galasko D, Kosaka K, *et al*. Consensus guidelines for the clinical and pathologic diagnosis of dementia with Lewy bodies (DLB): Report of the consortium on DLB international workshop. *Neurology* 1996; **47**: 1113–24.

Orrell RW, Wade JPH. Clinical diagnosis: How good is it and how should it be done?. In: Prohovnik I, Wade J, Knezevic S, Tatemichi T, Erkinjuntti T (eds.). *Vascular dementia. Current concepts.* Chichester. John Wiley & Sons, 1996.

Philpot M P, Burns A. Reversible dementias. In Katona C L (ed.) *Dementia disorders. Advances and prospects.* London New York: Chapman and Hall, 1989: 142–59.

Román GC, Tatemichi TK, Erkinjuntti T, *et al.* Vascular dementia: Diagnostic criteria for research studies. Report of the NINDS-AIREN international workshop. *Neurology* 1993, **43**: 250–60.

Sahakian BJ. Depressive pseudodementia in late life. *International Journal of Geriatric Psychiatry* 1991; **6**: 453–8.

Skoog I. Blood pressure and dementia. In: Hansson L, Birkenhäger WH (eds.). *Handbook of hypertension.* Vol. 18. Assessment of hypertensive organ damage. Amsterdam, Elsevier Science BV., 1997.

Smith JS, Kiloh LG. The investigation of dementia: results in 200 consecutive admissions. *Lancet* 1981; **1**: 824–7.

*Walstra GJ, Teunisse S, van Gool WA, van Crevel H. Reversible dementia in elderly patients referred to a memory clinic. *Journal of Neurology* 1997; **244**: 17–22.

Weatherall DJ, Ledingham JG, Warrell DA. *Oxford Textbook of Medicine* (3rd edn). Oxford University Press, 1996.

*Wells CE. Pseudo-dementia. *American Journal of Psychiatry* 1979; **136**: 895–900.

Victor M. Alcoholic dementia. *Canadian Journal of Neurological Science* 1994; **21**: 88–99.

5 Psychiatric assessment

C. Ballard and R. Eastwood

Introduction

Since the first memory clinics were established in the United States in the mid 1970s, there has been a massive expansion in memory clinic services throughout Europe and North America. Indeed, there are now more than 30 memory clinics in the United Kingdom and mainland Europe (Wright and Lindesay 1995; Verhey *et al.*, 1993; Walstra *et al.*, 1992). The objectives of clinics are broadly similar, aiming to provide comprehensive specialist assessment of patients with mild memory disorders, specialist advice on the management of these disorders, and to identify patients who may be suitable for participation in pharmacological or other research projects. The majority of clinics are multidisciplinary, most commonly involving psychiatrists, geriatricians, psychologists, neurologists, nurses, speech therapists, and occupational therapists (Wright and Lindesay 1995). The tradition in North America is slightly different. Few North American studies have described the characteristics of memory clinic attendees (Hogan *et al.*, 1994) but many have utilized 'dementia clinics' or 'memory clinics' as a source of patients for research, focusing upon diverse subjects such as driving skills (Fitten *et al.*, 1995), neuroimaging (Wolfe *et al.*, 1995), and the validation of instruments to identify non-cognitive symptoms (Sultzer *et al.*, 1992).

This chapter concentrates on the role of the psychiatrist in the assessment of dementia as part of the comprehensive evaluation conducted by the team. Memory clinics have developed largely as a mechanism to facilitate standardized evaluation of patients with mild subjective or objective cognitive deficits. It is important, however, that a comprehensive assessment is undertaken for all dementia sufferers regardless of the severity of their disorder. It has long been recognized that there are numerous advantages in assessing elderly patients, particularly those who are confused, in their own homes. As a consequence many clinicians, particularly those in the United Kingdom, prefer to undertake assessments in the community. On occasions, factors such as the severity of disabilities, the level of problem behaviours, dangers in the home environment, the need for a detailed physical examination, or carer stress may necessitate a hospital or nursing home environment in which to conduct the evaluation.

Aims of memory clinics

Whatever the setting of the assessment, a standardized approach with appropriate physical examination and investigation will improve symptom identification and provide a detailed baseline against which improvement can be measured. In addition, the use of validated instruments will result in greater consistency of reporting between different services and offer the opportunity for widespread research collaborations. Priorities will, however, differ slightly between memory clinics and community clinical services. Patients seen by clinical assessment services often have more severe cognitive impairment, with the identification of concurrent psychiatric morbidity assuming greater importance.

Depression, anxiety, and age-associated memory impairment as primary diagnoses

Diagnosis of psychiatric disorders

The accurate diagnosis of dementia is becoming increasingly important as new treatments are developed. Other essential aspects of assessment are, however, sometimes neglected. A substantial proportion of patients assessed in memory clinics do not suffer from dementia. This varies from 3 to 85 per cent in different United Kingdom clinics, with a mean of 25 per cent (Wright and Lindesay, 1995), and a mean of approximately 6 per cent in North American studies (Hogan et al., 1994; Weiner et al., 1991). The most common alternative diagnoses are 'worried well', minimal cognitive impairment, depression, and other psychiatric disorders. The prevalence of depression as a main diagnosis has varied from 0 per cent (Cohen et al., 1994) to 15.3 per cent (Nicholl et al., 1995), with most studies finding prevalence rates between 5 and 10 per cent (Skerrit et al., 1996; Ames et al., 1992).

Diagnostic criteria

Diagnostic procedures for depression have varied widely from expert diagnosis and cut off scores on depression rating scales to operationalized criteria such as the Research Diagnostic Criteria (RDC) (Spitzer et al., 1978) and DSM-III-R criteria (American Psychiatric Association, 1987) for major depression. Different assessment procedures probably explain some of the inconsistencies. Wright and Lindesay (1995) reported that only 45 per cent of United Kingdom memory clinics used standardized instruments to evaluate mood disorders. The picture is similar for North American studies (Weiner *et al.*, 1991). Although it is less common for primary psychiatric disorders to present as an apparent dementia in clinical settings, they must still be considered as an important differential diagnosis.

Cognitive impairment in depression

Patients with depression have lower total scores on standardized cognitive assessments than the 'worried well' but higher scores than patients with dementia. For example in Nicholl *et al.* (1995), depressed patients had a mean score of 27.5 on the Mini Mental State Examination (MMSE) (Folstein *et al.*, 1975). Whilst the majority of patients with depression score above the standard cut off score indicative of dementia, some individuals fall below this threshold. This is illustrated by Ott and Fogel (1992), in whose study 10 per cent of patients received a diagnosis of amnesic disorder related to depression. Similarly, Pantel *et al.* (1996) showed that 7 out of 10 patients with late onset major depression scored less than 24 on the MMSE. The paucity of follow-up data limit our knowledge of the outcome that these patients could expect. Des Rosiers *et al.* (1995) compared 12 patients with major depression to 24 patients with mild dementia (12 of whom had concurrent major depression). The scores from 9 out of 11 cognitive screening instruments were significantly different between the two groups. The instruments which performed best in separating the groups were the Wechsler Logical Memory Test (a test of story recall: sensitivity .54, specificity 1.0) and the Kendrick Object Learning Test (sensitivity .71, specificity 1.0). For both instruments, some of the patients with dementia scored similarly to the patients with depression. Abas *et al.* (1990) found 70 per cent of depressed patients to have significant impairments on tests of memory, new learning, and visual attention from the CANTAB battery. One-third of these patients experienced persistent cognitive deficits on recovery from their mood disorder. Provisional evidence also suggests that certain neuroimaging indices, particularly hippocampal volumes measured from MRI scanning, may help discriminate between these groups of patients (O'Brien *et al.*, 1994; Pantel *et al.*, 1996). Although these distinctions may be helpful, depression and depression coexisting with mild dementia remain common reasons for misdiagnosis, particularly in memory clinic cohorts (Verhey *et al.*, 1993).

Depressive pseudodementia

The interaction of depression and dementia is complex. Dementia caused by depression has been referred to as 'pseudodementia' (Kiloh, 1961). In broad terms this category encompasses two types of patients. Firstly, those who perform badly on standardized tests of cognitive function largely due to a lack of interest, poor concentration, or lack of motivation. Secondly, a syndrome encompassing patients with a pattern of cognitive abnormalities which more closely resemble the deficits seen in patients with dementia. The symptoms are related to depression but are not entirely explained by poor concentration or lack of motivation. Although patients may on occasions give an excess of 'I don't know' answers, or may have an inconsistent pattern of deficits (Wells, 1979), Caine (1981) described three core elements: intellectual impairment related to psychiatric disorder; neuropsychological deficits similar to those seen in dementia; and reversibility of the impairments. Wells (1979) suggested a list of factors which may help identify these individuals: a distinct date of onset; a short duration of symptoms preceding referral; rapid progression; a past psychiatric history; and a clear awareness by the family of the severity of symptoms experienced by the patient. Many of these patients do not however, follow this typical pattern.

Although there are some differences in the pattern of deficits identified on neuropsychological testing between patients with depression and those with dementia (Abas et al., 1990), overlap exists. Patients with late onset depression have a degree of ventricular enlargement intermediate between that of normal older adults and those with dementia (Pearlson et al., 1989), indicating a degree of organicity. Provisional data suggest that approximately 15 per cent of patients with resolved depressive pseudodementia go on to develop dementia over 2 years of follow-up (Alexopoulos et al., 1991). The small numbers preclude firm conclusions at this point.

The information currently available does not give a detailed breakdown of the cognitive performance of depressed individuals. Information regarding consistency of deficits and the effort made by the individual during testing are essential for the accurate interpretation of apparent cognitive deficits in an individual with a depressive disorder. Given the substantial proportion of memory clinic patients suffering from depression, follow-up data from these cohorts would provide invaluable information. Provisional data suggest that the cognitive deficits in depressed patients do resolve with appropriate treatment (Walstra et al., 1992), The evaluation of depression in mild dementia will be discussed in more detail later on in the chapter. It is, however, important to bear in mind that approximately 20 per cent of individuals with dementia will experience concurrent depression (Burns, 1991). Perhaps the most important recommendation should be a re-evaluation of cognitive performance after the depression has been treated, which should be combined with longer-term monitoring of cognitive function. Only a minority of United Kingdom (Wright and Lindesay, 1995) and North American (Williams et al., 1995; see also Chapter 2) memory clinics offer routine follow-up to patients. Regular follow-up visits are routine practice for community clinical services, but standardized information is not usually collected.

Self-referring patients

The majority of memory clinics and dementia services focus primarily on referrals from medical practitioners, although some accept referrals from other health-care professionals and self referrals. Barker *et al.* (1994, 1995) suggested that individuals who self refer are particularly likely to exhibit symptoms of depression. Fifty percent of these patients also have a past history of depression and may have mild depressive symptomatology at the time they are seen, with a mean Geriatric Depression Scale score of 4.4 in Barker *et al.*'s (1995) study. Barker *et al.*'s patients were also distressed about their perceived memory difficulties, despite scoring well within normal limits on tests of cognitive function. Despite the fact that few of these patients were diagnosed with major depression at the time of assessment, they are none-the-less a vulnerable group of individuals. One might expect that reassurance from a specialist following a comprehensive assessment would ease distress. It may also be that, at least in some cases, the individuals themselves were more sensitive to real and early changes in their functioning; changes which the cognitive assessments used were insufficiently sensitive to pick up. Further study of the course of their depression or distress would have been helpful. This is an important area for further research.

Other psychiatric diagnoses

Few other studies have reported data pertaining to primary diagnosis other than depression. Almeida *et al.* (1993) found that 5 per cent of their 418 patients had a main diagnosis of 'neurotic disorder other than depression' and one patient had a diagnosis of schizophrenia. One of the 100 patients attending Ames *et al.*'s (1992) clinic had a primary diagnosis of RDC Generalized Anxiety Disorder (Spitzer *et al.*, 1978). Given the high level of concern expressed by a number of patients with subjective memory complaints, it might be expected that primary anxiety disorders would be quite common and this again requires further investigation. Coen *et al.* (1994) identified two out of 81 patients with primary aphasia and one out of 81 with an isolated area of frontal lobe infarction.

Outcome of psychiatric disorders

The long-term consequences of depression or anxiety and their effects on cognition in patients without a primary dementia needs further study. This important research topic will benefit from more widespread collection of standardized information.

Summary

Most memory clinics use standardized criteria to diagnose dementia, usually based upon a detailed clinical assessment, physical examination, neuro-psychological evaluation, and neuroimaging. Rather less care is taken to diagnose primary conditions other than dementia. Twenty-five percent of patients attending memory clinics do not suffer from dementia, a fifth of whom suffer from a depressive disorder. A significant proportion may also suffer from anxiety disorders or have mild depressive symptomatology. There is a need for memory clinics to introduce routine screening for depression and anxiety symptoms with standardized schedules and to apply standardized criteria to make operationalized psychiatric diagnoses. Standardized evaluation and diagnosis are less widely used by community clinical services, although the benefits are similar.

Psychiatric symptoms and behaviour problems in patients with dementia

Prevalence of depression in patients with dementia

Depression occurs in a significant proportion of patients with dementia. Prevalence rates have varied from 0 per cent (Burns *et al.*, 1990) to 52 per cent (Pozzi *et al.*, 1993) in standardized clinical studies. The mean prevalence rate is 20 per cent (Burns, 1991; Ballard *et al.*, 1996a). There is a significant body of evidence to suggest that depression is more prevalent in patients with less severe cognitive impairment (Ballard *et al.*, 1996a), an important con-sideration in dementia patients attending a memory clinic. The symptoms of depression in these patients are similar to those occurring amongst individuals suffering from depression in the absence of cognitive impairment. They include: sadness; loss of interest, sleep, and appetite disturbances; psycho-motor changes; guilt feelings; anxiety; and suicidal thoughts (Ballard *et al.*, 1996a). Depression in individuals with dementia not only causes distress to the patients (Burns, 1991) but it may also further impair cognitive function (Ballard *et al.*, 1996a), as well as instrumental activities of daily living (Fitz and Teri, 1994). Life expectancy may also be reduced (Burns *et al.*, 1991). In addition, depression in patients causes distress to their carers (Ballard *et al.*, 1996a).

Depression is, therefore, an important disorder which adds to the disability experienced by patients with dementia and it is common in individuals attending a memory clinic. Cohen *et al.* (1994), Ott and Fogel (1992), Sultzer *et al.* (1992), Ballard (1995), and Weiner *et al.* (1991) have all reported depression in memory clinic patients. Although the proportions varied considerably between the five studies, it is evident that a substantial number of patients with dementia suffered from a concurrent depressive disorder, sufficiently severe to meet standardized diagnostic criteria. A detailed breakdown of these studies is given in Table 5.1. Summary data pertaining to concurrent depression from community dementia services are presented in Table 5.2.

Insight into the dementing illness per se has not been found to be associated with the occurrence of depression (Ott and Fogel, 1992). Nevertheless, it is not surprising that patients attending a memory clinic, who may expect to be told they are suffering from dementia, are susceptible to mood disorders. Retained insight and dysphoria are common presenting symptoms in memory clinic attendees (Williams *et al.*, 1995).

Table 5.1 Depression in memory clinic attendees

Study	Number of patients	Prevalence of significant depression (%)	Assessment instrument
Cohen *et al.*, 1994	514	25	Hamilton depression scale
Ott and Fogel, 1992	50	44	DSM-III-R
Sultzer *et al.*, 1992	61	26	Neurobehavioural rating scale
Ballard, 1995	25	8	RDC major depression
Weiner *et al.*, 1991	192	2	DSM-III-R

Table 5.2 Summary of psychiatric symptoms in patients with dementia

	*Number of standardized studies	Overall mean prevalence (%)	Main associations
Depression	20	20.6	Mild cognitive impairment Vascular dementia
Anxiety	3	40.6	Mild cognitive impairment
Psychosis	22	46.5	Moderate or severe cognitive impairment Deafness or visual impairment Dementia with Lewy bodies

*Definition and data from Ballard, 1995.

Outcome of depression in individuals with dementia

Two intervention studies (Reifler *et al.*, 1989; Roth *et al.*, 1996) and a naturalistic follow up study (Ballard *et al.*, 1996b) suggest that there is a high rate of spontaneous resolution of depression in individuals with dementia. In Ballard *et al.*'s (1996b) study, more than 80 per cent experienced resolution of depressive symptoms within 6 months and approximately 30 per cent experienced resolution within 3 months. There is a paucity of specific data available for memory clinic cohorts, although Williams *et al.* (1995) found dysphoria to be a less common problem at 3-year follow-up. Even though depression can be disabling for people with dementia, it is therefore inappropriate to instigate treatment in all newly incident cases. However, one double blind, controlled trial of antidepressant medication has been shown to be significantly more efficacious than placebo (Roth *et al.*, 1996).

The role of memory clinics in managing patients with depression and dementia

Memory clinic patients, in general, have relatively mild dementia which facilitates identification of concurrent depression. These clinics provide an ideal opportunity to assess the course of depression and whether it resolves, following the initial diagnosis together with associated advice and counselling. They also provide an opportunity to assess ongoing symptoms of depression in addition to changes in cognitive performance and to commence treatment for more persistent mood disorders. Depression is, however, also common in community clinical settings, where it can be more difficult to recognize in patients with more marked cognitive impairment. A standardized approach which incorporates an informant interview becomes even more valuable in such settings.

Anxiety in dementia

Anxiety disorders are also common in patients with dementia. Wands *et al.* (1990) used the Hospital Anxiety and Depression Scale to investigate anxiety amongst 50 patients with mild dementia, 38 per cent of whom had possible or probable anxiety disorder. Ballard *et al.* (1994) found 31 per cent of patients with dementia in contact with a day hospital fulfilled RDC criteria for Generalized Anxiety Disorder (Spitzer *et al.*, 1978). This study suggested that those with mild dementia were most at risk of experiencing anxiety symptoms. Ballard *et al.* (1996c) reported anxiety symptoms in 109 patients with DSM-II-R diagnosed dementia from the Leicester Memory Clinic. Table 5.3 shows the pattern of anxiety symptoms. Summary data are presented in Table 5.2.

    The limited information available does suggest that concurrent anxiety

Table 5.3 Anxiety symptoms experienced by patients with dementia (Ballard *et al.*, 1996c)

Anxiety symptom	Percentage of patients
Subjective anxiety	22
Autonomic anxiety	11
Tension symptoms	39
Situational anxiety	13
Panic attacks	2

symptoms are highly prevalent in patients attending a memory clinic and those seen by community dementia services. Little is known about the natural course of these disorders or what additional disability they may confer. Again, memory clinics provide the ideal opportunity to investigate these issues in more detail. Of particular interest is whether the initial diagnosis and associated counselling procedures have any impact on the level of anxiety symptoms. No intervention trials have so far been conducted.

Psychosis in dementia

'Psychosis' has often been used to describe a broad range of behaviour disturbance in older adults with dementia. Fortunately, more rigorous definitions limiting the term to describe delusions and hallucinations in clear consciousness have been used in the majority of recent studies. Psychotic symptoms in patients with dementia cause a great deal of distress both to the patients and to carers (Ballard, 1995), and are associated with a number of behaviour difficulties (Rockwell *et al.*, 1994). In addition, they reduce the likelihood of people continuing to live in their own homes (Steele *et al.*, 1990). All of these factors emphasize the importance of identifying concurrent psychosis in patients with dementia.

Prevalence and treatment of psychosis in dementia

Standardized studies focusing on clinical samples have suggested a prevalence rate for psychosis in excess of 60 per cent (Devanand *et al.*, 1992; Ballard, 1995). The general consensus is that hallucinations are associated with a more severe degree of cognitive impairment and that delusions are more common in patients with dementia of moderate severity (Ballard *et al.*, 1991; Jeste *et al.*, 1992; Ballard, 1995). Nevertheless, patients with milder cognitive impairment do experience these symptoms. For example, in Ballard *et al.*'s (1991) study, 50 per cent of patients with minimal CAMDEX dementia (Roth *et al.*, 1986) and 29 per cent of patients with mild CAMDEX dementia met the CAMDEX

Table 5.4 Psychosis in memory clinic samples

Study	Number of patients	Psychosis overall (%)	Prevalence of hallucinations (%)	Prevalence of delusions (%)	Assessment instrument
Cohen et al., 1994	514	na	11.1	11.6	Clinical interview
Ballard, 1995	25	64	22	48	Burns' symptom checklist

criteria for Paranoid Disorder. A meta-analysis of treatment trials suggests that neuroleptic agents are significantly better than placebo for the treatment of psychosis in dementia, although the response rate was only 20 per cent better than placebo (Schneider et al., 1990).

In memory clinic studies, Sultzer et al. (1992) identified a 'psychosis' component from a principal components analysis and Williams et al. (1995) found delusions to be a frequent presenting problem. Cohen et al. (1994) and Ballard (1995) have reported prevalence data which are presented in Table 5.4.

In many cases, the symptoms will be fleeting or unobtrusive but some may require treatment. As the symptoms cause distress to patients and their carers, identification is important and is best facilitated by a standardized schedule. The advantages of a standardized approach are clear when one considers that case note studies only identify 30 per cent of psychotic symptoms (Ballard, 1995).

Personality change in dementia

A commonly described characteristic of dementia is personality change, which is a feature of diagnostic criteria. This concept is a difficult one in the context of dementia, given the assumption that personality reflects a lifelong pattern of characteristics and responses for a particular individual. Whether the individual's behaviour represents actual personality change or alterations in behaviour patterns is an important subject with which psychiatrists must grapple. One study does focus on personality changes in patients attending a dementia clinic (Bozzola et al., 1992). Eighty patients were assessed, 33 (41 per cent) of whom displayed increased rigidity in thinking, 31 (39 per cent) had reduced regard for the feelings of others, 21 (26 per cent) expressed increased egocentricity, and 29 (36 per cent) had coarsening of affect. These findings are likely to be more prominent in patients with frontal lobe dementias. Although this is an important area for study, greater clarity of the concepts is required before progress can be made.

Behaviour problems in dementia

Rapp *et al.* (1992) summarized the main non-cognitive symptoms experienced by dementia sufferers, including behaviour problems such as agitation, abnormal eating patterns, shouting/screaming, restlessness, wandering, rage/violence, sleep–wake disturbances, and inappropriate sexual behaviours. These are all common symptoms which add considerably to carer burden. They are considered in more detail in Chapter 19.

Standardized schedules

In an unstructured interview it is all too easy to omit crucial questions if a patient does not appear to be depressed or anxious or to have behavioural or personality changes. Scales such as the Cornell Depression scale, the Montgomery Asberg Depression Rating Scale (Montgomery and Asberg, 1979) and the Hospital Anxiety and Depression Scale (Kenn *et al.*, 1987) ask focused questions of clinical relevance. They improve the consistency of symptom ratings and ensure that enquiries are made about key symptoms. The majority of these instruments take only 10 or 15 minutes to administer, a similar time commitment to a detailed clinical enquiry about affective symptoms and behaviour problems.

Evaluating depression

The instrument of choice for the evaluation of depression is the Cornell Depression Scale (CDS) (Alexopoulos *et al.*, 1988). The CDS is the only depression screening instrument which has been designed and validated specifically for the evaluation of depression in patients with dementia. The scale uses patient and informant reports with the evaluator arbitrating for discrepancies. It also has specific rules to clarify the importance of loss of interest in patients suffering with dementia; a key element in diagnosis. A score of 10 or more is indicative of significant depression and the items facilitate the application of operationalized diagnostic criteria.

Evaluating anxiety

In the absence of any scales validated for the assessment of anxiety in individuals with dementia, it is difficult to recommend any particular standardized instrument. A standardized inventory for identifying anxiety symptoms in patients without dementia should be chosen as a symptom checklist. Indeed, no criteria have been validated specifically for the identification of anxiety disorders in dementia sufferers. Instruments used for symptom identification include the Hospital Anxiety and Depression Scale (Kenn *et al.*, 1987), the anxiety section of the CAMDEX schedule (Roth *et al.*, 1986), and a checklist of anxiety symptoms based upon the RDC (Spitzer *et al.*, 1978). There are no clear advantages to any of these methods over any other.

Instruments for measuring psychosis in dementia

A number of schedules have now been described. The best validated brief schedules are the BEHAVE-AD (Reisberg *et al.*, 1987) and the CUSPAD (Devanand *et al.*, 1992). Both rely on informant accounts and cover a checklist of common psychotic symptoms, taking 10 to 20 minutes to administer. The BEHAVE-AD also asks questions about problem behaviours.

Summary

The main reason for setting up a memory clinic is to facilitate the accurate diagnosis of early or complex dementias with a view to early intervention, treatment studies, and other research, as well as providing opportunities for detailed monitoring of the progression of cognitive impairment. The majority of clinics use standardized criteria to diagnose dementia and standardized neuropsychological tests. The assessment of psychiatric symptoms, however, has received less attention. This is particularly surprising in the United Kingdom where 75 per cent of memory clinics involve psychiatrists, a substantial minority of patients have a primary diagnosis other than dementia, and a large group of patients with dementia experience psychiatric or behavioural problems. As depression and anxiety are particularly common in patients with mild dementia, memory clinics have an obligation to diagnose and monitor these symptoms. Community clinical dementia services, on the whole, assess patients with more severe cognitive impairment, when the main focus is often on the assessment of concurrent psychiatric morbidity, although differential diagnosis from other primary psychiatric disorders remains important.

It is proposed that a standardized psychiatric assessment package should be adopted by memory clinics and other dementia services. This should include standardized schedules to assess depression, anxiety, psychosis, and behavioural problems. The importance of follow-up to monitor the course of these symptoms is also stressed. Psychiatrists within multidisciplinary teams have the responsibility for the diagnosis of primary psychiatric conditions, as well as psychiatric problems and behavioural disturbances in the context of dementia. In addition, they should provide a standardized psychiatric assessment for the diagnosis of dementia.

References

Key references recommended by the authors are marked with an *.

Abas, M.A., Sahakian, B.J. *et al*. (1990). Neuropsychological Deficits and CT Scan. Changes in Elderly Depressives. *Psychological Medicine*, **20**, 507–520.

Alexopoulos, G.S. and Abrams, R.C. (1991). Clinical Presentation and Outcome of Geriatric Depressive 'Pseudodementia' (Abstract). *Psychiatric Bulletin*, **15** Suppl. 4,6.

Alexopoulos, G.S., Abrams, R.C., Young, R.C. and Shamoian, C.A. (1988). Cornell Scale for Depression in Dementia. *Biological Psychiatry*, **23**, 271–234.

*Almeida, O.P., Hill, K., Howard, R. *et al*. (1993). Demographic and Clinical Features of Patients attending a Memory Clinic. *International Journal of Geriatric Psychiatry*, **8**, 497–501.

American Psychiatric Association (1987). *Diagnostic and Statistical Manual of Mental Disorders*, Revised Third Edition. Washington, DC; American Psychiatric Association.

Ames, D., Flicker, L. and Helme, R.D. (1992). A Memory-Clinic at a Geriatric Hospital: Rationale, Routine and Results from the First 100 Patients. *Medical Journal of Australia*, **156**, 618–622.

Ballard, C.G. (1995). *Depression and Psychotic Symptoms in Dementia Sufferers*. MD Thesis, University of Birmingham.

Ballard, C.G., Chithiramohan, R.N., Bannister, C., Handy, S. and Todd, N. (1991). Paranoid Features in the Elderly with Dementia. *International Journal of Geriatric Psychiatry*, **6**, 155–157.

Ballard, C.G., Mohan, R.N.C., Patel, A. and Graham C. (1994). Anxiety Disorders in Dementia. *Irish Journal of Psychological Medicine*, **11**, 108–109.

Ballard, C.G., Bannister, C. and Oyebode, F. (1996a). Depression in Dementia Sufferers. *International Journal of Geriatric Psychiatry*, **11**, 507–515.

Ballard, C.G., Patel, A., Solis, M. *et al*. (1996b). A One Year Follow up Study of Depression in Patients with Dementia. *British Journal of Psychiatry*, **168**, 287–291.

Ballard, C.G., Boyle, A., Bowler, C. and Lindesay, J. (1996c). Anxiety Disorders in Dementia Sufferers. *International Journal of Geriatric Psychiatry*, in press.

Barker, A., Carter, C. and Jones, R. (1994). Memory Performance, Self Reported Memory Loss and Depressive Symptoms in Attendees at a GP Referral and A Self-Referral Memory Clinic. *International Journal of Geriatric Psychiatry*, **9**, 305–312.

Barker, A., Prior, J. and Jones, R. (1995). Memory Complaint in Attendees at a Self-Referral Memory Clinic: The Role of Cognitive Factors, Affective Symptoms and Personality. *International Journal of Geriatric Psychiatry*, **10**, 777–781.

Bozzola, F.G., Gorelick, P.B. and Freels, S. (1992). Personality Changes in Alzheimer's Disease. *Archives of Neurology*, **49**, 297–300.

Burns, A. (1991). Affective Symptoms in Alzheimer's Disease. *International Journal of Geriatric Psychiatry*, **6**, 371–376.

*Burns, A., Jacoby, R. and Levy, R. (1990). Psychiatric Phenomena in Alzheimer's Disease. *British Journal of Psychiatry*, **157**, 81–94.

Burns, A., Lewis, G., Jacoby, R. and Levy, R. (1991). Factors Affecting Survival in Alzheimer's Disease. *Psychological Medicine*, **21**, 363–370.

Caine, E.D. (1981). Pseudo-dementia: Current Concepts and Future Directions. *Archives of General Psychiatry*, **38**, 1359–1364.

Coen, R.F., O'Mahoney, D., Bruce, I., Lawlor, B.A., Walsh, J.B. and Coakley, D. (1994). Differential Diagnosis of Dementia: A Prospective Evaluation of the DAT Inventory. *Journal of the American Geriatrics Society*, **42**, 16–20.

*Cohen, D., Eisdorfer, C., Gorclick, P. *et al.* (1994). Sex Differences in the Psychiatric Manifestations of Alzheimer's Disease. *Journal of American Geriatric Psychiatry*, **41**, 229–232.

Des Rosiers, G., Hodges, J. and Berrios, G. (1995). The Neuropsychological Differentiation of Patients with Very Mild Alzheimer's Disease and/or Major Depression. *Journal of the American Geriatrics Society*, **43**, 1256–1263.

Devanand, D.P., Miller, L., Marder, K. *et al.* (1992). The Columbia University Scale for Psychopathology in Alzheimer's Disease. *Archives of Neurology*, **49**, 371–376.

Fitten, L.J., Perryman, K.M., Wilkinson, C.J., Little, R.J., Burns, M.M., Pachana, N., Mervis, J.R., Malmgren, R., Siembieda, D.W. and Ganzell, S. (1995). Alzheimer and Vascular Dementias and Driving. A Prospective Road and Laboratory Study. *Journal of the American Medical Association*, **273**, 1360–5.

Fitz, A.E. and Teri, L. (1994). Depression, Cognition and Functional Ability in Patients with Alzheimer's Disease. *Journal of the American Geriatrics Society*, **42**, 186–191.

Folstein, M.F., Folstein, S.E. and McHugh, P.R. (1975). Mini-Mental State— A Practical Method For Grading The Cognitive State of Patients for the Clinician. *Journal of Psychiatric Research*, **12**, 189–198.

*Hogan, D.B., Thierer, D.E., Ebly, E.M. and Parhad, I.M. (1994). Progression and Outcome of Patients in a Canadian Dementia Clinic. *Canadian Journal of Neurological Sciences*, **21**, 331–8.

Jeste, D.S., Wragg, R.E., Salmon, D.P. *et al.* (1992). Cognitive Deficits of

Patients with Alzheimer's Disease with and without Delusions. *American Journal of Psychiatry*, **149**, 184–189.

Kenn, C., Wood, H., Kucy, M., Watttis, J, and Cunane, J. (1987). Validation of the Hospital Anxiety and Depression Rating Scale (HADS) in an elderly psychiatric population *International Journal of Geriatric Psychiatry*, **2**, 189–193

Kiloh, L.G. (1961). Pseudo-Dementia. *Acta Psychiatrica Scandinavica*, **37**, 336–351.

Montgomery, S.A., and Asberg, M. (1979). A New Depression Scale designed to be sensitive to change *British Journal of Psychiatry*, **134**, 332–9.

Nicholl, C.G., Lynch, S., Kelly, A. *et al.* (1995). The Cognitive Drug Research Computerised Assessment System in the Evaluation of Early Dementia— Is Speed of the Essence? *International Journal of Geriatric Psychiatry*, **10**, 199–206.

O'Brien, J.T., Ames, D. and Schweitzer, I. (1994). The Differentiation of Depression from Dementia by Magnetic Resonance Imaging. *Psychological Medicine*, **24**, 633–640.

Ott, B.R. and Fogel, B.S. (1992). Measurement of Depression in Dementia: Self vs. Clinical Rating. *International Journal of Geriatric Psychiatry*, **7**, 899–904.

Pantel, J., Dech, D., Essig, M. *et al.* (1996). Differential Diagnosis of Depression and Dementia in Geriatric Patients by Quantitative Magnetic Resonance Image. (Abstract). *European Psychiatry*, **11** Suppl 4, 2775.

Pearlson, G.D., Rabins, P.V., Kim, W.S. *et al.* (1989). Structural Brain CT Changes and Cognitive Deficits in Elderly Depressives with and without Reversible Cognitive Impairment (Pseudo-dementia). *Psychological Medicine*, **19**, 573–584.

Pozzi, D., Golimstock, A., Migliorelli, R. *et al.* (1993). Quantified Electroencephalographic Correlates of Depression in Alzheimer's Disease. *Biological Psychiatry*, **34**, 386–391.

Rapp, M.S., Flint, A.J., Herrmann, N. and Proulx, G.B. (1992). Behavioural Disturbances in the Demented Elderly—Phenomenology, Pharmacotherapy and Behavioural Management. *Canadian Journal of Psychiatry*, **37**, 651–657.

Reifler, B.V., Teri, L. and Raskind, M. *et al.* (1989). Double Blind Trial of Imipramine in Alzheimer's Disease Patients with and without Depression. *American Journal of Psychiatry*, **146**, 45–49.

Reisberg, G., Borenstein, J., Salob, S. *et al.* (1987). Behavioural Symptoms in Alzheimer's Disease: Phenomenology and Treatment. *Journal of Clinical Psychiatry*, **48** 5 (Suppl), 9–15.

Rockwell, E., Jackson, E., Vilke, G. and Jeste, D.V. (1994). A Study of Delusions in a Large Cohort of Alzheimer's Disease Patients. *American Journal of Geriatric Psychiatry*, **2**, 157–164.

Roth, M., Tym, E., Mountjoy, C., Huppert, F., Hendrie, H., Verma, S. and

Goddard, R. (1986). CAMDEX: A standardised instrument for the diagnosis of mental disorder in the elderly with special reference to the early detection of dementia. *British Journal of Psychiatry*, **149**, 698–709.

Roth, M., Mountjoy, C.Q., Amerin R. and The International Collaborative Study Group (1996). *British Journal of Psychiatry*, **168**, 149–157.

Schneider, L.S., Pollock, V.E. and Lyness, S.A. (1 990). A Meta Analysis of Controlled Trials of Neuroleptic Treatment in Dementia. *Journal of the American Geriatric Society*, **38**, 553–563.

Skerrit, U., Pitt, B., Armstrong, S. *et al*. (1996). Recruiting Patients for Drug Trials: A Difficult Task! *Psychiatric Bulletin*, **20**, 708–710.

Spitzer, R.L., Endicott, J. and Robins, E. (1978). Research diagnostic criteria, rationale and reliability. *Archives of General Psychiatry*, **35**, 73–82.

Steele, C., Rovner, B., Chase, G.A. and Folstein, M. (1990). Psychiatric Symptoms and Nursing Home Placement of Patients with Alzheimer's Disease. *American Journal of Psychiatry*, **147**, 1049–1051.

Sultzer, D.L., Levin, H.S., Mahler, M.E., High, W.M. and Cummings, J.L. (1992). Assessment of Cognitive, Psychiatric and Behavioural Disturbances in Patients with Dementia: The Neurobehavioral Rating Scale. *Journal of the American Geriatrics Society*, **40**, 549–55.

Verhey, F.R.J., Rozendaal, N., Ponds, W.H.M. and Jolks, J. (1993). Dementia, Awareness and Depression. *International Journal of Geriatric Psychiatry*, **8**, 851–856.

Walstra, G.J., Derix, M.M., Hijdra, A. and Van Crevel H. (1992). An Outpatient Clinic for Memory Disorders: Initial Experiences. *Nederlands Tideschrift voor Geneeskunde*, **136**, 328–32.

Wands, K., Merskey, H., Hachinski, V.C., Fishman, M., Fox, F. and Boniferro, M. (1990). A Questionnaire Investigation of Anxiety and Depression in Early Dementia. *Journal of American Geriatric Society*, **36**, 535–538.

Weiner, M.F., Bruhn, M., Svetlik, D., Tintner, R. and Hom, J. (1991). Experiences with Depression in a Dementia Clinic. *Journal of Clinical Psychiatry*, **52**, 234–8.

Wells, C.E. (1979). Pseudo-dementia. *American Journal of Psychiatry*, **136**, 895–900.

Williams, G.O., Gjerde, C.L., Haugland, S., Darnold, D., Simonton, L.J. and Woodward, P.J. (1995). Patients with Dementia and Their Caregivers 3 Years After Diagnosis. A Longitudinal Study. *Archives of Family Medicine*, **4**, 512–7.

Wolfe, N., Reed, B.R., Eberling, J.L. and Jagust, W.J. (1995). Temporal Lobe Perfusion on Single Photon Emission Computed Tomography Predicts the Rate of Cognitive Decline in Alzheimer's Disease. *Archives of Neurology*, **52**, 257–62.

*Wright, M. and Lindesay, J. (1995). A Survey of Memory Clinics in the British Isles. *International Journal of Geriatric Psychiatry*, **10**, 379–385.

6 Investigations—laboratory, radiological, and neurophysiological

Kim A. Jobst, Rodolfo Suarez, and Bruce L. Miller

Introduction

Dementia is a clinically-defined syndrome. It may be caused by a plethora of conditions (see Chapters 4, 14, and 15). Making the diagnosis of dementia is important because some causes are treatable, and because accurate diagnostic information can help patients and their families to plan for the future and come to terms with their condition (Jobst 1996; Smith *et al.* 1988). Since it is obviously impractical to exclude all possible causes of dementia in each case, the specific and differential diagnosis of dementia is a challenge to the astute clinician. If the memory disorders team is to be clinically effective and financially viable, good clinical judgement is the cornerstone upon which to determine which laboratory tests and special investigations should be requested (Larson *et al.* 1986; Terry *et al.* 1994).

It is essential first to exclude potentially treatable disorders. Acquiring meticulous medical and psychiatric histories is essential to determining whether the patient is medically ill, has taken medications or recreational drugs, herbs, or other substances which could affect cognition and brain function, or whether there may be a psychiatric cause which may exacerbate cognitive dysfunction, particularly in the early stages of dementia. A comprehensive physical examination should be performed, to search for signs of systemic illness and focal neurological signs, since the distinction between delirium and dementia can be subtle, and brain function in elderly people can be particularly vulnerable to mild metabolic, toxic, or infectious insults and also to alterations in mood such as occur in depression and psychosis. Any of these conditions may occur in combination so whenever possible the history should be corroborated by a relative or close friend.

Laboratory tests and special investigations in dementia

Arguably one cannot exclude many of the causes listed above with clinical history and examination alone, thus routine laboratory tests, designed to identify potentially treatable conditions, are necessary when the initial evaluation is not diagnostic. Judicious use of tests based on sound clinical judgement can defray between 25 and 34 per cent of costs (Larson *et al.* 1986). A comprehensive baseline biochemical and haematological profile on entry to the clinic permits comparative evaluations, if there is a need for reassessment, and data collection for longitudinal evaluation, if the memory team has a research agenda.

The basic laboratory evaluation at baseline in dementia should include:

♦ A full blood count:

haemoglobin level and mean cell volume;

white cell count and possibly differential white count;

platelet count;

erythrocyte sedimentation rate (ESR)/ blood viscosity.

This will detect anaemias, myeloproliferative disorders, infection, inflammatory, and autoimmune conditions. Further investigation with specialized tests such as autoantibody screens, immunoglobulin levels, bone-marrow sampling, abdominal ultrasound, serum iron and total iron binding capacity, investigation for sources of blood loss, evaluation of alcohol consumption, and other causes of macrocytosis will then follow.

♦ Baseline electrolytes and biochemistry:

urea;

creatinine;

sodium and potassium;

calcium, phosphate, and albumin;

liver enzymes.

These simple indices will reveal whether basic renal, hepatic, cardiac, and bone function are within normal limits. Furthermore, any abnormalities will flag the need for careful re-evaluation of the history for other possible causes of metabolic dysfunction if there is no evidence of a primary cause in any of the major organ systems. Potassium levels are particularly relevant in the presence of cardiac or renal disease.

Hyper- and hypoparathyroidism are often forgotten as causes of cognitive dysfunction and mood disturbance and, although rare, are rewarding to treat. The distinction between primary and secondary disease, and even pseudo-parathyroid disease, can be taxing but should be remembered when abnormalities are discovered.

Less common metabolic disorders, such as lead and organophosphorous poisoning and porphyria, may need to be considered. However, by far the most important cause of metabolic disturbance in the elderly population is iatrogenic drug toxicity: the importance of a careful drug history cannot be over stressed.

Blood sugar level

Diabetes, hypoglycaemia, and hyperglycaemia are important possible causes of an organic brain syndrome, not only in themselves but it is thought also as a result of long-term microvascular change within the central nervous system (Pirttila *et al.* 1992; Croxson and Jagger 1995). Thus baseline blood glucose levels should routinely be assessed, particularly if there is a history of fluctuating symptoms, weight loss or gain, dysrhythmias, postural hypotension, repeated infections, alterations in bowel or drinking habits, or peripheral sensory disturbances.

Thyroid function tests

The clinical symptoms of both hyper- and hypothyroidism may be subtle, with the primary cognitive manifestations ranging from depression and mild mental slowing to severe dementia (Shetty and Duthie 1995). Furthermore, in elderly people the manifestations of both conditions may easily be confused and biochemical confirmation should always be sought (Cummings and Benson 1992). Although some doubt its routine value, most would agree that baseline assessment of thyroid function is mandatory since neurodegenerative dementia does not prohibit concomitant hypo- or hyperthyroidism, either of which may exacerbate cognitive dysfunction. Since levels of tri-iodothyronine (T3) may be high in the presence of normal levels of thyroxine (T4), the thyroid stimulating hormone (TSH) level is recommended as the initial test, since this will be low despite a normal T4. Clearly this will not reveal secondary hypothyroidism but if there is clinical evidence free-T4 and free-T3 levels should be measured. Elderly patients may be more sensitive to only mildly or moderately raised T3 so the threshold for remeasuring, further investigating with a radio-iodine thyroid scan, and treating abnormal levels should perhaps be lower in old age.

Vitamin B$_{12}$ and folic acid levels

The relationship of serum vitamin B$_{12}$ and folic acid with dementia and cognitive dysfunction is controversial (Riggs *et al.* 1996; Joosten *et al.* 1997).

Red cell folate may be normal in the presence of low serum folate so it is sensible to measure both. If only one test is to be carried out, it should be the red cell folate assay. Distinct correlations between low levels and dementia have been shown (Riggs *et al.* 1996), as has improved cognitive function with treatment of the deficiencies by vitamin supplementation, but others have failed to confirm this (Crystal *et al.* 1994). However, there is a possibly causal relationship between cognitive dysfunction and low folate and vitamin B_{12} levels (Joosten *et al.* 1997), and even to confirmed Alzheimer's disease (Clarke *et al.* 1998). Whether this is due to the toxic effects of the consequent high serum homocysteine levels remains to be established, but increasingly it is suggested that in elderly people low to normal vitamin B_{12} or folate levels may represent a functionally significant metabolic deficiency, for which reason the best markers of excessively low levels are the serum levels of their metabolites, homocysteine and methymalonic acid (Joosten *et al.* 1997). Since treatment with either vitamin B_{12} or folic acid supplementation has been shown to be beneficial in dementia and other psychiatric diseases, serum vitamin B_{12} and folic acid levels should be requested in elderly patients with atypical dementias and in those with anaemia, neuropathies, or long-tract spinal cord signs (Nilsson *et al.* 1994; Carney 1995; Refsum *et al.* 1998).

Testing for Apolipoprotein E4 (ApoE4) genotype and other genetic tests

There has been much debate over the diagnostic value of testing for the presence of ApoE4 in Alzheimer's disease. Although some have claimed that it can increase specificity to 100 per cent in cases of clinically diagnosed NINCDS 'probable Alzheimer's disease' (Saunders *et al.* 1996), others have failed to confirm this in subjects more representative of memory clinic populations with a wide range of diagnoses (Smith *et al.* 1996). Not only is the ApoE4 genotype not confined to Alzheimer's disease, (that is it is found in non-Alzheimer's disease dementias) but it is also found in completely normal elderly people without any cognitive dysfunction and without central nervous system pathology at post-mortem (Jobst *et al.* 1998).

Other autosomal dominant genes have also been shown to give rise to Alzheimer's disease, notably on chromosomes 21, 14, and 1. However, they account for a very very small proportion of all Alzheimer's disease dementias. There are also genetic associations in non-Alzheimer's disease dementias. In the differential diagnosis of dementia, genetic testing should only be undertaken with the full back up of genetic counselling and support services, and after due consultation with relevant family members (Lovestone 1996) .

Other tests

The electrocardiogram

A baseline electrocardiogram is recommended since it may reveal evidence of conduction disturbances not detectable clinically. This has management implications since treatment of cardiac dysrhythmias, pacemaker insertion, and anticoagulation may diminish the risk of progressive cerebrovascular dysfunction. Appropriate treatment may increase well being and thus cognition. If rhythm disturbances are identified and there is a clinical suspicion of cerebrovascular disease, echocardiography should be performed. Some commonly used antifailure, antihypertension, and antidysrhythmia drugs are contraindicated in some arrhythmias, for example the deleterious effects of calcium antagonists on re-entrant phenomena in Wolff–Parkinson–White syndrome.

Chest radiographs and other radiographs

Only rarely are changes demonstrated in baseline chest radiographs which would alter management without prior clinical evidence. Now that CT, MRI, and functional brain scanning techniques are available there is no longer any indication for skull radiographs, unless fractures are suspected.

Doppler ultrasonography

Doppler ultrasonography is used to evaluate carotid patency and cerebrovascular status. It should be considered whenever there is a strong suspicion of occlusive cerebrovascular disease and has been shown to help in distinguishing between Alzheimer's disease and vascular dementias (Sattel *et al.* 1996), although in both significant changes in cerebrovascular blood flow were seen. In the future, Doppler ultrasonography is likely to play a greater role in establishing the risk profile of patients with vascular disease since it is cheap and effective.

Electroencephalography (EEG)

EEG detects brain electrical activity and event related potentials (ERP). Brain wave amplitude and frequency are recorded by scalp electrodes which, being closest to the cerebral cortex, directly reflect cortical activity and only indirectly subcortical activity. Whilst temporal resolution is high, regional specificity is imprecise as a result of the diffuse regional connectivity of the neuronal networks (Hegerl and Möller 1997). In general, focal disease generates focal EEG changes and vice versa for diffuse disease. The dominant frequency of normal awake individuals is called alpha (8–13 cycles per second). In diseased brain, there is typically a global decrease in alpha and beta activity, with increased delta and theta activities and P300 and other specific ERP latencies.

EEG in dementia

In dementia the sensitivity of EEG is inversely proportional to its specificity; neither being high. However, an abnormal EEG is very unlikely to be found in normal ageing or 'functional' cognitive impairment, for example pseudo-dementia, pointing instead to an organic cause. However, in mild dementia the EEG may remain entirely normal.

Seizures

Seizures are common in dementia and may cause acute changes in behaviour. Although the investigation of choice for diagnosing seizures, EEG is rarely indicated for organic dementia but is useful when distinguishing between diffuse neurodegeneration and temporal lobe status epilepticus.

EEG in delirium

In delirium the EEG typically shows dramatically diffuse slowing, which may be of value in some patients. In acute and potentially reversible conditions bursts of rhythmic delta and theta activity with frontotemporal localization occur; something rarely seen in Alzheimer's disease.

EEG in other dementias

However, in frontotemporal dementia (FTD), even when severe, the EEG is often normal, which helps to distinguish between FTD and Alzheimer's disease. The EEG may be diagnostic in Creutzfeldt–Jakob disease and prion dementias, revealing a characteristic triphasic pattern with sharp waves occurring with a one per second perfect periodicity, often triggered by acoustic stimuli. If Creutzfeldt–Jakob disease is considered, an EEG is mandatory and should be repeated at regular intervals since a positive diagnosis has implications for the handling of brain tissue and body fluids, and in particular for notifying the appropriate authorities so as to rule out the human form of bovine spongiform encephalopathy. Whilst the periodic triphasic wave pattern is highly specific for Creutzfeldt–Jakob disease and is uncommon in Alzheimer's disease, it may become evident only late in the disease (Bortone *et al.* 1994).

EEG in the future

Arguably, quantitative EEG and spectral analysis is as diagnostically accurate in dementia as single photon emission computed tomography (SPECT) scanning. If substantiated, its low cost may make it clinically significant (Sloan *et al.* 1995; Hegerl and Möller 1997).

Lumbar puncture

A lumbar puncture to examine cerebrospinal fluid for cells and opening pressure must be performed to search for evidence of infection, inflammation, and appropriate antigens whenever such diagnoses are suspected, particularly in atypical cases. Lumbar puncture has very low morbidity in elderly patients if performed by those skilled in the technique (Hindley *et al.* 1995).

Electromyography

Myopathy may accompany neurodegenerative diseases, which can also give rise to dementia. However, the most common indication in the memory team setting will be for fasciculation, most often due to motor neurone disease, itself well recognized to occur with other dementias, most notably fronto-temporal dementia (FTD) and sometimes Alzheimer's disease. Amyotrophic lateral sclerosis may sometimes be associated with dementia. Electromyography in these cases is confirmatory but may also suggest upper motor neurone dysfunction from multiple sclerosis, cerebrovascular disease, and metabolic conditions such as hyperparathyroidism and severe hyponatraemia. Nerve conduction studies should be undertaken when peripheral neuropathies are suspected. In the more rare and esoteric conditions leading to dementia, such as the mitochondrial encephalomyopathy with lactic acidosis and stroke-like episodes syndrome (MELAS), electrophysiology may help to confirm the diagnosis (Grunwald *et al.* 1990). Almost invariably, however, simpler tests will reveal the diagnosis.

Bowel (jejunal) biopsy

This is indicated in Whipple's disease, a rare multisystem disorder caused by a bacilliform bacterium, which should be considered in patients with weight loss, diarrhoea, malabsorption, lymphadenopathy, arthralgias, and cognitive impairment (Adams *et al.* 1987).

Serum antibody testing

This is indicated in Lyme disease, caused by the spirochete *Borrelia bergdorferae*, which typically presents with arthralgias, rash, chronic meningitis or meningoencephalitis, malaise, and chronic fatigue. Rarely, however, as in multiple sclerosis, dementia may be the only early manifestation of the illness (Fallon and Nields 1994). Neurosyphilis is now rare, and is most likely to occur in immune-deficient individuals (Powell, *et al.* 1993). AIDS dementia complex is often, but by no means always, a late manifestation of infection with human immunodeficiency virus (HIV), and should be considered in all atypical cases and at-risk individuals. Other meningitides are more likely in HIV-positive cases, for example cryptococcal, mycobacterial, treponemal, pseudomonas, and various viral infections (Price 1996).

White cell enzyme studies

These are virtually never indicated in the memory clinic setting. However, awareness of the situations when they should be considered, and the patient sent for specialized investigations, will distinguish the clinic of excellence from its counterparts elsewhere (Miller *et al.* 1995).

Urine testing

Urinary tract infections are a frequent cause of cognitive decline and delirium in cognitively normal elderly people or those with borderline cognitive dysfunction or incipient dementia.

Skin biopsy

Sarcoid and other granulomatous conditions may be diagnosed by skin biopsy.

Summary

Clinical history and physical examination are the cornerstones of dementia diagnosis and differential diagnosis but laboratory tests are essential to identify the specific differential diagnosis and exclude potentially reversible conditions, which may be primary or contributory to the dementia. The choice of tests should be determined by an experienced clinician. Only in cases with an atypical presentation or progression is more exhaustive investigation required.

Neuroimaging tests in dementia

The various imaging modalities and their individual contributions to diagnosis in dementia will be briefly described and then a discussion of their relative merits for application in the clinic setting will follow.

Computed tomography (CT)

Using the ionizing radiation of X-rays, CT translates tissue density into a two-dimensional visual image of brain structure with a resolution of 1.5 to 2.0 mm.

Contrast enhancement with radiodense media improves CT detection of intracerebral pathology, making it the investigation of choice to rule out neoplastic, vascular, or traumatic brain lesions in many parts of the world where MRI is not widely affordable (DeCarli *et al.* 1990).

Much has been written about the use of CT in the differential diagnosis of dementia. Semiquantitative subjective parameters, linear, planimetric, and even tissue density assessments have all been shown to be reliable and useful in detecting regional and global brain atrophy. Such indices, especially in experienced hands, may contribute usefully to assessing significant atrophy in at-risk individuals. However, all show extensive overlap with normal elderly people (DeCarli *et al.* 1990).

However, when attention is focused on the hippocampal formation, the site of maximum pathology in Alzheimer's disease, and CT scans are performed using the temporal-lobe-oriented scan angle, Alzheimer's disease can be reliably differentiated from normal ageing and other dementias (Jobst *et al.* 1998). This is the case using semiquantitative visual assessment of the hippocampal formation and hippocampal fissure dilatation (DeLeon *et al.* 1997), or using the simple linear measurement of the minimum medial temporal lobe width derived either from the CT hard copy using hand held callipers or on screen (Smith and Jobst 1996; Jobst *et al.* 1998). If frontal atrophy, leucencies in grey and/or white matter, and other regional atrophic changes are taken into account in consecutive necropsy-confirmed dementias, CT can reliably differentiate frontotemporal dementia, Alzheimer's disease, multi-infarct dementia, and other dementias (Jobst *et al.* 1998). These techniques have been replicated and can readily be applied in busy clinical practice (Pasquier *et al.* 1994; Frisoni, Trabuchi, and Beltramello 1996; Frisoni *et al.* 1996; O'Brien 1996).

Furthermore, medial temporal lobe (MTL) atrophy precedes cognitive dysfunction, and may be useful to monitor rate of change in treatment trials (Jobst *et al.* 1994b; Smith and Jobst 1996), findings which have been confirmed with MRI in living subjects (Fox *et al.* 1996). Moreover, those at risk of Alzheimer's disease, whether with age-associated memory impairment or mild cognitive impairment, and even in those still cognitively normal with only subjective memory loss, show significant hippocampal formation atrophy and a greater rate of MTL thinning than those who do not progress.

CT is simple to carry out and can greatly improve the detection of organic dementias, in particular limiting the number of patients in whom treatable brain lesions such as tumour and subdural haematoma are missed. The limited resolution of CT means that small subcortical areas of ischaemia may be missed, as may be white matter lesions, isodense tissue changes such as subdural haematomas, and small temporal lobe tumours. However, whilst MRI volumetric and planimetric measures are taxing and time consuming, the simple measure of minimum MTL width is easily learned and applied (Smith and Jobst 1996; Jobst *et al.* 1998).

Magnetic resonance imaging (MRI)

MRI exploits the propensity of the nucleus of an atom to precess when placed in a magnetic field, and in so doing to generate a resonant signal which can be transformed to generate an image of tissue structure and content. Thus, in the brain, protons (primarily water) generate the energy required to reconstruct an image as they relax to their original positions having been subjected to a magnetic field (Truwit and Lempert 1994). The digital acquisition of volumetric data enables easy reconstruction of the images in any plane with a spatial resolution of about 1.0 to 1.5 mm. T_1-weighted scans are best for delineating brain anatomy and show cerebrospinal fluid as dark and brain tissue as white. T_2-weighted scans are better for detecting pathologic conditions and show brain as grey and water and cerebrospinal fluid (and therefore inflammation) as white. Other protocols may be used further to enhance differentiation.

Arguably, in the dementias the main advantage of the anatomical resolution of MRI is in the detection of grey and white matter changes, particularly leucencies, believed to be indicative of ischaemia and/or inflammation (Erkinjuntti *et al.* 1984; George *et al.* 1986; Johnson *et al.* 1987). However, white matter change is not confined to cerebrovascular disease and is found in a significant proportion of Alzheimer's disease cases (Amar *et al.* 1995). It still remains to be determined exactly how much white matter change accompanies normal ageing (George *et al.* 1986), but evidence of white matter leucency should not exclude a diagnosis of Alzheimer's disease.

In the dementias, MRI evaluation of the temporal lobes, and in particular the hippocampal formation, reveals qualitative and quantitatively similar changes to linear measures on CT (DeLeon *et al.* 1997). MRI is particularly valuable for demonstrating small vascular or other intracerebral lesions, and it is better than CT for precisely delineating areas like the temporal lobes and brainstem located against bone (Victoroff *et al.* 1994). Nevertheless, whether the routine use of MRI in the memory clinic setting has any significant advantage over CT, given the greater cost of MRI, remains to be established. There is complete agreement, however, that the grey–white matter junction is better delineated with MRI than with CT.

Claustrophobia is more likely to occur with MRI due to the longer time required for imaging and the greater constriction of the subject's space, particularly now that spiral CT has been introduced (Butler *et al.* 1995). However, new open scanners are being developed which alleviate claustrophobia and faster scanning techniques have shortened the time required for MRI.

Magnetic resonance angiography (MRA)

MRA permits comparable visualization of the cerebral vasculature to conventional angiography. Although many still maintain conventional angiography is necessary to delineate surgically significant vascular lesions (such as carotid stenosis or aneurysms), MRA can add valuable anatomical information about cerebral vasculature (Schima *et al.* 1996). With continued technological development MRA will supersede angiography, although it is unlikely to impact on memory clinic function for some time.

Functional/ diffusion and perfusion MRI

Functional MRI allows the detection and imaging of brain metabolism during brain activation, the principle being that blood flow increases to brain regions that are metabolically active (Toga and Mazziotta 1996).

Diffusion MRI is an MR-based technique which detects brain ischaemia many hours before changes appear on CT. This is likely to have significant application in acute stroke services, particularly with the advent of acute thrombolysis.

Cerebral blood volume can be evaluated using gadolinium-enhanced MRI, so-called 'perfusion MRI'. Cerebral blood volume strongly correlates with cerebral blood flow, yielding information similar to single photon emission computerised tomography (SPECT) but with better resolution. It is unlikely to impact on routine memory clinic function in the foreseeable future.

Magnetic resonance spectroscopy (MRS)

MRS is non-invasive. It enables identification and quantification of the concentration of various intracellular molecules and metabolites within brain parenchyma currently being explored as potential diagnostic markers for the differential diagnosis of dementia, and also for monitoring the course of the dementia. It remains largely a research tool (Gonzalez *et al.* 1996).

Single photon emission computed tomography (SPECT)

SPECT uses single photon gamma emitters tagged to lipophilic agents which cross the blood–brain barrier, permitting visual images of regional cerebral blood flow to be generated. The three most common agents used are the gas Xenon-133, 99m-Technetium hexa-methyl-propyleneamineoxime (HMPAO), and 99m-Technetium Biscisate (ECD) (Greenberg and Lassen 1994; Waldemar 1995). With the new SPECT cameras it is now possible to achieve 3 to 4 mm spatial resolution with HMPAO and ECD, approximating that of positron emission tomography (PET).

Because for the most part regional cerebral blood flow and regional cerebral metabolism are coupled, SPECT may be of diagnostic use in the degenerative dementias where brain function is altered in specific regions. SPECT has helped define certain dementia syndromes such as frontotemporal dementia (Miller *et al.* 1997) and is used by many to confirm the diagnosis of Alzheimer's disease and increase specificity (Waldemar 1995; Jobst *et al.* 1998). New tracers which permit visualization of specific brain receptors are likely to assume greater importance in the immediate future and to impact on the memory clinic not only in determining diagnostic but also assessment protocols for responses to treatment, particularly in the dementias involving specific neurochemical systems such as Parkinson's dementia complex.

Positron emission tomography (PET)

PET is a highly sophisticated functional imaging method using radionuclides capable of emitting high energy radiation, permitting quantification of regional cerebral blood flow, oxygen utilization, or other neuronal metabolic processes, and also receptor density (Miller *et al.* 1995; Kuhl *et al.* 1996). Whilst PET offers better resolution than SPECT, it is vastly more expensive and is usually only available in research centres.

The use of neuroimaging to diagnose dementia

Degenerative dementias

Alzheimer's disease
Structural imaging
Brain imaging now has a clear role in the diagnosis of Alzheimer's disease (DeLeon *et al.* 1997; Jobst *et al.* 1998). Until the advent of specific temporal lobe views, both structural and functional neuroimaging served only to exclude tumours and strokes, and as indicators of hydrocephalus or congenital anomalies. However, there is now indisputable evidence that there is significant detectable MTL atrophy in the earliest, and even presymptomatic, stages of Alzheimer's disease. The presence of MTL atrophy supports a clinical diagnosis of dementia of Alzheimer type (DAT), its absence making Alzheimer's disease less likely. Thus, the use of the simple measurement of MTL atrophy visualized on temporal-lobe-oriented sections on CT (Jobst *et al.* 1992) or MRI (DeLeon *et al.* 1997), the minimum MTL width measured at the level of the brainstem, midway between the rostral and caudal limits, can enhance diagnostic accuracy in confirmed cases of Alzheimer's disease (Jobst *et al.* 1998) and in the memory clinic setting (Pasquier *et al.* 1994; Fox *et al.* 1996; DeLeon *et al.* 1997). Furthermore, the evidence of rapidly progressing atrophy in the MTL by CT or MRI has led to proposals that change over time

could be used not only to confirm a clinical diagnosis of Alzheimer's disease, but also as a marker for the disease (Fox *et al.*, 1996; Jobst 1996; Smith and Jobst 1996).

However, not only is MTL atrophy not unique to Alzheimer's disease, but other areas of focal cortical atrophy occur, particularly in atypical presentations of the disease (Caselli *et al.* 1992; Jobst 1996). Longitudinal studies now reveal that MTL atrophy occurs significantly earlier in Alzheimer's disease (i.e. at minimal to mild severity) than it does in non-Alzheimer's disease dementias (i.e. only when moderate to severe) (Jobst 1996; Jobst *et al.* 1998). This is important if only structural imaging (CT or MRI) is available to the memory clinic. Neuroradiologists need to be made aware of these early and prognostic focal changes in Alzheimer's disease and how best to visualize them—most importantly how to distinguish reliably between the dementias and that to make the diagnosis the scan should be early in the course of the disease.

Functional imaging

When it is not possible to distinguish between Alzheimer's disease and other dementias such as FTD, by focal cortical changes, the combination of structural and functional imaging becomes relevant. In Alzheimer's disease there is characteristic parietotemporal hypometabolism and hypoperfusion. The diagnostic accuracy of these changes is approximately the same as for MTL atrophy on CT or MRI (Jobst *et al.* 1994a; Waldemar 1995). However, as with MTL atrophy, parietotemporal hypoperfusion does not occur in all cases and is not specific to Alzheimer's disease. Other conditions can give rise to the same pattern as a result of local parietotemporal pathology, such as strokes, tumours, gliosis or post-traumatic atrophy, and also following damage to distant regions which project to it. This phenomenon is known as diaschisis (Feeney and Baron 1986; Waldemar *et al.* 1994). In a series of 118 post-mortem-confirmed cases the diagnostic sensitivity and specificity of SPECT were 89 per cent and 80 per cent respectively and 84 per cent accurate (Jobst *et al.* 1998).

Combined structural and functional imaging

In difficult cases of NINCDS 'possible Alzheimer's disease' or complex dementia cases, combining structural and functional imaging permits the most accurate diagnosis to be made. Not only does the combination of MTL atrophy and parietotemporal hypoperfusion enhance diagnostic accuracy in Alzheimer's disease, but if other SPECT changes, and changes in the white matter, grey matter, or focal atrophic changes on CT are taken into account, the false positive rate in the differential diagnosis of dementias falls to under 5 per cent (Jobst *et al.* 1998).

What to do in practice

Should brain imaging be used in every case and should both CT or MRI and SPECT be undertaken on all occasions? The answer must be a qualified 'no!'.

Ultimately, how best to use brain imaging remains a matter of clinical judgement in each individual case. Although SPECT is slightly more accurate in identifying Alzheimer's disease than MTL atrophy on CT, we would not advise first-line use of SPECT except when FTD is the major differential diagnosis. Only CT or MRI will reveal the tumours, strokes, haemorrhage, hydrocephalus, inflammation, cysts, and ischaemia which might otherwise be missed. Initially, therefore, it is advisable to consider a structural scan, CT or MRI, and to assess MTL width or volume. If MRI is chosen, then it is advisable to request a rapid volumetric acquisition so that reconstructions in any plane can be performed.

Requesting a SPECT scan should be reserved for those cases where MTL atrophy is minimal or mild, or where the clinical picture prohibits clear differentiation from Alzheimer's disease, especially when the differential diagnosis is between FTD and Alzheimer's disease or where diffuse regional ischaemia is suspected. In FTD, SPECT is diagnostic (Miller *et al.* 1997) and in ischaemia, SPECT may reveal discrete deficits when either CT may be normal or MRI reveals excessive white matter leucencies (Miller *et al.* 1995).

Combining structural and functional imaging is the most effective means of arriving at an accurate diagnosis in cases other than NINCDS 'probable Alzheimer's disease'. It is the addition of the information from the SPECT image to the structural information which significantly improves specificity (Jobst *et al.* 1998). With the advent of specific drug therapies for Alzheimer's disease, diagnostic accuracy is no longer merely an academic nicety. Treatments may have side-effects and precise case identification will minimize this in those without the disease. Furthermore, it is likely to be of relevance to memory-clinic-based patient recruitment for therapeutic trials where it may be argued that the relative cost of the investigations is outweighed by the increased diagnostic certainty. In one centre of excellence in the United Kingdom, it has been calculated that the neuroimaging component of dementia assessment (both CT and SPECT) approximates only 2 per cent of total assessment costs (Vivien, G. 1994. Total cost of neuroimaging investigations in dementia assessment in Plymouth and Cornwall. Personal communication).

However, many clinicians remain innocent of these simple diagnostic tools. Whilst almost every general hospital will have a SPECT camera, not all will know how to process brain images, and few GPs will have direct access to imaging services. Nevertheless, the technology is not prohibitively expensive and enquiry of the specialist services may stimulate interest and activity. Diagnostic certainty affects the relationships between physician, patient, and family, and in some cases may be cause enough to request an additional scan in difficult cases. Ultimately clinical acumen, wisdom, and experience are the best arbiters of when to request brain scans in Alzheimer's disease.

Frontotemporal dementia (FTD)

FTD reflects dysfunction in the anterior frontal and temporal lobes and should be suspected when the first clinical manifestations are behavioural (Gustafson 1987). Once thought to be indistinguishable from Alzheimer's disease in life, FTD is now recognized to account for up to 25 per cent of presenile dementias (Snowden *et al.* 1996; Miller *et al.* 1997) and diagnostic accuracy approximates 90 per cent in clinics which specialize in this disorder (Brun 1993). With the use of a careful clinical evaluation focusing upon neuropsychiatric manifestations and SPECT neuroimaging, FTD can reliably be diagnosed early in the disease when structural imaging may still be unrevealing (Miller *et al.* 1997).

Whilst, CT or MRI may show focal frontal and/or temporal atrophy, often extending to the medial temporal lobes later in the disease (Jobst 1996), most investigators agree that SPECT is necessary to confirm the diagnosis (Miller *et al.* 1997). It is the evidence of blood flow changes very early in the disease, when structural imaging may still be normal which makes SPECT the investigation of choice to distinguish between clinically similar presentations of pathologically distinct dementias (Jobst 1996). Thus, if after a history, examination, and cognitive testing, the differential is between Alzheimer's disease and FTD and the routine CT is normal, the diagnostic investigation would be a SPECT scan.

Lewy body disorder

Patients with a combination of dementia and parkinsonism defy easy classification, but are now known to represent up to 20 per cent of all dementias. Accurate diagnosis is of immediate practical significance since not only are Lewy body disorder patients exquisitely sensitive to neuroleptics which may precipitate life threatening neuroleptic sensitivity syndrome (McKeith *et al.* 1992), they are also believed to be more responsive to cholinomimetics such as the anticholinesterases (Kaufer *et al.* 1996). There are distinct features which separate Lewy body disorder from classical Alzheimer's disease clinically. Specifically, they show more parkinsonian features, greater psychiatric symptomatology (particularly visual hallucinations), and fluctuating cognitive dysfunction. They are characterized neuropathologically by eosinophilic cortical neuronal inclusions (Lewy Bodies) (Galasko *et al.* 1994; McKeith *et al.* 1994; Perry *et al.* 1996).

The alternate diagnosis most closely resembling Lewy body disorder is cerebrovascular ischaemia; it is well known that many patients with sub-cortical white matter and basal ganglia ischaemia and infarctions, can present with mixtures of parkinsonism and dementia (McKeith *et al.* 1994). SPECT studies suggest that many Lewy body disorder patients show similar changes to Alzheimer's disease (Miller *et al.* 1996), although this may simply reflect mixed pathology. Where there is no Alzheimer's disease pathology at post-mortem, imaging showed less parietotemporal hypoperfusion and less MTL atrophy in life than is found in Alzheimer's disease (Jobst 1996). Future SPECT studies with dopaminergic receptor ligands are very likely to enable accurate diagnosis of Lewy body disorder in life. Until then, a high index of suspicion and clinical acumen will remain the mainstays of diagnosis. Brain imaging should therefore be used to exclude confounding diagnoses, particularly ischaemia.

Other degenerative disorders

There are a variety of degenerative disorders in which brain scanning can help significantly in diagnosis in suspected, incipient, or frank dementia. These include Creutzfeldt–Jakob disease, metachromatic leukodystrophy, progressive supranuclear palsy, and mitochondrial disorders.

Patients with Creutzfeldt–Jakob disease typically have normal CT scan images, especially in the early stages and even during the rapid progressive phase, whereas SPECT may show a 'moth-eaten' appearance due to the presence of multiple areas with diminished metabolism; perfusion deficits reflecting localization of the pathology and its associated diaschisis (Markus *et al.* 1992). MRI may reveal leucencies reflecting inflammation in grey and white matter but equally may be normal, as with CT. SPECT therefore is the investigation of choice to reveal the metabolic disturbances, which may significantly precede manifest cognitive dysfunction. This is of particular relevance in evaluating intervention with therapeutic agents such as Zidovudine in the earliest stages of the disease.

Adult-onset metachromatic leukodystrophy patients show large subfrontal white matter lesions on CT or MRI (Skomer *et al.* 1983), with accompanying deficits and often substantial diaschisis with functional imaging. The same is true of other leucoencephalopathies.

Some patients with progressive supranuclear palsy may show significant atrophy of the colliculi in the midbrain, prominent ambient cisterns, third and fourth ventricles, and cerebral aqueduct (Ambrosetto 1987). However, in the early stages, structural imaging may look normal. On the other hand, functional imaging with SPECT typically demonstrates hypoperfusion of the superior frontal regions with sparing of inferior frontal areas (Testa *et al.* 1988; Johnson *et al.* 1991). Thus the combination of structural and functional imaging may help in suspected progressive supranuclear palsy, especially since it may be confused with Lewy body disorder clinically. Both, however, show reduced dopamine receptor density. In the future, therefore, SPECT using specific ligands may prove diagnostic.

Imaging findings in mitochondrial disorders are variable, and although SPECT findings may be confused with those of Alzheimer's disease, some show lesions in the basal ganglia on CT or MRI which can help to distinguish them from Alzheimer's disease (Barkovich *et al.* 1993).

Presymptomatic hypometabolism of the basal ganglia, sometimes with concomitant atrophy of the head of the caudate nucleus may be found in Huntingdon's disease. Regional atrophy and hypometabolism is also specific to olivopontocerebellar atrophy. Metachromatic leukodystrophy may look like vascular dementia on CT or MRI and where the diagnosis is suspected, nerve biopsy should be performed to reveal loss of myelinated fibres and characteristic intracellular lamellar inclusions (Zhao 1992).

Vascular dementias

The term 'vascular dementia' subsumes a highly heterogeneous group of 'diseases' (Erkinjuntti and Hachinski 1993). The misdiagnosis rate for patients with the clinical diagnosis of vascular dementia is high. However, even with sophisticated neuroimaging a misdiagnosis can occur (Galasko et al. 1994). Clearly, not all patients with a stroke on CT or MRI have vascular dementia and vice versa, and patients with slowly progressive dementia and stroke on CT or MRI may be demented due to other causes. Some have large cortical infarctions, often due to cardiac embolic disease or carotid occlusion. Some arise from small infarcts, often subcortical, whilst others are believed to result from diffuse arteriosclerotic disease causing widespread white matter change, subcortical microinfarcts, and generalized hypoperfusion, known as Binswanger's disease (Babikian and Ropper 1987). Further complicating the diagnosis of vascular dementia is the finding that small infarctions in critical areas such as the left angular gyrus (Benson et al. 1982) or the left dorsomedial nucleus of the thalamus (Guberman and Stuss 1983) can lead to dementia syndromes, while multiple strokes in the basal ganglia do not always lead to serious cognitive impairment (Liu et al. 1992). Obviously what is important clinically is the location of the vascular lesion which will determine the clinical presentation (Joseph 1990).

MRI permits greater visualization of white matter changes than CT, especially smaller subcortical lesions. Larger areas of ischaemia or infarction are well detected by both CT and MRI. However, the clinical significance of the white matter changes seen in many normal elderly people remains controversial. Furthermore, white matter changes may not be due only to vascular disease, nor are they necessarily irreversible. Histopathological correlations with white matter leucencies have been shown with demyelination, cystic changes, glial accumulations, and perivascular dilatation (Leifer et al. 1990).

Beyond a certain threshold they are indicative of significant pathology, an increased risk of cognitive dysfunction, cerebrovascular disease, and stroke (DeCarli et al. 1995a, b). Clinical manifestations will depend on the volume and location of white matter changes (Amar et al. 1995, 1996). Thus, whilst MRI reveals leucoencephalopathy more often than CT, the significance of the changes seen is far from clear (Fazekas 1989). Of relevance to the memory clinic is the clear evidence that the strongest correlations with cognitive function are those leucencies detected by CT (Lopez *et al.* 1995), that is if seen on CT, and more than mild in extent, it is probably significant. Where the picture is unclear and there is a possibility of either a mixed diagnosis (e.g. mixed Alzheimer's disease and vascular dementia) functional imaging may help to differentiate between them.

Concluding remarks

Much more work needs to be undertaken to assess the utility of possible diagnostic tests in the light of the prior probability of the diagnosis, the degree of clinician confidence in the diagnosis prior to ordering investigations, and the impact that the diagnosis may have upon further management (Van Gool and Van Crevel 1996). Assessment of the effects of false positives and false negatives on management and outcome is also required. Cost, clinical impact, likelihood, and management implications must all be assessed in each case for the available investigations (Weytingh *et al.* 1995; Walstra *et al.* 1997). The routine use of neuroimaging remains controversial. However, all are agreed that blood tests to detect indicators of treatable disease must be requested and are cost effective. While the syndrome of dementia remains a clinical diagnosis in many cases, its aetiological differential diagnosis depends on laboratory and radiological testing. There is now an impressive amount of evidence showing high sensitivity and specificity for neuroimaging parameters in diagnosing the cause of dementia. The uptake of such measurements, however, remains limited, not so much by availability but by lack of education and knowledge. Perhaps studies showing how neuroimaging adds to the differential diagnosis, particularly in cases of clinical uncertainty, will accelerate the appropriate evaluation and uptake of these modalities (Jobst *et al.* 1998).

References

Key references recommended by the authors are marked with an *.

Adams, M., P. A. Rhyner, J. Day, *et al.* 1987. Whipple's disease confined to the central nervous system. *Annals of Neurology* **21**:104–8.
Amar, K., T. Lewis, G. K. Wilcock, M. Scott, and R. S. Bucks. 1995. The relationship between white matter low attenuation on brain CT and vascular risk factors: a memory clinic study. *Age and Ageing* **24**:411–15.
*Amar, K., R. S. Bucks, T. Lewis, M. Scott, and G. K. Wilcock. 1996. The effect of white matter low attenuation on cognitive performance in dementia. *Age andAgeing* **25**:443–8.

Ambrosetto, P. 1987. CT in progressive supranuclear palsy. *American Journal of Neuroradiology* **8**:849–51.

Babikian, V., and A. H. Ropper. 1987. Binswanger's Disease: A review. *Stroke* **18**:2–12.

Barkovich, A. J., W. V. Good, T. K. Koch, *et al.* 1993. Mitochondrial disorders: Analysis of their clinical and imaging characteristics. *American Journal of Neuroradiology* **14**:1119–1137.

Benson, D. F., J. L. Cummings, and S. Y. Tsai. 1982. Angular gyrus syndrome simulating Alzheimer's disease. *Archives of Neurology* **39**:616–20.

Bortone, E., L. Bettoni, C. Giorgi, M. G. Terzano, G. R. Trabattoni, and D. Mancia. 1994. Reliability of EEG in the diagnosis of Creutzfeldt-Jakob disease. *Electroencephalography and Clinical Neurophysiology* **90**:323–30.

Brun, A. 1993. Frontal lobe degeneration of non-Alzheimer type revisited. *Dementia* **4**:126–31.

Butler, R. E., D. C. Costa, A. Greco, P. J. Ell, and C. L. E. Katona. 1995. Differentiation between Alzheimer's disease and multi infarct dementia: SPECT vs. MR imaging. *International Journal of Geriatric Psychiatry* **10**:121–28.

Carney, M. W. P. 1995. Neuropsychiatric disorders associated with nutritional deficiencies. *CNS Drugs* **3**:279–90.

Caselli, R. J., C. R. Jack, R. C. Petersen, H. W. Wahner, and T. Yanagihara. 1992. Asymmetric cortical degenerative syndromes: clinical and radiologic correlations. *Neurology* **42**:1462–8.

Clarke, R., A. D. Smith, K. A. Jobst, H. Refsum, L. Sutton, and P. M. Ueland, (1998). Folate, vitamin B$_{12}$ and serum total homocysteine levels in confirmed Alzheimer's disease. *Archives of Neurology*. In Press.

Croxson, S. C. M., and C. Jagger. 1995. Diabetes and cognitive impairment: a community-based study of elderly subjects. *Age and Ageing* **24**:421–4.

Crystal, H. A., E. Ortof, W. H. Frishman, A. Gruber, D. Hershman, and M. Aronson. 1994. Serum vitamin B12 levels and incidence of dementia in a healthy elderly population: a report from the Bronx Longitudinal Aging Study. *Journal of the American Geriatric Society* **42**:933–6.

*Cummings, J. L., and D. F. Benson. 1992. *Dementia: A Clinical Approach*. Boston, MA: Butterworth-Heinemann.

*DeCarli, C., J. A. Kaye, B. Horwitz, and S. I. Rapoport. 1990. Critical analysis of the use of computer-assisted transverse axial tomography to study human brain in aging and dementia of the Alzheimer type. *Neurology* **40**:872–83.

DeCarli, C., D. G. M. Murphy, A. R. McIntosh, D. Teichberg, M. B. Schapiro, and B. Horwitz. 1995a. Discriminant analysis of MRI measures as a method to determine the presence of dementia of the Alzheimer type. *Psychiatry Research* **57**:119–30.

DeCarli, C., D. G. M. Murphy, M. Tranh, C. L. Grady, J. V. Haxby, J. A.

Gillette, J. A. Salerno, A. Gonales-Aviles, B. Horwitz, S. I. Rapoport, and M. B. Schapiro. 1995b. The effect of white matter hyperintensity volume on brain structure, cognitive performance and cerebral metabolism of glucose in 51 healthy adults. *Neurology* **45**:2077–84.

*DeLeon, M. J., A. E. George, J. Golomb, C. Tarshish, A. Convit, A. Kluger, S. De Santi, T. McRae, S. H. Ferris, B. Reisberg, C. Ince, H. Rusinek, M. Bobinski, B. Quinn, D. C. Miller, and H. M. Wisniewski. 1997. Frequency of Hippocampal Formation Atrophy in Normal Aging and Alzheimer's Disease. *Neurobiology of Aging* **18**:1–11.

*Erkinjuntti, T., and V. C. Hachinski. 1993. Rethinking vascular dementia. *Cerebrovascular Diseases* **3**:3–23.

Erkinjuntti, T., J. T. Sipponen, M. Iivanainen, L. Ketonen, R. Sulkava, and R. E. Sepponen. 1984. Cerebral NMR and CT imaging in dementia. *Journal of Computer Assisted Tomography* **8**:614–18.

Fallon, B. A., and J. A. Nields. 1994. Lyme disease: a neuropsychiatric illness. *American Journal of Psychiatry* **151**:1571–83.

Fazekas, F. 1989. Magnetic resonance signal abnormalities in asymptomatic individuals: their incidence and functional correlates. *European Neurology* **29**:164–8.

Feeney, D. M., and J. C. Baron. 1986. Diaschisis. *Stroke* **17**:817–30.

Fox, N. C., P. A. Freeborough, and M. N. Rossor. 1996. Visualisation and quantification of rates of atrophy in Alzheimer's disease. *Lancet* **348**:94–7.

Frisoni, G. B., M. Trabuchi, and A. Beltramello. 1996. Hippocampal atrophy measurement in Alzheimer's disease. *International Journal of Geriatric Psychiatry* **11**:81–3.

Frisoni, G., A. Beltramello, C. Weiss, C. Geroldi, A. Bianchetti, and M. Trabuchi. 1996. Usefulness of simple measures of temporal lobe atrophy in probable Alzheimer's disease. *Dementia* **7**:15–22.

Galasko, D., L. A. Hansen, R. Katzman, W. Wiederholt, E. Masliah, R. Terry, L. R. Hill, P. Lessin, and L. J. Thal. 1994. Clinical-neuropathological correlations in Alzheimer's disease and related dementias. *Archives of Neurology* **51**:888–95.

George, A. E., M. J. de Leon, A. Kalnin, L. Rosner, A. Goodgold, and N. Chase. 1986. Leukoencephalography in normal and pathologic aging. II. MRI of brain leucencies. *American Journal of Neuroradiology* **7**:567–70.

Gonzalez, R. G., A. R. Guimaraes, G. J. Moore, A. Crawley, L. A. Cupples, and J. H. Growdon. 1996. Quantitative in vivo p-31 magnetic resonance spectroscopy of Alzheimer disease. *Alzheimer's Disease and Associated Disorders* **10**:46–52.

Greenberg, J. H., and N. A. Lassen, eds. 1994. 99mTc-Bicisate (ECD) and SPECT. *Journal of Cerebral Blood Flow and Metabolism* (Supplement 1) **14**:S1–S120.

Grunwald, F., S. Zierz, K. Broich, S. Schumacher, A. Bockisch, and H. J.

Biersack. 1990. HMPAO-SPECT imaging resembling Alzheimer-type dementia in mitochondrial encephalomyopathy with lactic acidosis and stroke-like episodes (MELAS) [Case Report]. *Journal of Nuclear Medicine* **31**:1740–2.

Guberman, A., and D. Stuss. 1983. The syndrome of bilateral paramedian thalamic infarction. *Neurology* **33**:540–6.

Gustafson, L. 1987. Frontal lobe degeneration of non-Alzheimer type. II. Clinical picture and differential diagnosis. *Archives of Gerontology and Geriatrics* **6**:209–23.

Hegerl, U., and H.-J. Möller. 1997. EEG as a diagnostic instrument in dementia: review and perspectives. *International Psychogeriatrics* **9**(Suppl 1):237–46.

Hindley, N. J., K. A. Jobst, E. King, L. Barnetson, A. Smith, and A.-M. Haigh. 1995. High acceptability and low morbidity of diagnostic lumbar puncture in elderly subjects of mixed cognitive status. *Acta Neurologica Scandinavica* **91**:405–11.

Jobst, K. A. 1996. *Neuroimaging in Alzheimer's disease: a prospective, longitudinal, clinicopathological study.* DM Thesis, Bodleian Library, Oxford University, Oxford, UK.

Jobst, K. A., A. D. Smith, M. Szatmari, A. Molyneux, M. M. Esiri, E. King, A. Smith, A. Jaskowski, B. McDonald, and N. Wald. 1992. Detection in life of confirmed Alzheimer's disease using a simple measurement of medial temporal lobe atrophy by computed tomography. *Lancet* **340**:1179–83.

Jobst, K. A., N. J. Hindley, E. King, and A. D. Smith. 1994a. The diagnosis of Alzheimer's disease: a question of image? *Journal of Clinical Psychiatry* **55**:22–31.

Jobst, K. A., A. D. Smith, M. Szatmari, M. M. Esiri, A. Jaskowski, N. Hindley, B. Mcdonald, and A. J. Molyneux. 1994b. Rapidly progressing atrophy of medial temporal lobe in Alzheimer's disease. *Lancet* **343**:829–30.

*Jobst, K. A., L. P. D. Barnetson and B. J. Shepstone, on behalf of OPTIMA. 1998. Accurate prediction of histologically confirmed Alzheimer's disease and the differential diagnosis of dementia: The use of NINCDS-ADRDA and DSM III-R criteria, SPECT, x-ray CT and ApoE4 in medial temporal lobe dementias. *International Psychogeriatrics* **10**(3):271–302.

Johnson, K. A., K. R. Davis, F. S. Buonanno, T. J. Brady, T. J. Rosen, and J. H. Growdon. 1987. Comparison of magnetic resonance and roentgen ray computed tomography in dementia. *Archives of Neurology* **44**:1075–80.

Johnson, K. A., R. A. Sperling, B. L. Holman, J. S. Nagel, and J. H. Growdon. 1991. Cerebral perfusion in progressive supranuclear palsy. *Journal of Nuclear Medicine* **33**:704–9.

*Joosten, E., E. Lesaffre, R. Riezler, V. Ghekiere, L. Dereymaeker, W. Pelemans, and E. Dejaeger. 1997. Is metabolic evidence for vitamin B12 and folate deficiency more frequent in elderly patients with Alzheimer's disease? *Journal of Gerontology. Medical Sciences* **52A**:M76–9.

Joseph, R. 1990. *Neuropsychology, Neuropsychiatry, and Behavioural Neurology*. London. UK: Plenum Press.

Kaufer, D. I., J. L. Cummings, and D. Christine. 1996. Effect of Tacrine on behavioural symptoms in Alzheimer's disease: an open-label study. *Journal of Geriatric Psychiatry and Neurology* **9**:1–6.

Kuhl, D. E., S. Minoshima, and J. A. Fessler. 1996. In vivo mapping of cholinergic terminals in normal aging, Alzheimer's disease, and Parkinson's disease. *Annals of Neurology* **40**:399–410.

Larson, E. B., B. V. Reifler, S. M. Sumi, C. G. Canfield, and N. M. Chinn. 1986. Diagnostic tests in the evaluation of dementia: a prospective study of 200 elderly outpatients. *Archives of Internal Medicine* **146**:1917–22.

Leifer, D., F. S. Buonanno, and E. P. J. Richardson. 1990. Clinicopathologic correlations of cranial magnetic resonance imaging of periventricular white matter. *Neurology* **40**:911–18.

Liu, C. K., B. L. Miller, J. L. Cummings, M. D. Mehringer, M. A. Goldberg, S. L. Howng, and D. F. Benson. 1992. A quantitative MRI study of vascular dementia. *Neurology* **42**:138–43.

*Lopez, O. L., J. T. Becker, C. A. Jungreis, C. Rezek, C. Estol, F. Boller, and S. T. Dekosky. 1995. Computed tomography—but not magnetic resonance imaging—identified periventricular white matter lesions predict symptomatic cerebrovascular disease in probable Alzheimer's disease. *Archives of Neurology* **52**:659–64.

Lovestone, S. 1996. The genetics of Alzheimer's disease—new opportunities and new challenges. *International Journal of Geriatric Psychiatry* **11**:491–7.

Markus, H. S., L. W. Duchen, E. M. Parkin, A. B. Kurtz, H. S. Jacobs, D. C. Costa, and M. J. Harrison. 1992. Creutzfeldt-Jakob disease in recipients of human growth hormone in the United Kingdom: a clinical and radiographic study. *Quarterly Journal of Medicine* **82**:43–51.

McKeith, I., A. Fairbairn, R. Perry, P. Thompson, and E. Perry. 1992. Neuroleptic sensitivity in patients with senile dementia of Lewy body type. *British Medical Journal* **305**:673–8.

McKeith, I. G., A. F. Fairbairn, R. H. Perry, and P. Thompson. 1994. The clinical diagnosis and misdiagnosis of senile dementia of Lewy body type (SDLT). *British Journal of Psychiatry* **165**:324–32.

*Miller, B. L., I. Mena, and J. L. Cummings. 1995. Neuuroimaging in Clinical Practice. In *Comprehensive Textbook of Psychiatry*. 6th edn, ed. H. I. Kaplan and B. J. Sadcock, 257–76. Baltimore Md: Williams and Wilkins.

Miller, B. L., L. Chang, R. Booth, *et al.* 1996. The clinical and functional imaging characteristics of Parkinsonian-Dementia. In *Lewy Body Dementia*, ed. E. K. Perry, I. McKeith, and R. Perry. Cambridge,UK: Cambridge University Press.

Miller, B. L., C. Ikonte, M. Ponton, M. Levy, K. Boone, A. Darby, N. Berman,

I. Mena, and J. L. Cummings. 1997. A study of the Lund-Manchester research criteria for frontotemporal dementia: clinical and single photon emission CT correlations. *Neurology* **48**:937–42.

Nilsson, K., L. Gustafson, R. Fäldt, A. Andersson, and B. Hultberg. 1994. Plasma homocysteine in relation to serum cobalamin and blood folate in a psychogeriatric population. *European Journal of Clinical Investigation* **24**:600–6.

O'Brien, J. T. 1996. Hippocampal atrophy in Alzheimer's disease. *International Journal of Geriatric Psychiatry* **11**:83.

Pasquier, F., L. Bail, F. Lebert, J. P. Pruvo, and H. Petit. 1994. Determination of medial temporal lobe atrophy in early Alzheimer's disease with computed tomography. *Lancet* **343**:861–2.

*Perry, E. K., I. G. McKeith, and R. Perry, eds. 1996. *Lewy Body Dementia*. Cambridge. UK: Cambridge University Press.

Pirttila, T., R. Jarvenpaa, P. Laippala, and H. Frey. 1992. Brain atrophy on computerised axial tomography scans -interaction of age, diabetes and general morbidity. *Gerontology* **38**:285–91.

Powell, A. L., A. C. Coyne, and L. Jen. 1993. A retrospective study of syphilis seropositivity in a cohort of demented patients. *Alzheimer Disease and Associated Disorders* **7**:33–8.

Price, R. W. 1996. Neurological complications of HIV infection. *Lancet* **348**:445–52.

Refsum, H., P. M. Ueland, O. Nygard, and S. E. Volllset. 1998. Homocysteine and caridiovascular disease. *Annual Review of Medicine* **49**:31–62.

Riggs, K. M., A. Spiro, K. Tucker, and D. Rush. 1996. Relations of vitamin B-12, vitamin B-6, folate, and homocysteine to cognitive performance in the Normative Aging Study. *American Journal of Clinical Nutrition* **63**:306–14.

Sattel, H., H. Forstl, and S. Biedert. 1996. Senile dementia of Alzheimer type and multi-infarct dementia investigated by transcranial doppler sonography. *Dementia* **7**:41–6.

Saunders, A. M., C. Hulette, K. A. Welsh-Bohmer, D. E. Schmechel, B. Crain, R. J. Burke, M. J. Alberts, W. J. Strittmatter, J. C. S. Breitner, C. Rosenberg, S. V. Scott, P. C. J. Gaskell, M. A. Pericak-Vance, and A. D. Roses. 1996. Specificity, sensitivity, and predictive value of apolipoprotein-E genotyping for sporadic Alzheimer's disease. *Lancet* **348**:90–3.

Schima, W., A. Mukerjee, and S. Saini. 1996. Contrast-enhanced MR imaging. *Clinical Radiology* **51**:235–44.

Shetty, K. R., and E. H. Duthie. 1995. Thyroid disease and associated illness in the elderly. *Clinics in Geriatric Medicine* **11**:311–25.

Skomer, C., J. Stears and J. Austin. 1983. Metachromatic leukodystrophy (MLD):XV. Adult MLD with focal lesions by computed tomography. *Archive of Neurology* **40**:354–5.

Sloan, E. P., G. W. Fenton, N. S. Kennedy, and J. M. MacLennan. 1995.

Electroencephalography and single photon emission computed tomography in dementia: a comparative study. *Psychological Medicine* **25**:631–8.

Smith, A. D., and K. A. Jobst. 1996. Use of structural imaging to study the progression of Alzheimer's disease. *British Medical Bulletin* **52**:575–86.

Smith, A. D., K. A. Jobst, C. Johnston, C. Joachim, and Z. Nagy. 1996. Apolipoprotein-E genotyping in diagnosis of Alzheimer's disease. *Lancet* **348**:483–4.

Smith, A., E. King, N. Hindley, L. Barnetson, J. Barton and K. A. Jobst. 1998. The experience of research participation and the value of diagnosis in dementia: Implications for practice. *Journal of Mental Health* **7**(3):309–21.

Snowden, J. S., D. Neary, and D. M. A. Mann. 1996. *Fronto-temporal Lobar Degeneration: Fronto-temporal Dementia, Progressive Aphasia, Semantic Dementia*. New York: Churchill Livingstone.

*Terry, R. D., R. Katzman, and K. L. Bick, eds. 1994. *Alzheimer Disease*. New York: Raven Press.

Testa, H. J., J. S. Snowden, D. Neary, R. A. Shields, A. W. Burjan, M. C. Prescott, B. Northen, and P. Goulding. 1988. The use of [99mTc]-HM-PAO in the diagnosis of primary degenerative dementia. *Journal of Cerebral Blood Flow and Metabolism* **8**:S123–6.

Toga, A. W., and J. C. Mazziotta. 1996. *Brain Mapping: the Methods*. San Diego CA: Academic Press.

Truwit, C. L., and T. E. Lempert. 1994. *High Resolution Atlas of Cranial Neuroanatomy*. Baltimore: Williams and Wilkins.

Van Gool, W. A., and H. Van Crevel. 1996. Impact on management of new diagnostic tests in Alzheimer's disease. *Lancet* **348**:961.

Victoroff, J., W. J. Mack, S. T. Grafton, S. S. Schreiber, and H. C. Chui. 1994. A method to improve interrater reliability of visual inspection of brain MRI scans in dementia. *Neurology* **44**:2267–76.

*Waldemar, G. 1995. Functional brain imaging with SPECT in normal aging and dementia. *Cerebrovascular and Brain Metabolism Reviews* **7**:89–130.

Waldemar, G., P. Bruhn, M. Kristensen, A. Johnsen, O. B. Paulson, and N. A. Lassen. 1994. Heterogeneity of neocortical cerebral blood flow deficits in dementia of the Alzheimer type: a [99mTc]-d,l-HMPAO SPECT study. *Journal of Neurology Neurosurgery and Psychiatry* **57**:285–95.

Walstra, G. J. M., S. Teunisse, W. A. Van Gool, and H. Van Crevel. 1997. Reversible dementia in elderly patients referred to a memory clinic. *Journal of Neurology* **242**:17–22.

Weytingh, M. D., P. M. N. Bossuyt, and H. Van Crevel. 1995. Reversible dementia: more than 10% or less that 1%? A quantitative review. *Journal of Neurology* **242**:466–71.

Zhao, J. X. 1992. Later onset metachromatic leukodystrophy diagnosed by nerve biopsy. *Chung-Hua Shen Ching Ching Shen Ko Tsa Chih* **25**:271–316.

7 Neuropsychological assessment

Romola S. Bucks and David A. Loewenstein

Introduction

Neuropsychological assessment offers the clinician the means to measure an individual's cognitive performance in a standardized way using normative data gathered for persons of that age, education, gender, and cultural/ language background. It therefore forms an important means of quantifying the NINCDS-ADRDA (McKhann *et al.*, 1984) criteria for a diagnosis of *probable* Alzheimer's disease, which require that there is impairment in memory functioning plus at least one other cognitive domain such as language, praxis, perceptual skills, problem-solving abilities, attention, or orientation, supported by the Folstein Mini-Mental State Evaluation (MMSE) (Folstein *et al.*, 1975), Blessed Dementia Rating Scale (BDRS) (Blessed *et al.*, 1968), or a similar evaluation. These difficulties must interfere with everyday functional capacity. A diagnosis of *possible* Alzheimer's disease is rendered when a patient presents with only a single progressive cognitive deficit, an atypical presentation, or when there is a medical or neuropsychiatric condition that might account for observed deficits but is not considered to be the cause of the dementia.

Limitations of current diagnostic criteria

The NINCDS-ADRDA criteria as a whole possess a high degree of reliability in detecting the presence or absence of Alzheimer's disease when confirmed by autopsy findings (Kukull *et al.*, 1990; Tierney *et al.*, 1988). While the NINCDS-ADRDA neuropsychological criteria have considerable merit, there are some potential limitations of which the clinician should be aware (Loewenstein and Rubert, 1992). Firstly, the guidelines require that the individual fall at or below the fifth percentile in the eight areas of cognition (memory, language, praxis, perceptual skills, problem-solving abilities, attention, orientation, and functional abilities) relative to an appropriate normative comparative group. This stringent cut-off has considerable utility in ensuring **specificity**, that is observed cognitive deficits should be sufficiently severe to protect against *incorrect* classification of persons with otherwise normal variation in cognitive function or with age-related changes. However, there are some concerns that this might also lower **sensitivity**, that is exclude those Alzheimer's disease patients who are in the early stages of the illness, when new evolving psychopharmacological and psychosocial interventions may be of potential benefit. Further, there is often a **paucity of normative data** which are age, education, gender, and culturally appropriate, potentially leading to misdiagnosis in those individuals disadvantaged by culturally inappropriate tests (La Rue, 1987; Loewenstein *et al.*, 1994).

In addition, the criteria make assumptions both about **test sensitivity** and about **the equal importance of each cognitive domain** in arriving at a neuro-psychological diagnosis. So much of human cognition is measured or mediated by language that assessments which depend on language functioning tend to be more easily designed. For example verbal memory impairment, comprehension, and expression (syntax, semantics, and phonology) are affected by dominant hemisphere damage and are relatively simple to measure. On the other hand, non-dominant hemisphere damage, characterized by impairment of visual memory and prosodic characteristics of language (melody, tone, and intonation) are often more difficult to measure. Indeed, in the case of pure visual memory impairment, it is difficult to find a test which is not confounded by such factors as verbalization of different aspects of the stimuli which aid recall (Heilbronner, 1992).

Since Alzheimer's Disease involves both early bilateral medial temporal lobe deficits and cholinergic deficits (which are diffusely projected), evidence of bilateral damage should be found. But it may be easier to demonstrate dominant hemisphere effects than non-dominant. In addition, since cognitive domains such as memory and language (e.g. the ability properly to access the semantic lexicon) are usually affected first in Alzheimer's disease, deficits in these areas should probably be weighted differently than those in other domains such as perception, praxis, or executive function (Loewenstein and Rubert, 1992).

Finally, the NINCDS-ADRDA guidelines offer little guidance as to **the number of neuropsychological tests** which should represent a particular domain. For example one memory measure may be insufficient in and of itself for adequate coverage of the memory domain given all the different aspects of memory function, for example semantic and episodic memory impairments probably represent distinct areas of dysfunction (Leach and Levy, 1994). Conversely, countless numbers of tests administered in a domain may yield a positive but spurious result on one measure which might be of limited clinical or practical importance.

Less well validated diagnostic criteria, such as those for vascular dementia (Erkinjuntti, 1994) and for diffuse Lewy Body disease (McKeith *et al.*, 1996), suffer from similar drawbacks as those for Alzheimer's disease. Understanding some of the limitations of currently accepted neuropsychological criteria underscores the continuing need to develop new and modified criteria as well as more appropriate normative databases. Until then, neuropsychological assessment needs to focus on sensitive and specific measures of cognitive functioning which will best allow for diagnosis, whatever the currently accepted criteria.

Purposes of the assessment

Neuropsychological assessment enables the clinician to:

(1) determine the presence or absence of memory and/or other cognitive deficits;

(2) evaluate the nature and scope of observed deficits;

(3) assist in diagnostic determination;

(4) aid in treatment and management strategies;

(5) provide an objective baseline by which to measure change over time.

Neuropsychological assessment is not solely for diagnostic purposes. Because it involves detailed assessment of a broad range of cognitive skills, it allows the clinician to specify an individual's strengths as well as needs or weakness. This is especially helpful in setting up rehabilitation strategies (a topic explored in more detail in Chapter 18, Non-pharmacological approaches to treatment). Neuropsychological assessment is also useful in evaluating treatments and services, for legal purposes (see Chapter 19, Management of common problems), and for research (see Chapter 12, Research potential).

Who assesses cognitive function?

At present, in the United Kingdom as in most of Europe, neuropsychology is still a growing specialty. As a result, most European clinical teams do not have access to specialist neuropsychological input. In North America and Australia, where there are established training programmes for clinical neuropsychologists, this appears to be less of a problem. Historically, other professions have taken on the role of cognitive assessment including neurologists, psychiatrists, nurses, occupational therapists, and speech and language specialists. Many of these professionals rely on tests of cognitive function such as the Folstein MMSE to assess the presence or absence of dementia, or published batteries such as the CAMCOG (the cognitive section of the CAMDEX (Roth *et al.*, 1986)). Some others use computerized batteries (see Chapter 8, Computerized cognitive assessment).

A problem with the many published screening batteries is that they may be insensitive to impairment in the earliest stages of the disorder, or conversely may lead to inappropriate diagnosis because of sensory deficits or cultural/language differences. Huff *et al.* (1987) found that of their patients with Alzheimer's disease, 19 per cent had a MMSE score of 27 or above, which would otherwise be considered normal. This problem is less likely with more extensive, standardized batteries such as the CAMCOG, although there will still be premorbidly bright individuals who will pass this assessment and yet have dementia (Huppert *et al.*, 1995). Further, published batteries may not include all of those cognitive functions which the diagnosis requires.

In addition, patient factors such as sensory impairments, depression, and test anxiety can influence neuropsychological test performance (Holden, 1995). Therefore, the neuropsychologist must account for these non-cognitive factors which may influence test-taking populations. Additionally, a neuropsychologist can supplement the assessment, if needed, with additional tests and will compare the results to appropriate standardized normative data. Estimated premorbid performance can be taken into account and sensory or other deficits that might affect test outcome can also be interpreted in accordance with obtained test behaviours. In the absence of a psychologist, the clinical team should consider asking a local neuropsychologist (perhaps from a nearby service) to train and to supervise the assessments carried out by the individual chosen to assess cognition.

The process of assessment

Introduction to and explanation of the testing process

One of the most important elements in neuropsychological assessment is to foster an atmosphere which will optimize the patient's performance and will therefore provide the most accurate representation of his or her current level of function. Introducing the patient to the neuropsychological assessment process is essential. An ideal introduction will include information about the assessor, the reasons that the patient has been asked to see them, and discussion of how long both the interview and test assessment will take. We have also found it beneficial to inform the patient that the tests that they will be administered tap different areas at different levels of difficulty. As such, the patient is told that some of the tasks may be relatively easy for them to perform while some others might be more challenging. The patient is encouraged to give their best effort, which is reinforced during the testing session as necessary. A series of sample introductory statements can be found in the box overleaf.

In the waiting room

'Hello, my name is .... I am a psychologist. I have been asked to see you by your GP. I will need to see you for about an hour. You will need your glasses if you wear them'.

(Walking to your office

Watch the patient's gait, awareness of his/her surroundings, talk to them about the weather, how long it took to get to the hospital, or about their home....)

In your office

'Please take a seat here. As I said before, my name is ....
and I am a psychologist. Do you know why I have been asked to see you today?'

'My job is to assess your thinking and memory skills. I am going to ask you some questions this afternoon. For example you will have to read some words and remember some pictures. Some of the questions may seem quite simple. I don't want you to feel insulted if I ask you an easy question. Some of the questions will be a little more difficult. Don't worry if you cannot do everything. If you are unsure please guess, guesses are often correct. Just have a go at everything. Is that OK?'.

'Do you have any questions?'

Begin with general information

'Can I start by checking that I have your name correctly? And your date of birth? How old were you when you left school? What did you do then? Hobbies?'

Optimizing performance and managing reactions in the neuropsychological examination

Test results are only valid if they are actually representative of the patient's current level of cognitive/neuropsychological performance. While some degree of anxiety is inevitable, this has to be kept within manageable levels. Careful attention to the feelings of the participant, avoidance of irrelevant or inappropriate questions, and recognition of the patient's concerns will help them to cope well with the testing situation. If individuals are treated with respect and are able to maintain their dignity then test results can be considered to be valid. Only valid results can be used meaningfully to infer current abilities.

A sensitive, friendly style is essential. If worried about being unable to answer a question and so appear foolish, a person may attempt to avoid giving a response. Self-punitive statements about test performance, anger towards 'these stupid tests', anxiety regarding whether relatives know about their whereabouts, and subtle humour ('you should ask my husband') are all

Table 7.1 Some possible responses to negative reactions in the testing situation

Acknowledge any criticisms, do not ignore them
Take a break
Provide reassurance but do not lie
If necessary abort the test
Ask the patient if they would mind trying a different test
Come back to the test later
Consider aborting the whole assessment

common responses made by older adults in the testing situation. Suggestions of how to deal with different patient reactions can be found in Table 7.1.

Feedback during testing

Many older adults will attempt to deal with the testing situation by asking for reassurance and feedback from the examiner. In general, it is useful to have made an introductory statement described above so that the patient can be reminded that some of the questions are more difficult than others. It is best that the patient receives no feedback as to whether they have made a correct or incorrect response. Occasionally, when a person is distressed or unco-operative, an examiner might reinforce a correct response sporadically using such words as 'good' or 'well done'. In general, however, effort rather than performance should be reinforced. This may often prove challenging when patients, particularly those with mild impairment, are painfully aware of their deficits. If pressed for an evaluation of performance on a specific test, it sometimes helps to tell the patient 'I am sorry, but I am not allowed to say'. At no time during the testing should conclusions be rendered by the examiner. Remarks such as 'I have not added that up yet' or 'we can discuss this at the end' (provided that you do) are appropriate responses to patient requests for conclusions. It is generally good practice to thank the patient for their effort and co-operation after the testing session and to be honest about having to look at the patient's performance relative to appropriate norms and carefully to examine test results relative to each other to give the patient accurate and meaningful feedback. Each clinician must be sensitive to the patient's con-cerns during and after testing, yet provide an objective, standardized method of evaluation so that meaningful results can be obtained.

Feedback after testing

Optimally, neuropsychological test results should be given to the patient in combination with results obtained by other specialists on the diagnostic team.

Important information can be provided to patient with regards to individual strengths and weaknesses on neuropsychological measures. It is essential, however, that the team designates those individuals who will be providing feedback for the patient and family. This feedback will include the overall results of the dementia evaluation, clinical diagnosis, and proposed interventions. Extensive review of the results of neuropsychological and other clinical/laboratory results may not be helpful The patient and family members are in need of specific but concise information. Ideally, this information should be summarized on an information sheet tailored to the individual which they can take away or even recorded on cassette tape at the interview.

Selection of neuropsychological test batteries

There is no blueprint for an ideal set of tests to use for the assessment of dementia. Issues such as the context in which tests are used (inpatient versus outpatient, in a clinic, or at the patient's home), the type of referrals and likely diagnoses, the resources available, and information derived from other team assessments will all affect the selection. Some of these administrative issues are discussed in Chapter 2.

Some teams operate a two stage assessment process, screening with the MMSE or other similar scale, in order to decide if full neuropsychological assessment is appropriate. Whilst conducting full assessment on those who score above a cut-off may be appropriate (see Wien Centre assessment on page 12) and is certainly a practical approach to managing the referral load, using an upper cut-off (say of 25 on the MMSE) to decide that the patient is normal will lead to failure to identify early or undifferentiated cases (Huff *et al.*, 1987). Moreover, given an emphasis on the early identification of cases, and that the diagnosis is generally less reliant on neuropsychological test performance in moderate or more advanced dementia, attention might best be focused on high performing individuals if resources do not permit neuropsychological testing for everyone.

In general, it is useful to assess the domains specified by the NINCDS-ADRDA neuropsychological criteria for a diagnosis of probable Alzheimer's disease and the DSM-IV criteria for dementia (American Psychiatric Association, 1994). These are:

◆ memory

◆ language

◆ praxis

◆ visuoperceptive skills

◆ higher order problem solving abilities

Table 7.2 Functions to assess with some additional functions to consider

Functions to assess	Additional functions
premorbid ability	calculation
attention	handling money
orientation	prospective memory
visual, auditory, and tactile recognition	
visuospatial skills	
perception	
language comprehension (oral and reading)	
language expression (repetition, fluency, naming, writing)	
recognition (verbal, non-verbal, spatial information)	
learning (verbal, non-verbal, spatial information)	
recall (cued recall) (verbal, non-verbal, spatial information)	
executive functioning	
cognitive speed	
praxis	

♦ attention

♦ orientation

♦ functional abilities.

More detailed analysis of memory and expressive/receptive language functions than set forth by the NINCDS-ADRDA working group is desirable and a minimum 'fixed core' of tests is recommended. Of course, each clinician should be able to combine this approach with a 'flexible' set of tests which can be added as clinically indicated. Table 7.2 contains a list of functions which should be assessed and some additional functions which clinics may wish to test.

How long should assessment take?

A brief survey of memory clinics in the United Kingdom and America suggests that assessment time can very between 45 minutes and 2 hours. Additional time will be needed for complex presentations. This may need to be divided into a couple of sessions to prevent patients becoming fatigued. Two factors seem to determine the amount of time an assessment takes:

(1) whether a neuropsychologist is available (if not then standard screening tools are often used which are shorter);

(2) how severely the patient is impaired.

As a general rule, more severe patients not only will need less testing to establish their deficits but will have lower tolerance. By contrast, very mildly impaired patients, particularly premorbidly bright ones or those with unusual presenting problems, will need more investigation. If the assessment takes place outside a clinic setting, the nature and duration of the testing procedure will be determined by factors such as who is undertaking the assessment, the portability of equipment, and the space available within which to test.

Established assessment batteries

To demonstrate the variability in assessment batteries three will be discussed here. All have in common the assessment of the same core domains though they differ in the tests chosen to assess those domains.

Consortium to Establish a Registry for Alzheimer's Disease (CERAD)

The Consortium to Establish a Registry for Alzheimer's Disease (CERAD) has developed a battery of neuropsychological assessments to be used in the clinical diagnosis of Alzheimer's disease (Morris *et al.*, 1989). This battery was validated in 354 patients with Alzheimer's disease and compared to 278 controls. The CERAD battery contains:

♦ Verbal Fluency (Animals);
♦ Modified Boston Naming Test;
♦ Mini-Mental State Examination;
♦ Tests of Constructional Praxis;
♦ Word List Memory Test;
♦ Word Recall List;
♦ Word List Recognition.

This collection of tests has been used successfully in many research and clinical centres. Many of these tests are desirable because of minimum ceiling and floor effects which allow for longitudinal follow-up over time (Welsh *et al.*, 1992). Welsh *et al.* have also shown that the tests of memory on the CERAD are sensitive to early Alzheimer's disease. However, there have been concerns that other tests may be more sensitive to incipient Alzheimer's disease, including the Fuld Object Memory Evaluation (Loewenstein *et al.*, 1995), the Hopkins Verbal Learning Test (Brandt, 1991), and Category Fluency (Monsch *et al.*, 1992). Moreover, the CERAD does not include tests of higher order problem-solving abilities, visuoperceptive skills, attention, or functional status which are domains specified by the NINCDS-ADRDA task force (McKhann *et al.*, 1984).

The Bristol Memory Disorders Clinic (BMDC)

Designed for a British context, the Bristol Memory Disorders assessment comprises a set of tests drawn up specifically for the Clinic, a programme of the University of Bristol Department of Care of the Elderly and Frenchay Healthcare National Health Service Trust. The multidisciplinary team includes geriatricians, psychiatrists, neuropsychologist, psychology assistants, and a nurse. In addition to the neuropsychological tests, patients undergo physical examination, laboratory, and anatomic or functional imaging (CT, and MRI or SPECT if clinically indicated). This set of neuropsychological assessments, which has been administered to over 500 patients, has been validated in 50 individuals (19 males and 31 females; mean age = 71.6 ± 6.8) with a diagnosis of probable Alzheimer's disease (DSM-III-R: American Psychiatric Association, 1994; McKhann *et al.*, 1984) who were matched on age, gender, and National Adult Reading Test (NART) predicted IQ with an equal number of normal older adults. Discriminant analysis provided 100 per cent correct classification of all cases. The assessment takes about 1 hour to complete. The BMDC tests include:

- Mini-Mental State Examination (MMSE, Folstein *et al.*, 1975);
- National Adult Reading Test (NART, Nelson and Willison, 1991);
- Digit Span (Wechsler Adult Intelligence Scale-Revised, WAIS-R) (Wechsler, 1981);
- Similarities (WAIS-R) (Wechsler, 1981);
- Picture Completion (WAIS-R) (Wechsler, 1981);
- Frenchay Aphasia Screening Test (Frenchay Aphasia Screening Test, FAST) (Enderby *et al.*, 1975);
- Story Recall: Immediate and Delayed (Adult Memory and Information Processing Battery, AMIPB) (Coughlan and Hollows, 1985);
- Visual Recognition (Middlesex Elderly Assessment of Mental State, MEAMS) (Golding, 1989);
- Hopkins Verbal Learning Test—Recall and Recognition (HVLT, Brandt, 1991);
- FAS Benton verbal fluency (Lezak, 1995);
- Weigl Colour Form Sorting (Grewal and Haward, 1984);
- Cube Analysis (Visual Object Space Perception Battery, VOSP) (Warrington and James, 1991);
- Digit Copying (Kendrick, 1985);
- Bristol Activities of Daily Living Scale (BADLS; Bucks *et al.*, 1996a) designed to assess activities of daily living in community dwelling adults with dementia by using informant report.

The Wien Center for Alzheimer's Disease and Memory Disorders

The Wien Center for Alzheimer's Disease and Memory Disorders, an affiliated program of the University of Miami Department of Psychiatry and Behavioural Sciences and Mount Sinai Medical Center, administers the following core battery for those individuals with a Folstein MMSE score of 18 or above. Research with hundreds of patients has shown that neuropsychological testing with these individuals produces the optimal yield of information for the multidisciplinary team, which includes an internist, neurologist, psychiatrist, social worker, and psychologist. Complete blood testing, electrocardiogram, and MRI of the brain is routinely administered to each individual.

- Fuld Object Memory Evaluation (Fuld, 1981);
- Immediate and Delayed Memory for Passages and Designs (Wechsler Memory Scale, WMS) (Wechsler and Stone, 1945);
- Orientation and Mental Control (WMS) (Wechsler and Stone, 1945);
- DAFS Delayed Memory for Groceries (Loewenstein, unpublished);
- Rey Osterrieth Complex Figure Test (copy, immediate recall, delayed recall) (Osterrieth, 1944);
- Boston Naming Test (BNT, Kaplan, *et al.*, 1983);
- Controlled Oral Word Association Test (COWAT, Lezak, 1995);
- Selected Subtests of the Boston Diagnostic Aphasia Examination (Goodglass and Kaplan, 1983);
- Wide Range Achievement Test-Revised (WRAT-R) Arithmetic (Jastak and Wilkinson, 1984);
- Benton Handedness Questionnaire;
- Vocabulary (WAIS-R) (Wechsler, 1981);
- Similarities (WAIS-R) (Wechsler, 1981);
- Digit Span (WAIS-R) (Wechsler, 1981);
- Block Design (WAIS-R) (Wechsler, 1981);
- Object Assembly (WAIS-R) (Wechsler, 1981);
- Trailmaking Test (TMT, Forms A and B) (Spreen and Strauss, 1991);
- Direct Assessment of Functional Status Scale (DAFS) (Loewenstein *et al.*, 1989).

Those scoring lower than 18 on the MMSE are administered a much briefer battery of tests since administration of the standard 2-hour battery is often unnecessary and overtaxing for these individuals. With liberal test breaks, these tests can easily be administered within one session.

Both the Bristol Memory Disorders Clinic and the Wien Centre use a broad array of other neuropsychological measures to provide more specific clinical information should these be required in complex presentations. There are many other published neuropsychological batteries for older adults and the reader is referred to La Rue (1992) and Zec (1993) for suitable alternatives.

Issues in the selection and interpretation of neuropsychological tests

Normative data

La Rue (1987; 1992) and Holden (1995) have eloquently discussed the limitations of many neuropsychological tests for use with older adults, principally that the test materials are not appropriate either by virtue of their size, the speed demands of the tests or their content. Further, La Rue has raised the issue of the lack of normative data for older adults on many commonly used neuropsychological tests. Normative data should be age appropriate and there have been increasing attempts to develop educational and gender specific norms, although there is much work to be done.

Normative data for those individuals who are 80 and above have been developed for the WAIS-R (Paolo and Ryan, 1995, Ivnik *et al.*, 1992a; Ryan *et al.*, 1990), WMS-R (Ivnik *et al.*, 1991, 1992b), California Verbal Learning Test (Delis *et al.*, 1991), Auditory Verbal Learning Test (Ivnik *et al.*, 1992c), CERAD Battery (Welsh *et al.*, 1994), Fuld Object Memory Evaluation (Fuld, 1981), COWAT, BNT, Multilingual Aphasia Examination Token Test, WRAT-R Reading, AMNART, STROOP, TMT and Judgement of Line Orientation (Ivnik *et al.*, 1996), and the DAFS Functional scale (Loewenstein *et al.*, 1989), and other tests described in the test batteries detailed above—even the MMSE (Bleecker *et al.*, 1988; Crum *et al.*, 1993). It should be noted, however, that many of these are North American norms. The United Kingdom, as in the rest of Europe, lags behind North America in producing adequate normative data for older adults, let alone for ethnic minority groups such as those from the Caribbean or the Indian subcontinent. Ideally, these tests would be properly translated by a native speaking psychologist, committee translated by a group of professionals and lay individuals who attempt to identify and correct potential errors in the translated version, and, finally,   backtranslated by a separate translator who takes the final version and translates it back into the original language of the test to insure that the translated version adequately captures the meaning of the original. The reader is referred to Loewenstein *et al.*, (1994) for a more detailed description of this intricate process.

Culturally appropriate tests

Despite proper translation of test instruments, a neuropsychological assessment must be reliable (yield a consistent measure) and valid (the test must measure the behaviour or construct that it is supposed to measure). For example Loewenstein *et al*. (1993) found that the comprehension subtest of the WAIS-R was not appropriate for Cuban–American Alzheimer's disease patients because the material was not salient or relevant to this population. Poorer performance on WAIS-R Comprehension, WAIS-R–Digit Span, and the FAS Controlled Oral word Association Test by Cuban-American, Spanish-speaking patients relative to cognitively matched English-speaking Alzheimer's disease patients was due to problems with the test content and format. Performance on the Memory for Passages of the Wechsler Memory Scale and Wechsler Memory Scale-Revised has been questioned as to the saliency of material for patients from Latin American and other Central American countries. In a recent study, Welsh *et al*. (1995) found when using the CERAD battery that black patients with Alzheimer's disease scored lower than whites on tests of visual naming, constructional praxis, and the MMSE. A thorough discussion of cross-cultural issues in the neuropsychological assessment of diverse cultural groups can be found in Loewenstein *et al*. (1994).

Educational issues

The MMSE and most neuropsychological tests are heavily influenced by educational and occupational factors. Low scores may merely reflect the lack of a formal education rather than being indicative of brain damage (Loewenstein *et al*., 1992; Loewenstein and Rubert, 1992; Marcopulos *et al*., in press). Serial testing in those patients with suspected Alzheimer's disease will usually determine whether there is a genuine progression of cognitive deficits. Loewenstein and colleagues (1995) have found that the Fuld Object Memory Evaluation, a selective reminding test for common household objects is culture-fair, with over a 0.95 sensitivity and specificity for both Cuban-American, Spanish-speaking and English-speaking Alzheimer's disease patients and controls. This test has also been successfully used for Japanese populations and has excellent potential as a more culture-fair test of dementia, although future studies with different ethnic/ language groups await (Fuld *et al*., 1988). This test is also promising in that retrieval scores have not been found to be correlated with level of educational attainment (Loewenstein *et al*., 1995).

Estimation of premorbid functioning

Many neuropsychologists make use of formulae based on age, level of education, gender, and level of occupational functioning to estimate premorbid IQs and level of premorbid function (see e.g. Crawford and Allan, 1997). A detailed history of academic achievement and level of function in the environment is also made by the clinician. This is of paramount importance, since bright individuals may be poorly detected because of their superior ability to compensate during cognitive assessment. In contrast, those with learning difficulties or poor educational attainment and literacy may be diagnosed as having an organic condition because they will have an unrealized lifetime difficulty with many of the cognitive assessments used in testing for dementia.

A commonly used measure of estimating premorbid performance is the National Adult Reading Test (NART) (Nelson and Willison, 1991). This test requires the individual to read 50 irregular nouns. The error score is used to predict WAIS-R Full Scale IQ. More recent studies suggest that the NART is not appropriate for use with individuals with poor literacy skills, dyslexia, or those with obvious speech impairments (Cipolotti and Warrington, 1995). In addition, O'Carroll *et al.* (1995) and Fromm *et al.* (1991), among others, have shown that performance on the NART is sensitive to dementia in moderate to severe stages and should therefore only be used with very mild to moderate cases. One other criticism of the NART is its length, which requires the patient to make 14 out of 15 consecutive failures before testing can be discontinued; this can be onerous. Beardsall and Brayne (1990) developed a short form of the NART which appeared to predict full NART scores very well. However, further validation in a memory disorders clinic sample demonstrated significant underestimation of full NART scores using the Short NART so that its use could not be recommended for clinical purposes (Bucks *et al.*, 1996a).

The NART is also problematic from a cultural perspective because it was designed for the British population. A number of North American researchers have amended the NART to make it more suitable for American (AMNART) (Grober and Sliwinski, 1991), Canadian/American (Blair and Spreen, 1989), and African-American patients (Boekamp *et al.*, 1995).

Two new alternatives are the Cambridge Contextual Reading Test (Beardsall and Huppert, 1994) which embeds the NART words into written sentences: a modification which the authors claim has significantly increased its predictive validity, and the Spot the Word Test (Baddeley *et al.*, 1993) which provides an estimate of premorbid ability based on the ability to choose between 50 pairs of words and non-words. In addition, Spot the Word has two alternate forms (A and B). The Spot the Word has the advantage that it does not require the individual to speak the words aloud and can therefore be used with people who have speech impairments such as dysarthria. Recent research with a modified form of the test (Spot-the Word C) has demonstrated good prediction of WAIS-R IQ scores as well as the NART and that inclusion of social class in the regression model significantly increases the variance predicted (Crawford and Allan, submitted).

Differential diagnosis

The most common reason for seeking an evaluation by a memory assessment team is that the patient and/or caregiver is concerned. In general, however, many of those who have suffered a stroke have already been identified, usually with sudden onset of gross and easily detectable difficulties such as hemiplegias, unilateral neglect or gross language, visuoperceptive, or reasoning deficits. They are therefore less likely to present to memory teams. As a result, patients referred to the team are likely to present with more subtle deficits. Neuropsychological testing is one of the most sensitive, objective means of detecting the earliest manifestations of these dementing disorders.

Neuropsychological assessment is the study of brain–behaviour relationships and is based on lesion studies as well as on theoretical formulations regarding cognition. An examination of the pattern of impairment on neuropsychological tests by a skilled neuropsychologist is therefore often particularly helpful in differential diagnosis.

Depression versus dementia

Neuropsychological assessment is perhaps the most effective method of teasing out the effects of depression and anxiety disorders from a primary degenerative dementia alone (such as Alzheimer's disease) or a primary degenerative brain disorder in which depression and/or anxiety may be comorbid features. Patients with depression alone may present themselves as experiencing greater deficits than their actual neuropsychological performance would indicate, relative to Alzheimer's disease patients without depression. They also exhibit primary difficulties with attention, concentration, and psychomotor slowing. Lack of effort or 'I don't know' responses may be observed, but are not in and of themselves diagnostic (see also Chapter 5 and Des Rosiers, 1992).

Localizing dysfunction

Patterns of language performance often provide a basis for localizing stroke, space occupying lesions, and other causes of damage. For example damage to the posterior third of the dominant frontal lobe, which controls motor speech, may produce non-fluent Broca's aphasia, whereas damage to the posterior third of the dominant temporal lobe, which controls more receptive speech comprehension, may result in a Wernicke's type aphasia. Similarly, different types of apraxia may be associated with different areas of impairment within the brain. Disinhibition and behavioural dyscontrol syndromes may relate to damage to the dominant (commonly left hemisphere) frontal lobe situated above the eye sockets (orbital region), whereas apathetic behaviour is more commonly associated with damage to the superior (dorsolateral) frontal lobes.

Given the complexity of each individual's presenting condition however, it does not seem appropriate to give general rules for differential diagnosis. The interplay between effort, sensory processes, and heterogeneity of disease argues against the use of one neuropsychological test or diagnostic rule, or even a battery of tests examined in isolation of medical, psychiatric, neuro-logical, and neuroimaging data. Development of interdisciplinary team models has allowed for neuropsychological, psychiatric, medical, neuro-logical, and psychosocial data to be integrated more meaningfully, resulting in better diagnosis and in the identification of comorbid conditions common in older adults, thus resulting in better patient management and treatment.

With the advent of newer, more sensitive diagnostic brain imaging tech-niques such as MRI, neuropsychological tests can be utilized as powerful tools in determining the extent to which hyperintensity or hypointensity, thought to be indicative of cerebral infarction (particularly outside of the periventricular white matter), is consistent with the nature, intensity, and scope of objective cognitive impairments. Neuropsychological assessment should also help to determine whether the changes noted on imaging are artefacts without clinical significance (for a review of imaging techniques and recent developments see Chapter 6.) Neuropsychological tests also provide important information about the effects of pharmacological and surgical treatments as well as other rehabilitative treatments for tumour, stroke, normal pressure hydrocephalus, epilepsy, and dementia.

Summary and conclusions

Neuropsychological assessment is an important part of the diagnostic and remediation process of adults presenting for suspected cognitive disorder. Current neuropsychological criteria, for example those for Alzheimer's disease, are quite stringent and conservative, rightly preventing an individual who is actually normal or has age-associated memory impairment from receiving an incorrect diagnosis. However, as suggested by Loewenstein and Rubert (1992), they could also benefit from changes which would increase sensitivity in earlier cases. These criticisms apply equally to criteria for other degenerative dementias such as vascular dementia (Erkinjuntti, 1994) and Diffuse Lewy Body disease (McKeith *et al.*, 1996).

It is advisable that neuropsychological tests selected for the assessment of the older adult have established reliability and validity for this population and that appropriate normative data by which to compare test performance is available. In our experience, it is not appropriate indiscriminately to administer a large neuropsychological battery to all patients presenting for evaluation. For those individuals who are significantly demented this only provides an unnecessary burden to the patient who may already be stressed, anxious, or in denial about his or her deficits.

While fixed batteries of tests for older persons who present with cognitive impairment are necessary, this by no means precludes adding additional tests when the case warrants (or in some cases, eliminating tests that are inappropriate given some particular sensory or language impairment). Another major issue concerns the use of neuropsychological tests for diverse cultural and ethnic groups. As with many assessment instruments before them, neuropsychological testing can be biased against those speaking different languages and belonging to different ethnic/cultural groups. It is also particularly difficult when evaluating the older adult in which there is often a paucity of normative data. If normative data is lacking, it is incumbent upon neuropsychologists to lead the way in developing adequate local norms for specific populations. Because the effects of education influence performance on so many neuropsychological tests, development of local norms, collection of epidemiological data, and multicentre trials would be a means of better serving groups for which normative data is lacking. One suggestion is that neuropsychological and geriatric advocacy groups work hand in hand with major test publishers to develop more standardized neuropsychological tests for different countries.

Clinical neuropsychologists are increasingly being asked to render opinions regarding an individual's ability to manage their finances, drive an automobile, or live independently. Objective behavioural-based assessments conducted within the clinical setting as well as good collateral reports by caregivers and other qualified informants can only improve the standard of evaluation and resultant patient care.

References

Key references recommended by the authors are marked with an *.

American Psychiatric Association (1994). *Diagnostic and Statistical Manual of Mental Disorders*, (4th edn.). Washington, DC.

Baddeley, A., Emslie, H. and Nimmo-Smith, I. (1993). The Spot-the-Word test: A robust estimate of verbal intelligence based on lexical decision. *Journal of Clinical Psychology*, **32**, 55–65.

Beardsall, L. and Brayne, C. (1990). Estimation of verbal intelligence in an elderly community: A prediction analysis using a shortened NART. *British Journal of Clinical Psychology*, **29**, 83–90.

Beardsall, L. and Huppert, F.A. (1994). Improvement in NART word reading in demented and normal older persons using the Cambridge Contextual Reading Test. *Journal of Clinical and Experimental Neuropsychology*, **16**, 232–242.

Blair, J.R. and Spreen, O. (1989). Predicting premorbid IQ: A revision of the National Adult Reading Test. *Clinical Neuropsychologist*, **3**, 129–136.

Bleecker, M.L., Bolla-Wilson, K., Kawas, C. and Agnew, J. (1988). Age-specific norms for the mini-mental state exam. *Neurology*, **38**, 1565–1568.

Blessed, G., Tomlinson, B. E., and Roth, M. (1968). The association between quantitative measures of dementia and of senile changes in the cerebral gray matter of elderly subjects. *British Journal of Psychology*, **225**, 797–811.

Boekamp, J.R., Strauss, M.E. and Adams, N. (1995). Estimating premorbid intelligence in African-American and white elderly veterans using the American version of the National Adult Reading Test. *Journal of Clinical and Experimental Neuropsychology*, **17**, 645–653.

Brandt, J. (1991). The Hopkins Verbal Learning Test: Development of a new memory test with six equivalent forms. *Clinical Neuropsychologist*, **5,** 125–142.

Bucks, R.S., Ashworth, D.L., Wilcock, G.K., and Siegfried, K. (1996a). Assessment of activities of daily living in dementia: Development of the Bristol Activities of Daily Living Scale. *Age and Ageing*, **25**, 113–120.

Bucks, R.S., Scott, M.I., Pearsall, T., and Ashworth, D.L. (1996b). The Short NART: Utility in a memory disorders clinic. *British Journal of Clinical Psychology,* **35**, 133–141.

Cipolotti, L. and Warrington, E.K. (1995). Neuropsychological assessment. *Journal of Neurology, Neurosurgery and Psychiatry*, **58**, 655–664.

Coughlan, A.K. and Hollows, S.E. (1985). *The Adult Memory and Information Processing Battery (AMIPB)*. AK Coughlan, St James's University Hospital, Leeds.

Crawford, J.R., and Allan, K.M. Estimating premorbid WAIS-R IQ: Development of regression equations for Spot-the-Word and comparison with the NART. Submitted.

Crawford, J.R. and Allan, K.M. (1997). Estimating premorbid WAIS-R IQ with demographic variables: regression equations derived from a U.K. sample. *Clinical Neuropsychologist*, **11**, 192–197.

Crum, R.M., Anthony, J.C., Bassett, S.S. and Folstein, M.F. (1993). Population-based norms for the Mini-Mental State Examination by age and educational level. *Journal of the American Geriatric Society*, **269**, 2386–2391.

Delis, D.C., Massman, P.J., Butters, N., Salmon, D.P., Cermak, L.S. and Kramer, J.H. (1991). Profiles of demented and amnesic patients on the California Verbal Learning Test: Implications for the assessment of memory disorders. *Psychological Assessment,* **3**, 19–25.

* DesRosiers, G. (1992). Primary or depressive dementia: Psychometric assessment. *Clinical Psychology Review*, **12**, 307–343.

Enderby, P., Wood, V. and Wade, D. 1975. *Frenchay Aphasia Screening Test (FAST)*. Test Manual, NFER-Nelson, Windsor.

Erkinjuntti, T. (1994). Clinical criteria for vascular dementia: the NINDS-AIREN criteria. *Dementia*, **5**, 189–192.

Folstein, M. F., Folstein, S. A., and Mc Hugh, P. R. (1975). Mini-mental state: A practical method for grading the cognitive state of patients for the clinician. *Journal of Psychiatric Research*, **12**, 196–198.

Fromm, D., Holland, A.L., Nebes, R.D. and Oakley, M.A. (1991). A longitudinal study of word-reading ability in Alzheimer's disease: Evidence from the National Adult Reading Test. *Cortex*, **27**, 367–376.

Fuld, P. A. (1981). *The Fuld Object Memory Evaluation*. Stoeling Instrument Company, Chicago.

Fuld, P.A., Muramato, O., Blau, A.D., Westbrook, L.E., and Katzman, R. (1988). Cross-cultural and multi-ethnic dementia evaluation by mental status and memory testing. *Cortex*, **24**, 511–519.

Golding, E. (1989). *The Middlesex Elderly Assessment of Mental State*. Thames Valley Test Company, Bury St Edmunds.

Goodglass , H. and Kaplan, E.F. (1983). *Boston Diagnostic Aphasia Evaluation (BDAE)*. Philadelphia: Lea and Febiger. Distributed by Psychological Assessment Resources, Odessa, Fl.

Grewal, B. and Harward, L. (1984). Validation of a new Weigl scoring system in neurological diagnosis. *Medical Science Research*, **12**, 602–603.

Grober, E. and Sliwinski, M. (1991). Development and validation of a model for estimating premorbid verbal intelligence in the elderly. *Journal of Clinical and Experimental Neuropsychology*, **13**, 933–949.

Heilbronner, R. L. (1992). The search for a 'pure' visual memory test: Pursuit of perfection? *Clinical Neuropsychologist*, **6**, 105–112.

* Holden, U.E. (1995). *Ageing, Neuropsychology and the 'New' Dementias: Definitions, Explanations and Practical Approaches*. Chapman and Hall, London.

Huff, F. J., Becker, J. T., Belle, S. H., Nebes, R. D., Holland, A. L., and Boller, F. (1987). Cognitive deficits and clinical diagnosis of Alzheimer's Disease. *Neurology*, **37**, 1119–1124.

Huppert, F.A., Brayne, C., Gill, C., Paykel, E.S., and Beardsall, L. (1995). CAMCOG—A concise neuropsychological test to assist dementia diagnosis: Socio-demographic determinants in an elderly population sample. *British Journal of Clinical Psychology*, **34**, 529–542.

Ivnik, R.J., Smith, G.E., Tangalos, E.G., Petersen, R.C., Kokmen, E. and Kurland, L.T. (1991). Wechsler Memory Scale: IQ-dependent norms for persons ages 65 to 97 years. *Psychological Assessment: A Journal of Consulting and Clinical Psychology*, **3**, 156–161.

Ivnik, R.J., Malec, J.F., Smith, G.E., Tangalos, E.G., Petersen, R.C., Kokmen, E. *et al.* (1992a). Mayo's older American normative studies: WAIS-R norms for ages 56 to 97. *Clinical Neuropsychologist*, **6 (Suppl.)**, 1–30.

Ivnik, R.J., Malec, J.F., Smith, G.E., Tangalos, E.G., Petersen, R.C., Kokmen, E. *et al.* (1992b). Mayo's older American normative studies: WMS-R norms for ages 56 to 94. *Clinical Neuropsychologist*, **6 (Suppl.)**, 49–82.

Ivnik, R.J., Malec, J.F., Smith, G.E., Tangalos, E.G., Petersen, R.C., Kokmen, E. *et al.* (1992c). Mayo's older American normative studies: Updated AVLT norms for ages 56 to 97. *Clinical Neuropsychologist*, **6 (Suppl.)**, 83–104.

Ivnik, R.J., Malec, J.F., Smith, G.E., Tangalos, E.G., and Petersen, R.C. (1996). Neuropsychological tests' norms above age 55: COWAT, BNT, MAE Token, WRAT-R Reading, AMNART, STROOP, TMT, and JLO. *ClinicalNeuropsychologist*, **10**, 262–278.

Jastak, S, and Wilkinson, S. (1984). *Wide-Range Achievment Test—Revised (WRAT-R)*. Wilmington, DE: Jastak Assessment Systems.

Kaplan, E.F., Goodglass, H., and Weintraub, S. (1983). *The Boston Naming Test* (2nd edn.). Lea and Febiger, Philadelphia.

Kendrick, D. (1985). *Kendrick Cognitive Tests for the Elderly*. NFER-NELSON, Windsor, England.

Kukull, W.A., Larson, E.B., Reifler, B.V., Lampe, T.H., Yerby, M.J. *et al.* (1990). The validity of three clinical diagnostic criteria for Alzheimer's disease. *Neurology*, **40**, 1364–1367.

La Rue, A. (1987). Methodological concerns: longitudinal studies of dementia. *Alzheimer Disease and Associated Disorders*, **1**, 180–192.

* La Rue, A. (1992). *Aging and Neuropsychological Assessment*. Plenum Press, New York.

Leach, J. and Levy, R. (1994). Reflections on the NINCDS/ADRDA criteria for the diagnosis of Alzheimer's disease. *International Journal of Geriatric Psychiatry*, **9**, 173–179.

* Lezak, M. D. (1995). *Neuropsychological Assessment* (3rd edn.). Oxford University Press, New York.

Loewenstein, D. A., Amigo, E., Duara, R., Guterman, A., Hurwitz, D., Berkowitz, *et al.*, (1989). A new scale for the assessment of functional status in Alzheimer's disease and related disorders. *Journal of Gerontology*, **4**, 114–121.

Loewenstein, D. A., Ardilla, A., Roselli, M., Hayden, S., Duara, R., Berkowitz, *et al.* (1992). A comparative analysis of functional status among Spanish-and English-speaking patients with dementia. *Journal of Gerontology: Psychological Sciences*, **47**, 142–149.

Loewenstein, D., Arguelles, T., Barker, W., and Duara, R. (1993). A comparative analysis of neuropsychological test performance of Spanish-speaking and English-speaking patient's with Alzheimer's disease. *Journal of Gerontology*, **48**, 142–149.

Loewenstein, D. A., Arguelles, T., Arguelles, S., and Linn-Fuentes, P. (1994). Potential cultural bias in the neuropsychological assessment of the older adult. *Journal of Clinical and Experimental Neuropsychology*, **16**, 623–629.

Loewenstein, D. A., Arguelles, T, Arguells and Duara, R. (1995). The uility of the Fuld Object Memory Evaluation in detection of Spanish-speaking and English-speaking patients with dementia. *American Journal of Geriatric Psychiatry*, **10**, 75–88.

Loewenstein, D. A. and Rubert, M. P. (1992). The NINCDS-ADRDA neuropsychological criteria for the assessment of dementia: Limitations of current diagnostic guidelines. *Behavior, Health, and Aging*, **2**, 113–121.

McKeith, I.G., Galasko, D., Kosaka, K., Perry, E.K., Dickson, D.W., Hansen, L.A. *et al.* (1996). Consensus guidelines for the clinical and pathological diagnosis of dementia with Lewy bodies (DLB). Report of the consortium on DLB international workshop. *Neurology*, **47**, 1113–1124.

McKhann, G., Drachman, D., Folstein, M., Katzman, R., Price, D., and Stadlan, E. M. (1984). Clinical diagnosis of Alzheimer's disease: Report of the NINCDS-ADRDA work group under the auspices of Department of Health and Human Services task force on Alzheimer's disease. *Neurology*, **34**, 939–944.

Marcopulos, B.A. *et al.* Cognitive impairment or inadequate norms? A study of healthy, rural, older adults with limited education. *Clinical Neuro - psychologist*. In press.

Monsch, A. U., Bondi, M. W., Butters, N., Salmon, D. P., Katzman, R., and Thal, L. J. (1992). Comparisons of verbal fluency tasks in the detection of dementia of the Alzheimer type. *Archives of Neurology*, **49**, 1253–1258.

Morris, J. C., Heyman, A., Mohs, R. C., Hughs, J. P., van Belle, G., Fillenbaum, G., and the CERAD investigators (1989). The consortium to establish a registry for Alzheimer's disease (CERAD). Part I. Clinical and neuropsychological assessment of Alzheimer's disease. *Neurology*, **39**, 1159–1165.

Nelson, H.E. and Willison, J. (1991). *National Adult Reading Test (NART). Test Manual Including New Data Supplement*. NFER-NELSON, Windsor, England.

O'Carroll, R.E., Prentice, N., Murray, C., Van Beck, M., Ebmeier, K.P. and Goodwin, G.M. (1995). Further evidence that reading ability is not preserved in Alzheimer's disease. *British Journal of Psychiatry*, **167**, 659–662.

Osterrieth, P.A. (1944). Le test de copie d'une figure complex. *Archives de Psychologie, 30,* 206–356.

Paolo, A.M. and Ryan, J.J. (1995). Selecting WAIS-R norms for persons 75 years and older. *Clinical Neuropsychologist*, **9,** 44–49.

Roth, M., Tym, E., Mountjoy, C.Q., Huppert, F.A., Hendrie, H., Verma, S., *et al.* (1986). CAMDEX: A standardised instrument for the diagnosis of mental disorder in the elderly with special reference to the early detection of dementia. *British Journal of Psychiatry*, **149**, 698–709.

Ryan, J.J., Paolo, A.M. and Brungardt, T.M. (1990). Standardisation of the Weschsler Adult Intelligence Scale—Revised for persons 75 years and older. *Psychological Assessment: A Journal of Consulting and Clinical Psychology*, **2**, 404–411.

Spreen, O. and Strauss, E. (1991). A *Compendium of Neuropsychological Tests*. Oxford University Press, New York.

Tierney, M.C., Fisher, R.H., Lewis, A.J. *et al.* (1988). The NINCDS-ADRDA workgroup criteria for the clinical diagnosis of probable Alzheimer's disease. *Neurology*, **38**, 359–364.

Warrington, E.K. and James, M. (1991). *The Visual Object Space Perception Battery*. Thames Valley Test Company, Bury St Edmunds.

Wechsler, D. (1981). *The Wechsler Adult Intelligence Scale-Revised*. The Psychological Corporation, New York.

Wechsler, D. and Stone, C. (1945). *Wechsler Memory Scale*. The Psychological Corporation, New York.

Welsh, K. A., Butters, N., Hughes, J. P., Mohs, R., and Heyman, A. (1992). Detection of abnormal memory decline in mild cases of Alzheimer's disease using CERAD neuropsychological measures. *Archives of Neurology*, **48**, 278–281.

Welsh, K.A., Butters, N., Mohs, R.C., Beekly, D., Edland, S., Fillenbaum, G., *et al.* (1994). The Consortium to Establish a Registry for Alzheimer's Disease (CERAD). Part V. A normative study of the neuropsychological battery. *Neurology*, **44**, 609–614.

Welsh, K. A., Fillenbaum, G., Wilkinson, W., Heyman, A., Mohs, R. C., Stern, *et al.* (1995). Neuropsychological test performance in African-American and white patients with Alzheimer's disease. *Neurology*, **45**, 2207–2211.

Zec, R. F. (1993). Neuropsychological functioning in Alzheimer's Disease. In: *Neuropsychology of Alzheimer's Disease and Other Dementias*. (Ed. R. W. Parks, R. F. Zec, and R. S. Wilson), pp. 3–80. Oxford University Press, New York.

8 Computerized cognitive assessment

Keith A. Wesnes, Kathleen Hildebrand, and Erich Mohr

Introduction

While many researchers in this field would reasonably believe that the automation of tests of mental capabilities would have started with the advent of the microcomputer in the late 1970s, this is by no means the case. Some may think the pioneering attempts of Gedye (1967) in the 1960s were the earliest attempts, or those with longer memories the introduction of the Continuous Performance Test in the 1950s (Rosvold *et al.*, 1956). However, to the knowledge of the authors, Clark Hull was one of the true pioneers in this field. Hull, better known for his later work on Classical Conditioning, actually conducted his PhD thesis on the effects of tobacco smoking on mental efficiency. In a publication of his thesis, Hull (1924) described a remarkable apparatus which included a reaction time measurement system, accurate to 1/300 second, and a voice key to facilitate the measurement of reading reaction times! The purpose of this chapter is to shed some light upon the intriguing question of *why,* for decades, some researchers have worked diligentlyto harness the latest technological advancements of the day in order to automate tests of mental capabilities, while their colleagues have been perfectly happy to make such assessments simply using pencil, paper, and sometimes, a stopwatch.

The rationale behind the automation of cognitive tests

This section will consider the motives behind the desire to automate cognitive tests. It will concentrate on the motives behind successful and practical attempts, and will ignore examples where automation has been conducted for frivolous reasons or where automation has made tests less sensitive, reliable, or valid. Some tests are not yet ready for automation, or at least full automation. Word recall, for example, has yet to be successfully automated. While the presentation of the words can now be automated by presenting them either visually, on a computer screen, or auditorily, via a speech synthesizer or in prerecorded form, the technology available for the collection of responses is still limited. They can be recorded on a tape recorder for later scoring, but in most cases are hand written. Typing them directly into a computer would be nonsensical for almost all patients, the exception being those with good keyboard skills. As yet, neither speech recognition technology nor screen-pads which recognize hand writing are sufficiently sophisticated, nor widely economically available, to permit general use.

There are four main reasons to automate test of cognitive function. The first is to improve the sensitivity, reliability, and standardization of the tests. The second is to facilitate the process of testing, thereby enabling more volunteers to be tested at any one time, increasing the speed of scoring and processing of data, and/or allowing non-specialists to administer tests. The third is to enable more definitive measurement of those aspects of cognitive function, such as attention, working memory, and recognition memory, which non-automated procedures cannot unequivocally assess. The fourth is to take advantage of the opportunities and facilities provided by the computer to develop the test in the first place (e.g. imagine a pencil and paper flight simulator).

To standardize test administration

The manner in which a test is administered can affect how it is performed. While professional test administrators are trained to administer tests in a consistent, pleasant but restrained, semi-impersonal manner, interpersonal interactions will necessarily affect the attitudes of both tester and patient to one another, and different testers will interact differently with the same patient. It must be acknowledged that different testers, no matter how professional, will adopt different styles when testing; variations in both voice tone and body language being the obvious but by no means the only aspects which will vary, not only between testers but also within an individual tester over different testing sessions. Also when information is presented by hand (such as pictures in recognition tests) variations in the time and/or rate of presentation may occur. Automation can minimize the influence of such factors on test performance, which will be important in circumstances where complete standardization is needed.

Nevertheless, regardless of any underlying cognitive deficits, not all patients react to computer technology in the same way. Moreover, it would be wrong to say that most automated tests do not still involve a degree of interpersonal interaction. Often, instructions must be presented by the tester, who must also be on hand to clarify matters if 'on-screen' instructions are not clear. Most properly automated procedures ensure that the test instructions and materials are presented in a controlled fashion, however. As such, they offer a great advantage to the standardization of test procedures.

To remove errors in test administration

Testers, being human, make mistakes. Sometimes instructions can be slightly garbled or stimulus cards dropped on the floor. Stop watches, particularly the multipurpose digital type, can be difficult to operate; and the tester may forget to start the stopwatch only to realize this when the patient has completed the test. Alternatively the tester may start the watch but become distracted and forget to stop the patient at the precise moment required by the test. If the tester is required to write down responses, some may be missed. Such .problems can largely be overcome with proper automation of tests using reliable equipment and programmes.

To make test administration easier

Testers, like patients, become tired. Automation can reduce the demands of testing in various ways. For example properly computerized test systems cue both tester and patient for the next test in sequence, and for repeated testing automatically select the appropriate parallel forms of the tests. Instructions can be presented on the computer screen, and the computer can control aspects of testing which are demanding for the tester. Also, by removing the requirement of the tester to record responses and score the test, test administration is further eased, allowing greater opportunity to make qualitative observations about the patient's performance. Improved standardization and reduced errors are both clear benefits of such automation.

To facilitate test administration

For large scale studies using volunteers, such as those of memory and ageing, multiple set-ups and testing groups in parallel can be achieved (e.g. Robbins, *et al.*, 1994; Ritchie, *et al.*, 1993). In clinical trials, a single administrator can generally supervise six to ten volunteers being tested in parallel. In memory clinics, such advantages are less applicable. The other main area of facilitation, though, is the speed of scoring and analysis of test performance. Test scores can be available immediately which may be of considerable benefit to memory disorders teams. In addition, numerous 'person-hours' which would otherwise be spent scoring tests may be saved. Automation also enables less-qualified personnel to administer the tests, something which can decrease the need for psychologists while enhancing the supervisory and interpretative role of those who are available.

In an excellent and comprehensive review of automated testing, Cull and Trimble (1987) outline a further, less obvious, advantage of the micro-computer:

'It does not get tired, angry or bored . . . It can work at any time of the day or night, every day of the week, every month of the year. It does not have family problems. It is never sick or hungover. Its performance does not vary from hour to hour or from day to day. It has no facial expression. It does not raise an eyebrow. It is very polite. It has a perfect memory. It need not be morally judgmental. It has no superior social status . . .' [Colby, 1980, cited by Cull and Trimble, 1987, p. 144].

To remove experimenter bias

We have considered errors of recording responses earlier, but in some procedures there are judgements to be made about whether or not responses are correct, which depend on how strictly (or accurately) criteria are applied. Different experimenters may apply the criteria with differing degrees of strictness (accuracy), and this will always be a source of potential variability, which is best removed, when possible, by automating the assessment.

To improve the accuracy and sensitivity of assessment

Most of these advantages help to reduce the variability associated with test administration, which improves the accuracy of the assessment. The ability to measure, to the nearest millisecond, the time of each response in relation to the test stimulus is one of the most significant advances in the quality of cognitive assessment over the last 30 years. In a continual recognition test for example, not only is each response definitively scored for its appropriateness, but the time taken to make each decision is also recorded. In attentional tests, the ability to detect target stimuli can be identified, as is the time taken to identify them. Further, by measuring response speed, test sensitivity is enhanced. In the first place, this aspect of performance is not always assessed in pencil and paper tests, and on some tasks cannot be measured on a response by response basis (e.g. letter cancellation, trail making).

Thus by adding the measurement of speed to that of accuracy, an additional opportunity to detect change is provided. When attempting to detect enhancements in cognitive function, speed offers the considerable advantage that it is never limited by the ceiling effects seen for accuracy scores in many tests. Certainly, in older adults and people with dementia, speed of cognitive processes can always improve.

To increase the range of parameters assessed

This follows on directly from the previous section. In a non-automated recognition test, for example, the correctness of the responses can be measured as can the types of errors made. In an automated procedure, however, the speed of each response can also be measured. Not only does assessment of both speed and accuracy allow calculation of 'speed–accuracy trade-offs', and thus some measure of changes in strategy, but changes to speed are just as valid, and potentially important, measures of the quality of functioning of cognitive processes as are changes to accuracy.

To prevent the 'back at school' reaction to being assessed

Many older people resent being tested by another, often younger, individual who records responses which they cannot see. This potential problem can be largely off set by the use of a computer. If tester and patient sit next to each other, the possible antagonism of the patient towards testing can soon evaporate, particularly if the tester makes it clear that the computer is making the assessments and it thus becomes obvious that an inanimate computer is the 'offender of the peace'.

To enhance the security/ integrity of data gathering

Over and above the advantages of ensuring that all responses are recorded accurately and their timing assessed precisely, some systems enable the data to be stored in encrypted files which cannot be accessed except by particular personnel. This can provide additional protection or privacy, and also help protect against fraud in clinical trials by preventing data being tampered with.

To permit the assessment of attention

The everyday importance of attention, its crucial role in overall cognitive function and the extent to which it plays a major role in, for example, the cognitive pathologies of the dementias has only been slowly recognized. The term 'memory clinics' makes this point. Yet there are clear and important attentional deficits in dementia (e.g. Mohr *et al.*, 1996; Simpson *et al.*, 1991), which are now being recognized in clinical trials of antidementia drugs (Ferris *et al.*, 1997). In fact, some recently discovered forms of dementia, such as dementia with Lewy bodies, may especially be characterized by attentional deficits (e.g. Ayre *et al.*, 1996). One important facet of attention is the ability to maintain concentration. Standardized paper and pencil tests are simply unable unequivocally to assess this aspect of attention, as they are only able to record the time taken to complete the test (or the number of targets identified in a given time) and subtle changes in attention may be missed by the assessor. Thus half way through a test, (unless the tester has the discretion to make such observations) the patient may become completely distracted for say 10 seconds, and then hurry on with the test to try to make up for the lapse. On a pencil and paper test this may be of little importance, but in everyday life it might have dramatic consequences, for example when driving a car. No such compensations are possible on properly constructed computerized vigilance tests. For example by having frequent targets and measuring the speed at which each target is detected, even a 10 second lapse would be seen as the failure to detect two or three consecutive targets, or as a large increase in the time taken to make the detections. If these crucial aspects of attention are to be assessed, as they should, then computerized testing offers an effective strategy.

Some testing procedures depend on automation

Much of the discussion above has concerned tests which have been automated from previous pencil and paper versions. However, some tests, for example the Mackworth Clock test, an automated procedure devised by the Canadian psychologist Norman Mackworth during the Second World War to simulate watching a radar screen (Wesnes, 1977), have always been automated. Other examples include: the classical pursuit rotor test; reaction time tests (e.g. simple and choice reaction time); and the now widely used rapid visual information processing test (Wesnes and Warburton, 1983). These clearly need to be computerized. Newer procedures, such as virtual reality, will also find their way into cognitive assessment in the future, and again, the question of automation will not be relevant to such tests.

Computerized systems for assessing cognitive function

The three most commonly used systems have emerged since the 1980's. Interestingly, the primary rationale behind the development of these systems was strikingly different. The Memory Assessment Clinic system (MAC: Crook, Salama, and Gobert, 1986) was developed using video disk technology, a touch screen and a telephone, to provide tests which closely simulated everyday tasks, both in order to improve their acceptability by patients, and to raise the perception by regulatory authorities of their relevance for everyday behaviour. The rationale behind the Cambridge Neuropsychological Test Automated Battery (CANTAB: Morris *et al.*, 1987) could not have been more different. In order to provide a link from behavioural testing in animals to man, the authors developed human equivalents of various long-established behavioural paradigms in rats and primates (e.g. delayed matching to sample), using PC and touch-screen technology. Thus, for example, from knowledge of behavioural deficits in animals produced by anatomical and neurochemical lesions, it is possible from measuring the extent to which various patient populations exhibit similar deficits, to use the lesion data to make speculations about the neuro-chemical/neuroanatomical bases of these disease states. The rationale behind the Cognitive Drug Research computerised assessment system (CDR: Wesnes, Simpson, and Christmas, 1987), was by incorporating the most sensitive and functionally specific tests currently available into a unified flexible software package in which all information is presented on computer screens and all responses gathered via YES/NO response modules, to provide a system which could be used in virtually any type of clinical trial.

Comparing computerized tests to traditional assessments

Among the limitations of traditional cognitive assessments are long administration times, lack of alternate forms to avoid practice effects, and inadequate depth of measurement of specific cognitive functions. Computerized cognitive testing has the potential to enhance the accuracy and standardization of measurements, provide numerous alternate forms, and measure with more detail and accuracy the speed and proficiency in specific aspects of cognitive function.

Four of the most widely used non-automated testing instruments in clinical research include the Mattis Dementia Rating Scale (DRS) (Mattis, 1989), the Mini-Mental State Examination (MMSE) (Folstein *et al.*, 1975), the Wechsler Memory Scale–Revised (WMS–R) (Wechsler, 1987), and the Alzheimer's Disease Assessment Scale (ADAS) (Rosen *et al.*, 1984). In a recent study (Mohr *et al.*, 1996), these measures were compared to the Cognitive Drug Research (CDR) computerized assessment system (Simpson *et al.*, 1991). The CDR system is a collection of automated test procedures designed to measure a range of aspects of cognitive function, particularly attention, working memory, and episodic (secondary) memory. The objective of this research was to examine the sensitivity of the four non-automated tests and the CDR system for identifying mild dementia, as well as to examine impairment of various specific neuropsychological domains in two different types of dementia.

The tests were administered to 15 normal controls and 30 patients with mild dementia, matched for education levels (mean 12 years). Fifteen patients had Alzheimer's disease and 15 had Huntington's disease. The two groups were matched for dementia severity (mean MMSE 24.5). Normal controls were matched on age to the Alzheimer's disease patients (mean 68 years).

The results of this study indicated that total scores in the various testing instruments were able to distinguish normal controls from demented patients, but were not able to differentiate the two types of dementia. A comparison of subtest results focusing on specific cognitive domains, however, showed more potential for distinguishing Alzheimer's and Huntington's disease patients, and this was particularly evident in the computerized battery. In the traditional tests, only Memory on the DRS, Attention/Concentration on the WMS-

R, and Orientation on the ADAS Cognitive Subscale differentiated the Alzheimer's patients from the Huntington's patients (no MMSE subtests did so). In the CDR system, normal controls performed significantly better than Alzheimer's patients on most delayed recognition subtests, while controls differed from Huntington's patients primarily on measures of speed of cognitive processing. In addition, Alzheimer's and Huntington's patient groups differed from each other on several delayed recognition subtests.

The results of a canonical discriminate analysis for this study indicated that, overall, 83 per cent of subjects were correctly classified using the CDR system, as opposed to 71 per cent with the DRS, 67 per cent with the MMSE, 67 per cent with the WMS-R, and 65 per cent with the ADAS. All of these tests were reasonably effective in classifying normal controls, ranging from 77 per cent to 87 per cent for individual tests. However, correct Alzheimer's disease patient classification was 77 per cent for the CDR system as opposed to 60 to 67 per cent for the other four tests.

It may seem surprising that the CDR system was more effective in identifying Alzheimer's patients than the ADAS (77 versus 67 per cent), a scale developed specifically for such patients, though one consideration here is the definitive assessment of attention in the CDR system, while the Cognitive Subscale of the ADAS does not contain an assessment of this major cognitive function. Indeed, there is a widespread and misplaced belief that attention is not disrupted in Alzheimer's patients, for example the DSM-IV (American Psychiatric Association, 1994) diagnostic criteria for Alzheimer's disease (in fact all dementias), does not even include an impairment of attention. However, the Alzheimer's patients in this study were impaired on choice reaction time, an attentional test, as well as the various memory tests. Certainly, there is much human evidence that the cholinergic system is involved in attention (e.g. Warburton and Wesnes, 1984), and cholinergic dysfunction is widely accepted as important in the cognitive decline in Alzheimer's disease. Thus the assessment of attention, and possibly other aspects of computerized assessment, could explain the superiority of the automated system to the ADAS in this study. The classification of Huntington's disease was likewise more effective with the CDR system, with 86 per cent being correctly classified versus 43 to 62 per cent for the other four tests. Here ADAS, with only 43 per cent accuracy, showed severe limitations. Other computerized testing protocols may also have similar benefits, for example the CANTAB (Cambridge Neuropsychological Automated Test Battery) (Sahakian et al., 1988) has been shown to discriminate between Alzheimer's and Parkinson's disease. Overall, the computerized system, which used measures of both speed and accuracy, was more effective than the four other widely used assessments—both in identifying early dementia and for the differentiation of Alzheimer's and Huntington's patient groups. The authors of the paper felt that the computerized administration of speed measures appeared to be particularly effective for identifying signs of early cognitive decline (Mohr *et al.*, 1996).

Consistently superior performance of automated tests has not been found in all studies, however. Youngjohn *et al.* compared test–retest reliability of automated and traditional memory tests. Both tests showed significant practice effects, but while test–retest reliability of the automated measures were equal or superior to traditional tests on recall tasks, they performed worse than traditional tests of attention and concentration (Youngjohn *et al.*, 1992a). This is clearly an area for further research.

The same group also compared automated and traditional tests in their ability to discriminate age-associated memory impairment from Alzheimer's disease. They noted that both types of tests performed reasonably well, although in both, false positive results were the most frequent classification errors. Overall, traditional tests had slightly higher accuracy (87.5 vs. 88.4 per cent) than computerized tests (Youngjohn *et al.*, 1992b).

Experience of using computerized tests in memory clinics

In a validation study, a version of the CDR system which was developed for use with demented patients was administered to 51 patients in a memory clinic (Simpson *et al.*, 1991). The results were very positive as evidenced by the following extract: 'The clinic staff were surprised at the extent to which physically disabled patients including those with Parkinson's disease and post-stroke patients were able to manage the response buttons. These patients did not appear to show any discomfort or stress, and in fact it was the impression of the researcher that patients of all abilities generally enjoyed performing COGDRAS-D more than the other tests, many commenting that they hoped they would be able to perform it on another occasion. The average completion time for the computerized system was under 15 minutes for the control group, indicating that assessments of vigilance, attention, information processing, picture and verbal recognition can be completed within this time' (Simpson *et al.*, 1991; p. 100).

The study found that the various submeasures of CDR system correlated well with a number of other procedures including the MMSE, the Kendrick tests, the Kew test, and the Stockton Behavioural Rating Scale (Simpson *et al.*, 1991). Some of the correlations were predictable as the CDR tests are aimed at identifying attention and memory, and thus would be expected to correlate generally with tests such as the MMSE and Kendrick. More surprising, perhaps, were the high correlations with the Stockton scale, which concerns the general capabilities of the patient, for example dressing and feeding. The Stockton was administered by ward staff not present when the computerized tests were conducted, yet there were high correlations between the scale and a number of the individual items from the CDR system, for example the ability to identify words correctly in a recognition test correlated at a level of 0.79 with the Stockton. Furthermore, two of the CDR measures, word recognition sensitivity and picture recognition sensitivity, were both able to differentiate the two populations with an overlap of only one patient, the same sensitivity as the MMSE, which was used to aid the assessment of dementia. Overall, this study confirmed the suitability, utility, and sensitivity of a computerized test system for use in a memory clinic. Whilst other researchers have also found such positive reactions to computerized testing with older people (Frydenberg, 1998), other work has been more equivocal. Ivnik *et al.*, (1996) evaluated 373 older normal people and rated their reactions to computerized testing versus traditional testing of cognition. The authors concluded; 'These findings suggest that it might be wrong to assume that normal elderly people, will react negatively to computer-based assessments . . . To the extent that slight differences might be present, older persons favoured traditional, person-to-person assessment procedures. However, in large part computers are generally as well received as working with another person (pp. 151)'. Overall, the data so far suggest that to the extent that elderly people enjoy having their cognitive function assessed in the first place, there is little to choose between their acceptance of traditional versions versus computerised tests. Age however, is not the only factor. In some cases cohort, educational, or cultural effects can also be determinants of local suitability of automated testing (Legg and Buhr, 1992). Though as computers become more widespread, lack of familiarity with the technology will cease to be a problem for acceptability.

Computerized tests or non-automated tests or both: the verdict

The space available in this chapter has not permitted a detailed description of the dos and do nots of computerized testing, nor a discussion of the various current systems available (Crook *et al.*, 1986; Fray *et al.*, 1996). However, the reader should now be in a position to evaluate tests and systems critically. Certainly, just as any novel pencil and paper test must be fully evaluated for its validity, utility, reliability, and sensitivity so should any computerized test or test system. Poorly automated procedures can nullify all of the potential benefits described in this chapter; while properly automating tests is always an extremely complex, lengthy, and costly business. Much of the current widespread persistence of use of pencil and paper techniques in clinical research is largely a consequence both of the limited numbers of automated procedures available and of the problems in developing customized automated tests. Undoubtedly, it is difficult to obtain computerized tests which have true sensitivity of assessment (true millisecond timing to response buttons achieved using machine-code sub-routines, not keyboard presses for example, which are only monitored every 40 milliseconds), and cost as well as availability must be considered when evaluating the benefits offered by automation.

Dementia is a major, expanding, and costly disease in society today. The ability to differentiate dementia from normality in early stages of disease and, further, to distinguish different types and aetiologies is essential. Accurate diagnostic assessment and the opportunity to follow either progression or regression of deficits is important both clinically and for the evaluation of the many new antidementia drugs that are currently being developed. Thus sensitivity and reliability are key issues in selecting tests and systems. The conclusion of this chapter is that computerized tests have a valuable role to play in cognitive assessment whether conducted within the context of a memory disorders team or within other services. Although few comparisons between automated and non-automated procedures for assessing cognitive function in various forms of dementia are available, most of those which have been undertaken reveal benefits to automation (e.g. Mohr *et al.*, 1996). The argument for not using such systems in dementia assessment may therefore relate to cost, availability, or reservations about new or unfamiliar approaches. Whether or not automated systems are employed, they *need not* be used exclusively at the expense of non-automated procedures, and both types of test can happily coexist in the investigator's armamentarium. However, in the opinion of the authors, solely using non-automated procedures cannot be recommended. Although a number of aspects of cognitive function can be soundly assessed using pencil and paper procedures (e.g. word recall, word fluency): properly implemented and validated computerised procedures offer the only definitive opportunities to measure functions like attention, while, for other functions like recognition, they permit speed-accuracy trade-offs to be identified which would otherwise be missed (e.g. Nicholl *et al.*, 1995). Overall, the authors believe that automation of tests is not only inevitable but ultimately desirable, particularly in offering definitive tests of automated speed of performance. The caveats, of course are that the automation must be conducted properly, and also that the process of automation does not invalidate the objective of the original test.

References

Key references recommended by the authors are marked with an *.

American Psychiatric Association (1994). Diagnostic and Statistical Manual of Mental Disorders, 4th Edition, Washington, DC.

Ayre G, McKeith IG, Wesnes K, and Sahgal A (1996). Psychological function in dementia with Lewy bodies and senile dementia of the Alzheimer's type. *Neurobiology of Aging* **17** (Suppl. 4S): 205–206.

Crook T, Salama M, and Gobert J (1986). A computerised test battery for detecting and assessing memory disorders. In: A. Bes *et al.* (eds), *Senile Dementias: Early Detection.* John Libbey Eurotext: 79–85.

Cull C and Trimble MR (1987). Automated Testing and Psychopharmacology in Hindmarch I and Stonier PD (eds.) Human Psychopharmacology: measures and methods Volume 1. Chichester, Wiley.

Ferris, S., Lucca, U., Mohs, R., Dubois, B., Wesnes, K., Erzigheit, H., Geldmacher, D., Bodick, N. (1997). Objective psychometric tests in clinical trials of dementia drugs. Position paper from the International Working Group on the Harmonisation of Dementia Drug Guidelines. *Alzheimer's Disease and Associated Disorders,* 11, Suppl 3, 34–8.

Folstein MF, Folstein SE, and McHugh PR (1975). Mini-mental state: a practical method for grading the cognitive state of patients for the clinician. *Journal of Psychiatric Research* **12**: 189–198.

Fray PJ, Robbins TW, and Sahakian BJ (1996). Neuropsychiatric applications of CANTAB. *International Journal of Geriatric Psychiatry* **11**: 329–336.

Frydenberg H (1988). Computers: Specialised applications for the older person. *American Behavioral Science* **31**: 595–600.

Gedye JL (1967). A teaching machine programme for use as a test of learning ability. In Unwin D and Leedham J (eds.), *Aspects of Educational Technology.* London: Methuin: 369–389.

Hull C (1924). The influence of tobacco smoking on mental and motor efficiency. *Psychological Monographs.*

Ivnik RJ, Malec JF, Tangalos EG, and Crook TH (1996). Older persons reactions to computerized testing versus traditional testing by psychometrists. *ClinicalNeuropsychologist* **10**: 149–151.

Legg SM and Buhr DC (1992). Computerized adaptive testing with different groups. *Educational Measurement Issues and Practice* **11**: 23–27.

Mattis S (1989). *Dementia Rating Scale.* Odessa, FL. Psychological Assessment Resources.

Mohr E, Walker D, Randolph C, Sampson M, and Mendis T (1996). The utility of clinical trial batteries in the measurement of Alzheimer's and Huntington's dementia. *International Psychogeriatrics* **3**: 397–411.

Morris RG, Evenden JL, Sahakian BJ, and Robbins TW (1987). Computer-aided assessment of dementia: comparative studies of neuropsychological deficits in Alzheimer-type dementia and Parkinson's disease. In Stahl SM, Iversen SD, and Goodman EC (Eds). Cognitive Neurochemistry. Oxford University Press, Oxford.

Nicholl CG, Lynch S, Kelly CA, White L, Simpson PM, Wesnes K, and Pitt BMN (1995). The cognitive drug research computerised assessment system in the evaluation of early dementia—is speed of the essence? *International Journal of Geriatric Psychiatry* **10**: 199–206.

Ritchie K, Ledésert B, and Touchon J. (1993). The Eugeria study of cognitive aging: Who are the 'normal' elderly? *International Journal of Geriatric Psychiatry* **8**: 969–977.

Robbins TW, James M, Qwen AM, Sahakian BJ, McInnes L, and Rabbitt P (1994). Cambridge neuropsychological test automated battery (CANTAB)—A factor-analytic study of a large-sample of normal elderly volunteers. *Dementia* **5**: 266–281.

Rosen WG, Mohs RC, and Davis KL (1984). A new rating scale for Alzheimer's disease. *American Journal of Psychiatry* **141**: 1356–1364.

Rosvold HE, Mirsky AF, Sarason BE, Bransome BE, and Beck LH, (1956) A continuous performance test of brain damage. *Journal of Consulting Psychology* **20**: 343–350.

Sahakian BJ, Morris RG, Evenden JL, Heald A, Levy R, Philpot M, and Robbins TW (1988). A comparative study of visuospatial memory and learning in Alzheimer type dementia and Parkinson's disease. *Brain* **111**: 695–718.

Simpson PM, Surmon DJ, Wesnes KA, and Wilcock GR (1991). The cognitive drug research computerised assessment system for demented patients: A validation study. *International Journal of Geriatric Psychiatry* **6**: 95–102.

Warburton DM and Wesnes K (1984). Drugs as research tools in psychology: Cholinergic drugs and information processing. *Neuropsychobiology* **11**: 121–132.

Wechsler D (1987). Wechsler Memory Scale—Revised. Psychological Corporation, New York.

Wesnes K (1977). The effects of psychotropic drugs on human behaviour. *Modern Problems of Pharmacopsychiatry* **12**: 37–58.

Wesnes K and Warburton DM (1983). Nicotine, smoking and human performance. *Pharmacology and Therapeutics* **21**: 189–208.

Wesnes K, Simpson PM, and Christmas L (1987). The assessment of human information processing abilities in psychopharmacology. In: Hindmarch I and Stonier PD (Eds.) Human Psychopharmacology: Measures and Methods Volume I. Chichester, Wiley, pp. 79–92

Youngjohn JR, Larrabee GJ, and Crook TH (1992a). Test-retest reliability of computerized, everyday memory measures and traditional memory tests. *ClinicalNeuropsychologist* **6**: 276–286.

Youngjohn JR, Larrabee GJ, and Crook TH (1992b). Discriminating age-associated memory impairment from Alzheimer's disease. *Psychological Assessment* **4**: 54–59.

9 The role of the speech and language therapist

Susan Stevens and Danielle Ripich

Introduction

Communication, defined as the sharing or imparting of information, is integral to the process of building and maintaining relationships. It can be verbal or non-verbal, and is often a combination of the two. Effective communication depends on shared language and semantic (knowledge) memory, adequate physical skills, and a common code of behaviour, including body language and gestures. Language as a cognitive function underpins many other aspects of cognition, including memory. Any breakdown in language is likely to affect both other cognitive skills and the ability to test those skills.

The four main components of language function are pragmatics (behaviour associated with communication, such as turn taking and appropriateness), semantics (meaning of words), syntax (grammatical structures), and phonology (sound system). All of these can be divided into functions of understanding and execution or expression. Within each area are more detailed divisions which can provide differential diagnostic information.

An individual's communication behaviour is influenced by a number of other considerations and/or skills. These relate principally to:

- educational background and literacy;
- first language and culture;
- sensory deficits, especially hearing;
- psychological state;
- communication requirements.

Background to language assessment

Development

Over the past 10 to 15 years, language research in early dementia, especially Alzheimer type, has concentrated on semantic breakdown. Performance on tasks such as confrontation naming (naming pictures) or word fluency (the listing of as many items as possible in a given category, in a limited period of time) provides information about early signs of cognitive deterioration (Hart *et al.* 1988; Stevens *et al.* 1992). These tasks relate closely to one of the most common early symptoms in individuals suffering from dementia—not being able to recall names, especially of people and places.

The focus of language assessment has extended to include a functional pragmatic perspective (Bates and MacWhinney 1979; Bayles and Kaszniak 1987; Terrell and Ripich 1989). Communication competence is regarded as more cogent than linguistic competence. Thus, pragmatics is viewed as central to communication assessment.

Heterogeneity

Whilst Alzheimer's disease is known to be heterogeneous in its age of onset, rate of decline, and patterns of loss of nervous and cerebral functions, there is marked variation in language function. For example Civil *et al.* (1993) have identified four main subgroups of dementia of Alzheimer type: benign, myoclonic, extrapyramidal, and typical. Although no two individuals present with exactly the same pattern of language breakdown, the most common sequence is shown in Fig. 9.1.

Although it may not be commonplace to find a speech and language

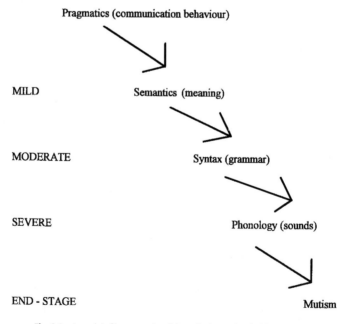

Fig. 9.1 A model of language breakdown in dementia of Alzheimer type.

therapist in a memory clinic or community team, assessment of communicative function provides valuable diagnostic information (Stevens *et al.* 1996), as well as being the basis for advice about strategies to maximize function and reduce related stress and anxiety (Ripich and Ziol, 1997).

Differential diagnosis

Because of difficulty in controlling many factors affecting the use of language in older adults, research into language function in normal elderly people has been limited. Bayles and Kaszniak (1987) produced a seminal work, which provided the basis for a standardized assessment battery, the Arizona Battery for Communication Disorders of Dementia (ABCD) (Bayles and Tomoeda 1993). In the United Kingdom, recent publication of a detailed analysis of language used by a group of elderly people has also informed debate (Maxim and Bryan 1994). These, and other more focused work, such as Van Gorp's on normal older adults' performance on the Boston Naming Test (Van Gorp *et al.* 1986) and Hart's work on Word Fluency (Hart *et al.* 1988), have provided a framework for comparison between normal and abnormal ageing. This is important when it comes to the diagnosis of language breakdown in early dementia.

Age-associated memory impairment

To date, the relationship of language function to the concept of age-associated memory impairment remains unclear. Indeed whether age-associated memory impairment is a precursor of pathology or a normal ageing process is a diagnostic question to which language assessment may contribute (Babakian *et al.* 1990; see also Chapter 13).

Alzheimer's and vascular dementia

Clinical diagnosis between dementia of Alzheimer type (DAT) and vascular dementia can be aided by assessment of the pattern and degree of language breakdown. Kontiola *et al.* (1990) found articulation, reading, and writing deficits and impaired speed of response in vascular dementia. However, as the tests used were not specified, comparisons with work relating to DAT are difficult. Stevens *et al.* (1996) found that those with vascular dementia had better understanding of sentences requiring inferences to be made than those with probable DAT. They took longer to carry out a reading comprehension task, possibly indicating a greater degree of insight or differences in the processing of the written word.

Progressive focal atrophy, Pick's disease, and frontal lobe dementia

Detailed documentation of patterns of language breakdown in individuals diagnosed as having semantic dementia (Hodges *et al.* 1992) or primary progressive aphasia (Poeck and Luzzatti 1988) has facilitated diagnosis in individuals whose language breakdown is comparatively greater than the breakdown in other cognitive functions. Those with a putative diagnosis of semantic dementia have a significantly greater deficit in language performance than in other areas of cognition. Some learning ability has been demonstrated in the early stages of the disease, together with intact procedural and other memory functions, insight, and personality (Hodges *et al.* 1992). The language deficit of semantic dementia is that of a fluent dysphasia characterized by severe anomia, reduced vocabulary, impaired single-word comprehension, but preserved comprehension of complex commands, syntax, and phonology. The impaired single-word comprehension indicates a breakdown in access to semantic memory.

Although there has been some delineation of language function in Pick's disease (Graf-Radford *et al.* 1990; Hodges and Gurd 1994) much of the knowledge gained has been too generalized to be of use to the clinical therapist. However, the disease is often characterized by non-fluent speech with a decrease in spontaneous output, differentiating it from the fluent speech and preserved quantity of output in DAT. Dysnomia and reading comprehension deficits are present in both pathologies. Ripich and Ziol (in press) have recently detailed language deficits in Pick's disease and frontal lobe type dementia.

The delineation of semantic and other language deficits in frontal lobe dementia is in its early stages, with diagnosis tending to be made at present on the basis of behavioural features (see Chapter 15). Language assessment may be highly informative in diagnosis however.

Dementia and depression

Another diagnostic problem is that of dementia and depression. Language assessment in depression has tended to concentrate on negative content and speed of response (Emery and Breslau 1989), both rarely assessed in those with probable DAT. Dessonville Hill *et al.* (1992) compared naming performance in the two groups, while Stevens *et al.* (1992, 1996) found that although there may be a slight reduction in the semantic language scores of those with depression compared to normal elderly individuals, scores are very much within normal ranges. Comparison with those with probable DAT shows clear-cut differences. The fact that a group with depression may include those with (1) reactive depression; (2) depression as an initial presenting sign of DAT; and (3) dysphoria, complicates the diagnostic picture. Reassessment over time may serve to confirm the original diagnosis; the patient with dementia showing deterioration in performance, while performance in depression is static or shows improvement.

Dementia and aphasia

A therapist's skills are of value when diagnosis between dementia and aphasia (Obler and Albert 1985) is in question. If the history is clear, diagnosis may be relatively uncomplicated but often there is no neurological examination at the time of onset or signs are absent, unrecorded, or very discrete. The type of errors seen on a confrontation naming test may differ markedly (Stevens 1989) with visual misinterpretation and semantic paraphasic errors being made by those with DAT, and word finding, circumlocution, and phonological errors by those with aphasia. The latter are more likely to use appropriate gesture to supplement responses. The diagnosis is important because aphasia may respond to appropriate treatment. Lack of early assessment and management can lead to anxiety and reduction of communicative function. However the language breakdown may be a sign of (1) primary progressive aphasia; (2) vascular dementia; or (3) a coexisting disorder (Ripich 1991). Other differential diagnostic differences are explored in Chapters 4, 14, and 15.

Assessment

Assessment provides a baseline for longitudinal review, a process which can confirm or refute the original diagnosis as well as providing the basis for optimum management. The course of different types of dementia grouped as Alzheimer's, let alone other pathologies, is varied (Becker *et al.* 1988).

Language assessment can be carried out in a hospital or community clinic setting, or a domiciliary environment. The extent of assessment will depend on the team's remit and philosophy. In the United States, some memory disorders services offer three-day, multidisciplinary assessment programmes, while in the United Kingdom individuals are seen over the period of a day at maximum, usually in a clinic, but sometimes as an outreach community service. Obviously the greater the amount of time available the more extensive and detailed can be the assessment. This is highly desirable for research purposes, but for most clinical services the additional information would not necessarily alter therapists' management and advice.

Although the focus of testing is likely to be on pragmatics and semantic language function, other assessments will provide pertinent information for differential diagnosis, advice, and review over time. The assessments selected depend on:

- severity of pathology;
- which other disciplines form part of the team (i.e. psychologist);
- focus of the clinic (i.e. assessment only, research, ongoing support);
- test availability (country and language of origin);

- patient's language/ educational background;
- the patient's tolerance of testing;
- site of testing (computerized testing may not be possible in all community settings).

Table 9.1 provides an overview of standardized assessments available. Most were designed for use with aphasic patients but have been, or are being, used with individuals with dementia (the definition of aphasia being an acutely acquired deficit in the ability to use language). As a result the validity of such tests may be questionable when used with individuals with dementia, and it is therefore important for therapists to evaluate performance qualitatively as well as quantitatively. When testing individuals with a possible dementia, it is important to use assessment to identify the process that is breaking down, rather than to attach an inappropriate label to the symptoms. The debate

Table 9.1 Standardized language and communication assessment measures

Level	Behaviour	Measure
I. Comprehensive	Receptive and expressive Oral and written language	*Arizona Battery for Communication Disorders of Dementia (Bayles and Tomoeda, 1993) Boston Diagnostic Aphasia Examination (Goodglass and Kaplan, 1983) Western Aphasia Battery (Kertesz, 1982)
II. Pragmatics and discourse	1. Schemata 2. Turn taking 3. Topic management 4. Conversational repair 5. Speech act use 6. Paralinguistic 7. Non-linguistic 8. Cohesion and coherence	*Discourse Abilities Profile (Terrell and Ripich, 1989)
III. Semantics	Lexical comprehension Confrontation naming Word fluency	Peabody Picture Vocabulary Test—Revised (Dunn and Dunn, 1981) Boston Naming Test (Kaplan et al., 1983) FAS Word Fluency Measure (Borkowski et al., 1967)
IV. Syntax	Sentence comprehension Sentence formulation	Shortened Token Test (DeRenzi and Faglioni, 1978) Reporter's Test (DeRenzi and Ferrari, 1978)
V. Phonology	Word production	Boston Diagnostic Aphasia Examination (Subtest III) (Goodglass and Kaplan, 1983)

*designed specifically for patients with dementia.

about whether the language breakdown in dementia is, or should be called, aphasia is on-going.

Comprehensive language tests

The recent standardization of the Arizona Battery for Communication Disorders of Dementia (ABCD) (Bayles and Tomoeda 1993) based on constructs of mental status, episodic memory, linguistic expression and competence, and visuospatial construction provides an excellent tool for use in the mild and moderate stages of dementia. The Battery takes from 45 minutes to an hour and a half to administer in its entirety, depending on fatigue and the number of subtests carried out.

In 1986, the therapist in the Hammersmith Hospital Memory Clinic, London, compiled an assessment battery taking about an hour to administer, covering many of the same fields as the ABCD. Although not standardized, the subtests are described in some detail in Stevens *et al.* (1996). Table 9.2 summarizes the breakdown of tests under construct headings.

The assessment of other cognitive functions is detailed in Chapter 7.

Pragmatics and discourse

The importance of pragmatics and discourse is their close relationship to functional communication, a skill most vulnerable to cognitive dissolution.

Table 9.2 Hammersmith memory clinic test battery

Construct	Subtest
Episodic memory	Story Retelling—Immediate
	Story Retelling—Delayed
	Word Learning—Free Recall
	Word Learning—Total Recall
	Word Learning—Recognition
Linguistic expression	Word Fluency—semantic
	Word Fluency—phonemic
	Written Picture—description
	Dictation Homophone Pairs
	What's Wrong—explanation
	Sentence Disambiguation—oral
	Confrontation Naming
Linguistic comprehension	Comparative Questions
	Paragraph Reading—factual
	Paragraph Reading—inferential
Visuospatial construction	What's Wrong—recognition
	Sentence Disambiguation—non-oral
	Unusual Angle Photographs

The Discourse Abilities Profile (DAP) (Terrell and Ripich 1989) assesses narrative discourse, procedural discourse, and spontaneous conversation. An example of narrative discourse would be, 'Tell me something that happened to you when you were growing up'. Performance relating to discourse features, information giving and turn taking, topic, and conversational repair skills, is rated, together with the type of speech acts used. It provides a useful basis for structuring interactions between therapist and patient, and/or patient and their partner or carer. Administration takes about 10 to 15 minutes and can be undertaken by trained health professionals as well as therapists. Although not standardized, it is helpful in differentiating normal and abnormal ageing.

Performance on the DAP demonstrated differences between groups of normal elderly people and those with early/ middle stage DAT. Narrative discourse was the most difficult activity for both groups who found the grammatical and hierarchic structures of the story hard to generate. The DAT group showed incomplete structure and poor narrative task performance. Conversation skills were more similar between the groups, perhaps because conversation involves a dialogue between two individuals—the second speaker's responses might have guided the subject's own contributions. Telling a narrative requires the subject to speak in a monologue which may have represented a more difficult task.

Semantics

Naming difficulty is one of the early features reported consistently by patients and their carers, who often comment on difficulty recalling names of people and places. Assessment of confrontation naming using the Boston Naming Test (Kaplan *et al.* 1983) can indicate deficits at a very early stage of cognitive decline (Stevens *et al.* 1992). Sometimes preceding deficits demonstrable on general cognitive measures.

Confrontation naming deficits can be due to problems accessing the semantic lexicon, or to the disappearance of words from the lexicon. Chenery's work (1996) indicates progressive decline, initially characterized by difficulty accessing words and then progressing to disappearance of words. A confrontation naming test may provide other significant diagnostic evidence when errors are categorized as semantic, phonemic, visual, or perhaps unrelated. Semantic errors can be further classified as paraphasias, generic category names, and perseverative responses. Error types give useful information concerning the type and extent of pathology. The type of circumlocution used is also informative; for example if the required word is 'chair', 'You sit on it' will be a targeted error, while 'That looks comfortable' would be tangential.

Semantic word fluency (or generative naming, commonly generating names of 'animals') is used in a number of tests; for example the Boston Diagnostic Aphasia Examination (Goodglass and Kaplan 1983) and Cambridge

Cognitive Examination CAMCOG (Roth *et al.* 1986). This timed task, taking one minute, requires no equipment and can be used with patients with sensory deficits. Work in the Hammersmith Clinic found considerable overlap between the scoring ranges of normal older adults and those with early DAT and vascular dementia. The generation of town and city names ('towns') appears to be a more sensitive measure in diagnostic terms (Hart *et al.* 1988; Stevens *et al.* 1996).

Other semantic tasks give useful information about early deterioration. Object Description tests the ability to provide factual information, while Concept Definition is helpful in assessing the amount of semantic information an individual can access. Note must always be taken of the possible effect of educational and cultural background on performance.

Writing tasks appear sensitive to early cognitive change. The Homophone Pairs Dictation task (see Table 9.2) focuses on the ability to use semantic knowledge to inform spelling performance, for example 'monk/nun : nothing/none' (Kempler 1987). Written Picture Description, whilst being more time efficient than oral description, provides information about discourse cohesion, inference, visuospatial, and semantic skills, as well as a base line for monitoring orthographic changes. These are often marked, and without any obvious physical pathology to account for them. An example of change in writing performance over time is shown in Box 9.1.

A What's Wrong test designed for the Hammersmith Clinic requires:

(1) recognition of a visual error in a simple coloured picture;

(2) meaningful description of that error.

It provides information about visuospatial and semantic skills, as does a Sentence Disambiguation (non-oral) task, where different pictorial interpretations of a sentence have to be identified; for example 'The duck is ready to eat'. All these tasks test expressive function, the breakdown of which usually precedes that of comprehension in dementia. Complex commands and comparative questions, both presented verbally, may detect some deficits but not often in early dementia.

Reading comprehension can also show early change. Many patients report a decline in both the amount and enjoyment of reading, with no obvious cause such as reduced visual acuity. Oral reading tends to remain intact until a moderate to severe stage of the disease (O'Carroll 1995), but the ability to make inferences from written text or retain such information may deteriorate early (Stevens *et al.* 1996).

None of these tests take more than ten minutes to administer.

Syntax and phonology

Both syntax and phonology are relatively well preserved in early dementia, although it is possible that those with vascular dementia may present with

---

Box 9.1 Written picture description

Patient: 83-year-old woman with possible mixed Alzheimer and vascular
           pathology.
The picture described is that of a family preparing to go on holiday.
The patient's written description of the picture is as follows:

At time 1

PACKING SUITCASE
GIRL WITH BUCKET AND SPADE
BOY WITH TWO SUIT CASES
CAR IN GARAGE
>   NB : Written in capitals
>   Phrase structure (mean length 3–5 words)
>   14 information units

At time 2   (13 months later)

CAR
WOMAN
CHILD
BOY
HANDBAG
COMB
DRAWER
CLOTHES-BRUSH
DRESSING TABLE
>   NB: Written in capitals (smaller than Time 1)
>   Single words (1 word units)
>   9 information units
>   Possible visual misinterpretation

---

such deficits (Powell *et al.* 1988). Syntactic comprehension can be assessed with the Sentence and Paragraph Comprehension subtests of the Boston Diagnostic Aphasia Examination (Goodglass and Kaplan 1983), The Reporters' Test (De Renzi and Ferrari 1978), or the shortened Token Test (De Renzi and Faglioni 1978). Written Picture Description will provide information about the ability to formulate correctly structured sentences. In early dementia it may be the complexity rather than the correctness of the structure which changes. Phonology can be assessed in the context of most of the expressive semantic tests, while the easy and quick to administer FAS fluency measure (Borkowski *et al.* 1967; Stevens *et al.* 1996) gives information about the phonological access route to the semantic lexicon.

Management

The role of the hospital, clinic, or community speech and language therapist in an integrated, multidisciplinary team is multifaceted. He/she participates collaboratively in identification and assessment of impairments, management intervention, and education. All should be updated in the light of continuing research. A full language assessment may take 90 minutes to 2 hours. Sessions of 1 hour to 90 minutes are optimal to avoid the influence of fatigue.

Options

Three management options are commonly considered. The first is to provide the patient, and if appropriate his/her carer(s), with information about the assessment findings. Clear delineation of the communication skills and deficits of an individual allows appropriate strategies to be discussed and tried with both the individual and those most concerned in his/her communication. Education and support can prevent anxiety and embarrassment about communication and help maximize function. The maintenance of adequate communication for as long as possible improves the quality of life and enhances satisfaction (Ripich 1994; Clark and Witte 1990). For example if an individual's naming difficulty is due to impaired vocabulary access, semantic and/or phonemic cueing may help. Encouragement in using compensatory strategies such as gestures and circumlocution can alleviate communication blocks.

While the management of distressing or antisocial behaviour in dementia has received attention, little has been written about the stressful aspects of communication breakdown. The Hammersmith Clinic produced two leaflets, one explaining the type of problems experienced in early dementia, the other advising about communication with those more severely impaired. Another useful booklet with pertinent cartoon drawings available in the United Kingdom is by Tanton (1993), while in the United States, the Alzheimer's Communication Guide, discussed in detail later, is a much more extensive information (and teaching) package for carers.

Secondly, a therapist may carry out a targeted course of intervention, perhaps when the diagnosis between language breakdown due to dementia and dysphasia (an acutely acquired language deficit due to neurological pathology) is unclear. If the problem is dysphasia the deficits may improve after therapy. Stress may also be reduced. In addition, a course of therapy provides the opportunity to get to know the patient better, facilitating more informed judgements about other cognitive skills such as memory and insight.

Thirdly, when functional communication between patient and carer, probably spouse or child, is markedly worse than the impairment warrants, intervention by a therapist may be helpful. An advantage of domiciliary visits is that social interactions can be observed, and therefore advice more accurately targeted. Outcome is often difficult to measure but anecdotally it is acknowledged as beneficial, with improved quality of life.

Whatever the intervention, reassessment within an agreed time frame is necessary and is a useful way of:

♦ confirming/ questioning the original (putative) diagnosis;
♦ updating information regarding change and the maintenance of competence;
♦ examining the focus of intervention and structure of case management;
♦ collecting longitudinal data on a variety of pathologies.

The following case histories illustrate some of these roles.

Case History 1

Mr C   **Dementia/aphasia**

Background information

An 88-year-old retired army officer, married. An 8-year history of cognitive decline and hearing loss in both ears.

Initial assessment

Mini Mental State Examination (max. 30) (Folstein *et al.* 1975)	24
Ravens Coloured Progressive Matrices (max. 36) (Raven 1956)	23 (Grade II)
Boston Naming Test (max. 60) (Kaplan *et al.* 1983)	9
Word Fluency (Towns) (Hart *et al.* 1988)	3
Story Retelling—immediate (max. 25) (Bayles and Tomoeda 1993)	12
Boston Diagnostic Aphasia Examination (Goodglass and Kaplan 1983)	
Comprehension (Complex Ideational Material) (max. 10)	7
Word Reading (max. 30)	29
Reading Sentences/Paragraphs (max. 10)	7
Responsive Naming (max. 30)	21

Although deficits were evident in general cognitive and some language tasks, performance was patchy with marked difficulty in confrontation naming. A hearing loss may have influenced some performance, but this would not apply to a confrontation naming task. Language performance showed some semantic breakdown, minor syntactic problems, and no phonological deficits.

The hypothesis was that the original presentation may have been an acute onset mild aphasia, although the history was unclear. His wife's impatience with Mr C's word-finding problems, together with increasing hearing loss, had caused a breakdown in their communication efficiency.

Treatment plan

♦ therapy sessions targeted at semantic language tasks;
♦ explanation of problems to Mr and Mrs C.;
♦ support for Mrs C. with suggested strategies.

Progress after three months

Boston Naming Test	20
Word Fluency (Towns)	8
Story Retelling (max. 25)	14

Some improvement was evident in semantic access, although it was still limited, while recall was marginally improved. Mr C was less distressed and handicapped by his impairments. He spoke fluently on the telephone and decided not to attend for further therapy.

Conclusion

The hypothesis of an original presentation of aphasia seemed probable. Lack of support originally may have created anxiety, while hearing loss and possibly increasing general cognitive impairment had led to communicative dysfunction greater than seemed warranted. Mr C. learnt to maximize skill, resulting in reduced stress for both him and his wife.

Case History 2

Mrs V   **Progressive aphasia**

Background information

A 70-year-old, right handed former college graduate, married, travelled extensively. Family history of memory problems (father had probable Alzheimer's disease, mother had possible Parkinson's disease). Active; shops, cooks, drives, keeps house, does banking, target shoots, fox hunts. Gradual, deteriorating language skills over 18months.

Neuropsychological evaluation suggested above average intelligence with no evidence of cognitive impairment in memory, executive function, perceptual, or abstract reasoning. An MRI scan showed mild parenchymal volume loss with focal parenchymal loss in the left frontal region (Broca's area).

Initial Assessment

Mini Mental State Examination (max. 30) (Folstein *et al.* 1975)	29
Boston Naming Test (max. 60) (Kaplan *et al.* 1983))	57
Word Fluency (Animals) (Hart *et al.* 1988)	22
Peabody Picture Vocabulary Test (max. 175) (Dunn and Dunn 1981)	167
Token Test (max. 78) (De Renzi and Faglioni 1978)	55
Boston Diagnostic Aphasia Examination (Goodglass and Kaplan 1983)	
Comprehension (Complex Ideational Material) (max. 10)	9
Sentence Reading (max. 10)	8
Sentence Repetition (max. 16)	14
Reading Comprehension (max. 10)	8

Breakdown was most evident in discourse as assessed in the DAP and a picture description task. Mrs V. was non-fluent with numerous hesitations and mazes (restarts, fillers, repairs). Language was telegraphic with omission of function words and with syntactic errors. A mild verbal apraxia was noted. Speech was monotonic, slow, and dysprosodic (impairment of rhythm and timing). Initiation was reduced and she was unable to expand or continue topics. Multidisciplinary assessment resulted in a diagnosis of progressive aphasia.

Treatment plan

♦ information about the disorder;

♦ to maintain communication skills as long as possible;

♦ counselling for Mrs V. and family;

♦ strategies to facilitate continued involvement in communication e.g. notebook in which 'cue' questions were noted to keep her socially involved;

♦ subscription to more visually-orientated magazines;

♦ drug intervention.

Progress and Treatment

Although cognitive testing showed minimal changes over two years, Mrs V's language deteriorated from mild to moderately-severe progressive aphasia. Motor speech became more impaired; discourse was agrammatic. Output was limited to single words which were frequently unintelligible. Compensatory strategies such as gestures, drawing, writing, use of the environment, and a communication notebook were presented in structured tasks. Alternative communication modalities and family education became more important as language deteriorated. Mr V. participated in several sessions for training as a communication partner. Although Mrs V. agreed that these options were helpful, she rarely used them spontaneously. She declined attending group sessions to practice strategies.

Conclusion

The primary role for the therapist was: to provide the team, patient, and family with information and support; to help maintain speech skills for as long as possible; to identify communication strengths; and to train in alternative modalities for communication.

Training

The teaching role for therapists provides an opportunity to highlight the importance of communication in the assessment and management of those with dementia. Arguably, it is the responsibility of professionals involved in the care of individuals with dementia to communicate as effectively as possible. For example using complex sentences which confuse a patient when discussing management may be unethical, when he/she could follow a discussion if simpler constructions were used. This places the bulk of the communication burden on the professional—the more competent communicator.

Training professionals and family carers in communication strategies could enhance quality of life for those with dementia, reducing frustration and improving competence in the delivery of care. Those who give 'front line' care can benefit from improved communication with their patients. Having strategies and techniques for dealing with communication would reduce the stress and burden experienced by carers. To improve communication for persons with dementia, Ripich and Wykle (1996) developed the Alzheimer's Disease Communication Guide: The FOCUSED Program for Caregivers.

The acronym FOCUSED identifies key techniques for communication maintenance. Based on an interactive discourse model for conversational exchanges (Terrell and Ripich 1989), the programme emphasizes seven strategies (F-face to face, O-orient to topic of conversation, C-continue the topic of conversation, U-unstick communication blocks, S-structure questions, E-exchange conversation, and D-direct, short sentences). The trainer's manual is divided into six modules and presents information about the characteristics, pathology, and stages of Alzheimer's disease, language components and processes, memory and ageing, depression, importance of communication, and how to use the communication strategies at each stage. An optional module for professional caregivers discusses cultural differences in caregiving and in the workplace. The programme can be presented over several sessions and includes role-play, discussion, and home assignments. Efficacy has been demonstrated with increased knowledge about Alzheimer's disease, improved attitude, and decreased stress and burden for professional and family carers (Ripich 1994; Ripich et al., in press).

Allowing other professionals to observe the therapist at work is another form of training. It is often a revelation to other professionals that someone who can apparently converse without great difficulty has such marked breakdown when it comes to specific types of language tasks.

Research

Many aspects of assessment and management of communication in dementia are, as yet, unknown. Twenty five years ago it was acceptable to compare a group of people with 'dementia' to those with dysphasia (Rochford 1971). Subsequently those with probable DAT were classified separately from those with multi-infarct or vascular dementia, while more recently other pathologies have been identified, such as semantic dementia (Hodges et al., 1992), which may or may not be a subgroup of Alzheimer's or Pick's disease. The increased availability of neuroimaging now provides opportunities for correlation with communication assessment, as well as contributing towards more precise diagnosis.

Because of the difficulties of controlling for all variables, group studies can be problematical, with relatively few 'clean' patients being available. Many papers report on groups of less than 20. But these studies are important, because over time cumulative trends become evident. Similarly, single case studies, although dismissed by some researchers, contribute towards meaningful bodies of data (Graf-Radford et al. 1990; Hodges and Gurd, 1994). They are particularly important as rarer pathologies are seen only occasionally, even in specialist clinics, and newer statistical techniques are being developed which make analysis of single cases more meaningful (see e.g. Diaconis and Efron, 1983).

Memory clinics or assessment teams may provide patients with access to research projects, or be undertaking research themselves. A specialized clinic is likely to be the only site of service provision where speech and language therapists have access to those with early cognitive impairment, which is particularly important for research, especially with new classes of drugs becoming available. Longitudinal studies (Chenery 1996), single case studies (Funnell 1992), and group studies comparing normal and abnormal ageing all depend on diagnosis early in the disease process.

Practical problems relate to time and funding. If a team is funded by research moneys, or as part of a research institution, neither may be difficult to solve, and may indeed be part of the employment remit. However, if the clinic or service has a clinical focus only and therefore relies on service contracts, research is unlikely to be part of the therapist's remit. Separate funding for research will need to be sought. It is still possible, however, to gather information on interesting cases, provided the standards of documentation are high enough.

Issues for present and the future

Communication is important in the diagnosis and management of dementia. It is often the area carers find most difficult to cope with, as its breakdown affects relationships. As the elderly population grows, so will the numbers with dementia. Whether it will be a priority, or even a part of speech and language therapy service provision, will depend on future health care purchasers. It may, therefore, be that work in this field will be research led; the research route being the only one through which funding can be obtained, and the effectiveness of such therapy demonstrated.

The focus of speech and language therapy in memory disorders teams is likely to remain assessment of semantic and pragmatic aspects of speech, as these are the areas most vulnerable to early cognitive change in dementia. The production of more standardized and refined tests specifically designed for, and validated with, people with dementia will improve diagnostic accuracy. The challenge to therapists working in community teams will be to select the most sensitive assessment tools for the type and severity of difficulties experienced by the individuals referred to them.

The increasing number of elderly people belonging to ethnic minorities within their countries who develop dementia will produce new challenges (see also Chapters 7 and 10). Does the rate and manner in which a second language breakdown differ from that of the first language? Is the pragmatic or semantic aspect of that breakdown the most obvious? What difference does the cultural bias of tests make to assessment findings (Worrall *et al.* 1995; Ripich *et al.*, 1997)? Other cultural issues, such as attitudes to care, may also be important (Brownlie 1991).

The philosophy and scope of the multidisciplinary team will dictate whether there is a therapist, and whether he/she only assesses or is also involved in targeted therapy and/or group work. Some therapists work with reminiscence, memory, or communication groups (Bender *et al*. 1987; Feil 1982). Involvement may be dictated by the availability and interests of other staff, for example psychologists or nurses, with the therapist feeling it appropriate to have an assessment and reassessment and/or planning role only.

Finally, ethical issues in the treatment of persons with dementia are a critical consideration. Quality of life and quality health care are rights of every individual, including those suffering from dementia. The components of quality of life include physical, mental, and spiritual health; cognitive ability; family and social relations; work and hobby activities; economic success and subjective well-being (Whitehouse and Rabins 1992). Social interaction and continuing interpersonal relations have been closely linked to quality of life (Larson 1978; Ishi-Kuntz 1990) and are affected by behavioural approaches to the treatment of dementia. Innovative and flexible management should address these quality of life issues.

Conclusion

It is important for therapists and other health care professionals to continue the shift from a more traditional medical model based on assessing pathology and restoring function, to a more holistic model based on maintaining function and preventing excessive response to disability (Clark 1995). There is a need for increasing involvement of the speech and language therapist in the assessment and management of persons with DAT and related disorders, helping to maintain functional communication for as long as possible, and improving both quality of life and quality of care (ASHA 1988).

Although the numbers of therapists available to work in this field may be relatively few, the specialist skills and knowledge in communication of a speech and language therapist may contribute towards more informed diagnosis, management, and training for professional and family carers.

Communication breakdown is one of the main areas of cognition causing distress to all concerned (Kinney and Stephens 1989). Developing communication skills of other professionals and carers can enhance the quality of life for the person with dementia. It is important for those who care for this increasing population to have adequate training to communicate with them effectively. The goal of quality caregiving, therefore, should clearly be to prolong and promote communication for as long as possible at the highest level possible. Professionals working with persons with dementia need to meet the challenge through teaching, research, and expanded clinical services to serve the complex needs of these individuals.

Acknowledgement

This manuscript was supported in part by the National Institutes of Health/National Institute on Aging (United States). Grant # AG-08012.

References

Key references recommended by the authors are marked with an *.

ASHA Committee on Communication Problems in Aging (1988). The roles of speech-language pathologists and audiologists in working with older persons. *ASHA*, **30**, 80–84.

Babakian VL, Wolfe N, Linn R, Knoefel JE and Albert ML (1990). Pattern of language impairment is different in Alzheimer's disease and multi-infarct dementia. *Brain and Language*, **38**, 364–383.

Bates E and MacWhinney B (1979). A functional approach to the acquisition of grammar. In Ochs S and Schiefflin B (eds.), *Developmental pragmatics*. Academic Press, New York.

*Bayles KA and Kaszniak AW (1987). *Communication and cognition in normal aging and dementia.* Taylor and Francis, London.

*Bayles KA and Tomoeda CK (1993). *Arizona Battery for Communication Disorders of Dementia.* Canyonlands Inc, Tuscon.

Becker JT, Huff FJ, Nebes RD and Holland A (1988). Neuropsychological function in Alzheimer's disease. *Archives of Neurology*, **45**, 263–268

Bender MP, Norris A and Bauckham P (1987). *Groupwork with the elderly.* Winslow Press, Bicester.

Borkowski JG, Benton AL and Spreen O (1967). Word fluency and brain damage *Neuropsychologia*, **5**, 135–140.

Brownlie J (1991). *A hidden problem? Dementia amongst minority ethnic groups.* Dementia Services Development, University of Stirling, Scotland.

Chenery H (1996). Semantic priming in Alzheimer's dementia. *Aphasiology*, **10,** 1–20.

Civil RH, Whitehouse PJ, Lanska DJ and Mayeux R (1993). The major categories of dementia. In Whitehouse PJ (ed.) *Dementia*. FA Davis Company, Philadelphia.

Clark LW (1995). Interventions for persons with Alzheimer's disease: Strategies for maintaining and enhancing communicative success. *Topics in Language Disorders*, **15**, 47–65.

*Clark LW and Witte K (1990). Nature and efficacy of communication management in Alzheimer's disease. In Lubinski R (ed.) *Dementia and communication*. BC Decker, Philadelphia, pp. 238–56.

De Renzi E and Faglioni P (1978). Normative data and screening power of a shortened version of the token test. *Cortex*, **14**, 41–49.

De Renzi E and Ferrari C (1978). The reporter's test : a sensitive test to detect expressive disturbances in aphasics. *Cortex*, **14**, 279–293.

Dessonville Hill C, Stondemine A, Morris R, Martino-Saltzman D, Markwalter HR and Lewison BJ (1992). Dysnomia in the differential diagnosis of major depression, depression related cognitive dysfunction and dementia. *Journal of Neuropsychiatry and Clinical Neurosciences*, **4**, 64–69.

Diaconis P and Efron B (1983). Computer-intensive methods in statistics. *Scientific American*, **247**, 96–129.

Dunn LM and Dunn LM (1981). *Peabody picture vocabulary test—revised*. American Guidance Service, Circle Pines, MN.

Emery OB and Breslau LD (1989). Language deficits in depression: comparisons with SDAT and normal aging. *Journal of Gerontology*, **44**, 85–92.

Feil N (1982). *Validation : the Feil method*. Edward Feil Productions, Cleveland.

Folstein MF, Folstein SE, and McHugh PR (1975). Mini Mental-State: a practical method for grading the cognitive state of patients for the clinician. *Journal of Psychiatric Research*, **12**, 189–98.

Funnell E (1992). Progressive loss of semantic memory in a case of Alzheimer's disease. *Proceedings of the Royal Society*, **249**, 287–291.

Goodglass H and Kaplan E (1983). *The assessment of aphasia and related disorders* (2nd edn). Lea and Febiger, Philadelphia.

Graf-Radford NR, Damasio AR, Hyman BT, Hart MN, Tranel D, Damasio H, Van Hoesen GW and Rezai K (1990). Progressive aphasia in a patient with Pick's disease : a neuropsychological radiologic and anatomic study. *Neurology*, **40**, 620–626.

Hart S, Smith CM and Swash M (1988). Word fluency in patients with early dementia of Alzheimer type. *British Journal of Clinical Psychology*, **27**, 115–124.

Hodges JR and Gurd JM (1994). Remote memory and lexical retrieval in a case of frontal Pick's disease. *Archives of Neurology*, **51**, 821–827.

*Hodges J, Paterson K, Oxbury S and Funnell E (1992). Semantic dementia : progressive fluent aphasia with temporal lobe atrophy. *Brain*, **115**, 1783–1806.

Ishi-Kuntz M (1990). Social interaction and social well-being. Comparison across stages of adulthood. *Aging and Human Development*, **30**, 15–35.

Kaplan E, Goodglass H and Weintraub S (1983). *Boston Naming Test*. Lea and Febiger, Philadelphia.

Kempler D, Curtis S and Jackson C (1987). Syntactic preservation in Alzheimer's disease. *Journal of Speech and Hearing Research*, **30**, 343–350.

Kertesz A (1982). *Western Aphasia Battery*. Grune and Stratton, New York.

Kinney JM and Stephens MAP (1989). Caregiver hassles scale : assessing the daily hassles of caring for a family member with dementia. *Gerontologist*, **29**, 328–332.

Kontiola P, Laaksonen R, Sulkava R and Erkinjuntti T (1990). Pattern of language impairment is different in Alzheimer's disease and multi-infarct dementia. *Brain and Language*, **38**, 364–383.

Larson R (1978). Thirty years of research on the subjective well-being of older Americans. *Journal of Gerontology*, **33**, 109–125.

*Maxim J and Bryan K (1994). *Language of the elderly*. Whurr, London.

Obler BA and Albert ML (1985). Language in the elderly aphasic and in the dementing patient. In Sarno M (ed.) *Acquired aphasia*. Academic Press, New York.

O'Carroll R (1995). The assessment of premorbid ability: a critical review. *Neurocase*, **1**, 83–89.

Poeck K and Luzzatti C (1988). Slowly progressive aphasia in 3 patients. *Brain*, **111**, 151–168.

Powell AL, Cummings JL, Hill MA and Benson DF (1988). Speech and language alterations in multi-infarct dementia. *Neurology*, **38**, 717–719.

Raven JC (1956). Coloured Progressive Matrices. HK Lewis and Co. Ltd, London.

Ripich DN (1991). Language and communication in dementia. In Ripich DN (ed.) *Handbook of geriatric communication disorders*. PRO ED, Austin.

Ripich DN (1994). Functional communication with AD patients : a caregiver training program. *Alzheimer disease and associated disorders*, **8**, 95–109.

*Ripich DN and Wykle ML (1996). *Alzheimer's disease communication guide: the FOCUSED programme for caregivers*. The Psychological Corporation, San Antonio.

Ripich DN and Ziol E (1997). Dementia : a review for the speech–language pathologist. In Johnson AF and Jacobsen BH (eds) *Medical speech–language pathology*. Theime Medical Publishers, New York.

Ripich DN, Carpenter B and Ziol E (1997). Comparison of African American and white persons with Alzheimer's disease on standardised language tests. *Neurology*, **48**, 781–3.

Ripich DN, Kercher K, Wykle M, Sloan D and Ziol E (in press). Effects of communication training on African American and white caregivers of persons with Alzheimer's disease. *Journal of Aging and Ethnicity*.

Rochford G (1971). A study of naming errors in dysphasic and demented subjects. *Neuropsychologia*, **9**, 437–443.

Roth M, Tym E, Mountjoy CS, Huppert F, Hendrie, H, Verma S and Goddard R (1986). CAMDEX : a standardised instrument for the diagnosis of mental disorder in the elderly with special reference to the early detection of dementia. *British Journal of Psychiatry*, **149**, 698–709.

Stevens SJ (1989). Differential naming difficulties in elderly dysphasic subjects and subjects with senile dementia of Alzheimer type. *British Journal of Disorders of Communication,* **24**, 77–92.

Stevens SJ, Pitt BMN, Nicholl CG, Fletcher AE and Palmer AJ (1992). Language assessment in a memory clinic. *International Journal of Geriatric Psychiatry,* **7**, 45–51.

Stevens SJ, Harvey RJ, Kelly CA, Nicholl CG and Pitt BMN (1996) Characteristics of language performance in 4 groups of patients attending a memory clinic. *International Journal of Geriatric Psychiatry,* **11**, 973–982.

Tanton M (1993). *Helping communication in the person with dementia.* (Published privately) Marsh Publications, Pudsey.

Terrell B and Ripich D (1989). Discourse competence as a variable in intervention. *Seminars in Speech and Language Disorders*, **24**, 77–92.

Van Gorp WG, Satz P, Kiersch ME and Henry R (1986). Normative data on the Boston Naming Test for a group of normal older adults. *Journal of Clinical and Experimental Neurology,* **8**, 702–705.

Whitehouse PJ and Rabins PV (1992). Quality of life and dementia. *Alzheimer's Disease and Associated Disorders,* **6**, 135–137.

Worrall LE, Yiu M-L, Hickson LMH and Barnett HM (1995). Normative data for the Boston Naming Test for Australian elderly. *Aphasiology,* **9**, 541–551.

10 Functional assessment

A. Carswell and R. Spiegel

Introduction

The measurement of function is integral to the assessment and diagnosis of individuals with suspected dementia (Blessed *et al.*, 1968). With the gradual decline in cognitive abilities, there is an accompanying decline in role, social, and physical abilities. Nevertheless, traditional mental status screening tools such as the Mini-mental State Examination (MMSE) (Folstein *et al.*, 1975) which focus on cognitive functions are not suited for monitoring the progression of the everyday manifestations related to cognitive impairment.

Useful and simple instruments for monitoring decline in functional abilities and thus the progression of dementia in all stages of the disease assess the ability of an individual to perform usual everyday tasks. The objective of a functional assessment is to determine the ability of individuals to complete successfully daily living tasks and live in their usual physical, social, and cultural environment.

The when and how for performing functional assessments depends upon the purpose to which the instrument is put, and for which it was developed. Daily living activities are often placed into three categories: activities of daily living (ADL), instrumental activities of daily living (IADL), and mobility related to walking and to managing stairs. ADL and IADL assessments are critical for establishing a diagnosis, monitoring the disease progression, determining the need for health services, and evaluating the efficacy of therapeutic interventions. Existing functional assessment tools differ as to the type of behaviours they assess, the nature of the observations that are made, and the scoring and scaling systems that are used. Therefore, the goal of this chapter is to discuss the appropriate selection and use of functional assessments in the evaluation of patients with dementia. More specifically the objectives are to:

(1) define functional assessment;
(2) discuss why a functional assessment is useful;
(3) identify the types of functional assessments;
(4) define two approaches to collecting information on function;

(5) discuss how to select an instrument for a functional assessment;

(6) present some useful measures;

(7) outline factors which affect a functional assessment;

(8) delineate a process of undertaking a functional assessment.

What is a functional assessment?

Before examining functional assessment in detail, it is relevant to discuss briefly the differences among psychometric screening, neuropsychological assessment, and functional assessment in the context of evaluating people with suspected dementia. Psychometric screening with such instruments as the MMSE, and the Dementia Rating Scale (DRS) (Mattis, 1976) provides an overall quantitative estimate of cognitive impairment. Cognitive impairment screens are fast and easy to perform and give an indication of whether further, more detailed assessments are necessary. Neuropsychological assessments (Lezak, 1996) provide detailed descriptions of specific sensory, motor, and cognitive impairments to explain further how these impairments affect IADL and ADL function, as well as guide more specific rehabilitation. Both psychometric screens and neuropsychological assessments are performed in a highly standardized, partly artificial setting, and comprise only a short observation period—usually less than half an hour.

One model for defining function has as its conceptual framework the WHO classification of impairment, disability, and handicap (WHO 1980). McDowell and Newell (1996) suggested that this model was appropriate to test alterations in functional ability with specific reference to disability and handicap. Disability is defined as 'any restriction or lack (resulting from an impairment) of (the) ability to perform an activity in the manner or within the range considered normal for a human being' (WHO 1980, p.141). Handicap encompasses both social and environmental influences and is defined as 'a disadvantage for a given individual, resulting from an impairment or a disability, that limits or prevents the fulfilment of a role that is normal (depending on age, sex and social and cultural factors) for that individual' (WHO 1980, p.183).

Therefore measures of function should accommodate both handicap and disability. The WHO model motivates the definition of a functional assessment and what items should be included in an instrument. It allows for measuring the deterioration in functional performance that accompanies dementia.

Within the context of this chapter, function is defined as the ability to perform usual, everyday tasks in a usual manner. It includes the ability to perform self-care tasks and to fulfil the social roles of everyday life. A distinction is usually made between two types of function—the ability to perform basic activities of daily living (ADL) such as eating and dressing, and the ability to perform more complex daily activities that allow for greater independence— for example housekeeping, home management, or budgeting. These are often labelled instrumental activities of daily living (IADL). ADL and IADL are two aspects of function thought to be hierarchical with IADL requiring a higher order of functioning than ADL.

ADL are basic activities of self-care and self-maintenance. They typically comprise washing, bathing, dressing, continence, eating, transferring (in and out of bed, on and off the toilet, or in and out of the bath tub/shower), grooming, and looking after one's person. ADL are hierarchical (Katz *et al.* 1963) with more complex activities such as dressing, bathing, and toileting being impaired before less complex activities such as eating or transferring. ADL are usually learned early in childhood, are performed habitually and are relatively free from biases related to culture and education (Loewenstein *et al.*, 1992).

The concept of IADL includes the basic skills reflected in ADL as well as more complex integrative skills that relate to roles adults assume in order to live independently within the community. Shopping, for example, requires being able to get out of bed, to get dressed, to leave the house, and to manage transportation. Additionally, it may involve organizational ability and money management. Because IADL are complex and include social, recreational, and occupational activities that greatly affect the quality of life, they are more likely to be affected by the environment, by social expectations, motivation, and dysfunction than are ADL. IADL are complicated and multifaceted, thus they are also more likely to be affected earlier in the dementia process than ADL (Green *et al.* 1993).

Measures of IADL typically include items such as preparing meals, shopping, managing money, using the telephone, doing light housework, doing heavy housework or household maintenance, managing means of transportation, taking medications reliably, and managing one's finances. IADL are influenced by a person's gender, profession, culture, and educational background to a greater degree than are the basic tasks of everyday living.

IADL also address one of the major concerns of family members of a person with dementia—that of safety inside and outside the home. Knowing whether a sufferer demonstrates appropriate judgement in possible dangerous situations is essential in planning whether, for example, a patient can continue to drive a car or to live at home. On the other hand, while slowing is often observed in mild dementia, measuring physical mobility is less relevant for functional assessment until very late in the progression of the disease and will not be discussed further, except to note that two useful measures are the timed 'Up and Go' test (Podsiadlo and Richardson, 1991) and the Balance Scale (Berg *et al.*, 1995).

In summary, functional assessments focus upon those skills that call upon previous life experiences that are also habitual. They reflect daily life activities and habits, and permit an estimate of independent functioning, usually in order of increasing dependency with some variation across the spectrum of instruments.

Why use a functional assessment?

A significant feature of dementia is functional decline demonstrated by the increasing loss of ability to perform IADL and ADL. A functional assessment enables the clinician to evaluate and consequently to manage the patient with dementia, and to guide caregivers appropriately.

The DSM-IV states that for a diagnosis of dementia to be made 'cognitive deficits in Criteria A1 and A2 (memory, language, praxis, gnosis, executive functions) each cause significant impairment in social and occupational functioning....' (American Psychiatric Association, 1994, p.135). Thus, for clinical practice and for research purposes it is necessary and useful to monitor changes in functional status. For many, the decline of functional ability may be the most problematic aspect of dementia, since the loss of ability to perform IADL, and later on ADL, results in the need for increased levels of assistance and care. Knowing the rate and impact of functional decline is helpful in planning for both the present and future. Functional assessments are also useful in determining the efficacy of treatment and intervention strategies (Carswell and Eastwood, 1993; Loewenstein *et al.*,1989; Patterson *et al.*, 1992; Tappen, 1994).

Neither physical health nor cognitive measures alone describe the degree of independent function. Functional skills combine motor, visual, and other perceptual skills, as well as cognitive competence in their performance, so that the effect of a decline in any *one* of these areas will impinge upon the ability to perform a functional task. A functional assessment that provides a hierarchical estimate of performance points the way to further evaluation of specific underlying perceptual or behavioural mechanisms of function, if this is required.

There are additional reasons for using a functional assessment in addition to other types of assessments. While there are a number of well known and psychometrically robust screening measures of cognitive impairment, there is evidence that their sensitivity and specificity are affected by educational and cultural biases (Kittner *et al.* 1986). Although Fillenbaum and her colleagues (1994) report that four items (day, date, recall of apple, and penny) of the MMSE appear to discriminate patients with mild dementia from normal controls, for the most part, the total scores of cognitive screening tests (such as the MMSE or the DRS) are not sensitive to identifying persons with a cognitive decline in the earlier stages of the disease (Johnston *et al.*, 1995;

Klein *et al.* 1985). Similarly, the CAMCOG, which forms part of the CAMDEX (Roth *et al.* 1986) is reportedly sensitive to early identification of dementia with well distributed total scores and no apparent ceiling effect (Huppert *et al.*, 1995; Lindeboom *et al.*, 1993). In any case, further detailed neuropsychological assessments are necessary to determine the underlying cognitive dysfunction.

Not infrequently, family members observe a decline in their relative's social, recreational, and occupational activities which may signal a decline in cognitive health, even though a simple cognitive screening tool does not indicate impairment. The sensitivity and specificity of cognitive screening tests are enhanced by the addition of IADL and ADL functional measures (Ashford *et al.* 1992; Green *et al.*, 1993; Warren, *et al.* 1989) although not necessarily in the very early stages of the disease (Fisk *et al.*, 1995). In the later stages of dementia, functional assessments are more meaningful tools for assessing the progression of the disease, because the traditional mental status measures and many specific neurological tests 'bottom out' in late stage patients (Auer *et al.*, 1994). In summary, functional assessments can be of particular use at both ends of the dementia severity spectrum where screening tools and neuropsychological assessments may lose their sensitivity, specificity, and applicability.

Declines in cognitive ability have a substantial impact on the capacity for independent living (Jagger, *et al.*, 1993; Roos and Havens, 1993). Several clinical studies have established that, as cognitive impairment increased, the impact upon functional abilities also increased (Carswell and Eastwood, 1993; Green *et al.* 1993; Hill *et al.*, 1995). Community residents who demonstrated mild-to-moderate cognitive impairment also demonstrated functional impairment, and within one year were dependent in at least one ADL (Gill *et al.*, 1995; Grenier *et al.* 1996).

Many people who suffer from dementia are aware that they are being cognitively tested and as a result they become defensive and agitated, affecting their performance. Observing the performance of a habitual activity tends to be less threatening to patients. Thus, a functional assessment can be a reliable means for determining overall ability (Ashford, *et al.*, 1992; Loewenstein *et al.*, 1989; Mahurin *et al.*, 1991). As well, behavioural observations may be a means of establishing a positive therapeutic relationship with the patient.

Two questions that may arise when examining the ability to perform functional tasks within an unfamiliar setting are: how do you observe highly personal tasks such as bathing or toileting and what is the effect of performing familiar tasks in an unfamiliar environment? Since people who suffer from dementia are likely to perform better in familiar surroundings than in an unfamiliar clinic with strangers, most functional assessments should be completed in an environment that is familiar to the individual and at a time that coincides with the usual performance of that activity. Patients can be asked to demonstrate how they get in and out of the bathtub, or on and off the toilet without removing their clothes.

Establishing a rapport with patients prior to testing function will facilitate performance, and conducting a functional assessment prior to a cognitive assessment is less threatening. Also, it is useful if the clinic has an area that simulates a usual bathroom, bedroom, and kitchen so that the opportunity to observe IADL and ADL behaviour is enhanced.

The alternative to asking patients to demonstrate their abilities is to ask about the capacity to perform activities of daily living. While it may not be as illuminating as observing the individual, caregivers are quite able accurately to report their relative's capacity to perform activities of daily living and there are a number of functional assessments which use caregiver report of capacity (Kiyak *et al.*, 1994; Rogers *et al.*, 1994).

The information gleaned through an assessment of a patient's ability to carry out activities independently, despite dementia, is of practical help to family and professional caregivers. For the most part, family caregivers want to know how to help their family member to become more independent, to be less of a burden, and to have an high quality of life.

One further reason to use a functional assessment is to address a major reason for caregiver concern—safety in the home. Community health care workers are aware that safety is dependent upon the patient's functional ability and it is essential to identify issues and concerns that can be easily transformed into recommendations for interventions and treatment (Oliver *et al.*, 1993).

Functional assessment scales

Traditionally, functional assessments use a rating scale with a range of ADL and IADL items (Lawton and Brody, 1969) or organize the stages of the disease process on the basis of both cognitive and functional abilities (Reisberg *et al.*, 1982). Recently, a third option is to focus on the actual process of IADL and ADL performance (Fisher, 1995).

Rating scales

There are two types of functional rating scales. Some instruments score a range of tasks based upon the successful completion of each task (Linn and Linn, 1982). Other instruments are scored according to the type and amount of assistance that is needed to complete the task (Lawton and Brody, 1969). Functional assessments which help to estimate the need for assistance are more immediately useful than those which simply define whether the sufferer is able or unable to complete a task.

Staging instruments

There are functional assessments that combine cognitive and functional abilities to distinguish phases (severity) of the disease process (Reisberg *et al.*, 1982; Burns *et al.*, 1994). These measures provide a global estimation of the severity of dementia and the need for community and institutional resources. Most global staging scales attempt to define a uniform order in which functional and cognitive abilities are lost. These scales assume that the progression of dementia has distinct steps which do not overlap. However, there is great heterogeneity in the decline of individual functions and many of the scales, developed from cross-sectional data, have not been validated in longitudinal studies (Cohen-Mansfield *et al.*, 1996).

The adequacy of functional assessments is related to their ability to provide useful information, not only for diagnosis or prognosis, but also for care and intervention (Katz and Stroud, 1990). Global scales do not provide an adequate estimate of the individual profile of disturbance nor the individual rate of the progression of the disease. They are not sufficiently sensitive to monitor the slow change in functional capacity over time, nor are they useful in assisting caregivers with specific intervention strategies for specific behavioural disabilities (Loewenstein *et al.*,1989).

Process scales

Another approach, relatively new in the literature, focuses on the process of performing an activity of daily living rather than whether an activity is or is not successfully performed (with or without assistance, aids, or adaptations) (Baum and Edwards, 1993; Burns *et al.*, 1994; Carswell *et al.*, 1995; Fisher, 1995). The objective of these process scales is to examine the underlying processes which affect the performance of a variety of tasks; the *how* of performance rather than the completion of an activity. Process skills typically include attention, organization, planning, sequencing, motivation, concentration, and motor ability as well as the effect of the environment upon performance. The specific activities that are observed are less important than the manner in which the individual performs the activity. Patients are observed while undertaking a typical task (say, dressing) and are evaluated not only on the performance (can they dress or not) but also upon the process that was used to undertake it (how did they dress or what impeded their performance). Process deficits affect the ability to complete a wide variety of IADL and ADL. For example if a patient demonstrates that sequencing is a problem in dressing, it is more than likely that sequencing will be a problem for many other activities. Thus, process scales are not comprised of items that measure whether a sufferer is able to complete IADL or ADL tasks, but of items which reflect the process of performance.

Functional assessment approaches

There are two fundamental approaches used to assess function. These include self-report and caregiver report of capacity (what *can* the person do?), and the direct observation of performance (what *does* the person do?).

Assessments of capacity

Self-report

A number of IADL and ADL scales rely upon self-report of capacity to perform. However, people who suffer from dementia frequently overestimate their functional capacity, particularly in IADL. Recent studies compared self-reports with family reports of functional abilities in persons with a cognitive impairment. Not unexpectedly, it was found that, although individuals with 'early' dementia were able to recognize that they had some functional deterioration, overall, patients with dementia tended to underestimate their dysfunction related to the degree of cognitive deterioration. (Rogers *et al.*, 1994; Zimmerman and Magaziner, 1994).

Caregiver report

Most ADL scales are completed by an evaluator based upon information obtained from caregivers' estimation of their relative's capacity. Although there are concerns about possible caregiver bias in reporting upon the capacity of a person with dementia (Kiyak *et al.*, 1994), caregiver reports are more accurately reflective of cognitive impairment and actual performance than self-reports (Rogers *et al.*, 1994) and are a preferred method of collecting data on functional capacity. Functional assessments which are either caregiver or self-report of performance capacity are found in Table 10.1.

Assessments of ability

Scales that require the person to perform actual tasks are useful when there is no consistent caregiver, when the clinician is concerned that the caregiver might not be able to provide an unbiased estimate of their relative's capacity, or if the clinician wishes to assess actual performance under more standardized conditions. Direct observation of function, usually in the natural setting of the person over an extended period of time, results in a reliable estimation of IADL and ADL ability. Functional assessments of performance ability are found in Table 10.2.

As with any psychometric testing, functional assessments provide a standard set of tasks—consequently the caveats for psychometric tests (the situational effects of the environment, time of day, and mood) also apply to

Table 10.1 Functional assessment instruments of capacity (self- and/or caregiver report)

Test	Items	Psychometric properties	Source	Comments
Bristol Activities of Daily Living Scale (BADLS)	20 items, four components IADL—drink preparation, telephone use, food preparation, housework, communication, shopping, eating. Self-care—dental care, hygiene, bathing, dressing, toileting, drinking Orientation—to space, games and hobbies, to time, driving or public transport, finances Mobility—transferring, mobility	Reliability—test–retest Validity—concurrent, construct	Bucks et al. (1996) UK	Sensitive to levels of dependence and independence Item selection based in part upon caregiver feedback Developed for clients with dementia Community residents
Disability Assessment for Dementia (DAD)	40 items in ten areas covering three dimensions of initiation, planning/organization, and performance ADL—hygiene, dressing, continence, eating. IADL—meal preparation, telephoning, going out, finance, mediation use, Leisure/housework.	Reliability -test-retest, inter-rater, internal consistency. Validity—content, concurrent, construct.	I. Gelinas (1994) School of physical and occupational therapy. McGill University 3654 Drummond St. Montreal, PQ H3G 1Y5 Canada	Developed for clients with dementia Validated in French and English Community residents Requires 20 min to complete.
Nurses Observation Scale for Geriatric Patients (NOSGER)	30 items in six dimensions ADL—grooming, toileting, cleanliness, dressing. IADL—television, shopping, hobbies orientation. Five levels per item.	Reliability—inter-rater, test-retest Validity—concurrent, predictive Sensitive to change	Spiegel et al. (1991); Tremmel and Spiegel (1993) Switzerland USA	In addition to ADL and IADL assesses memory, mood, social and disturbing behaviours Requires 20–30 min to complete.

Scale	Description	Reliability/Validity	Reference	Notes
				complete Institutional residents
Functional Dementia Scale	Affect—moaning, agressivity, mood changes. ADL —eating, grooming, continence Orientation—confusion, wandering, memory loss 16 items	Reliability—item, inter-rater Validity—concurrent	Moore et al. (1983) USA	Developed for clients with dementia Takes 5–10 min to complete
Physical Self-maintenance and Instrumental Activities of Daily Living Scales for Multilevel Assessment Instrument (MAI)	ADL—dressing, eating, grooming, transfers, toileting, bathing, ambulating IADL—finances, shopping, transportation, telephone, medication, food preparation, laundry housekeeping/handyman work Three to Four levels per item	Reliability—inter-rater, item, test-retest Validity—construct, concurrent	Lawton et al. (1982) USA	Primarily developed for frail and cognitively impaired older adults Takes 10–15 min to complete Community residents
Functional Activities Questionnaire (FAQ)	10 items Managing finances, shopping, leisure activity, meal preparation, current events, remembering appointments, travel from home Four levels of performance	Reliability—inter-rater Validity—concurrent, construct Sensitive	Pfeffer et al. (1982) USA	Developed for cognitively impaired community residents. Takes 20–30 min to complete
Parachek Geriatric Rating Scale	11 items Physical capabilities, self-care, social Five levels of performance	Reliability—inter-rater Validity, concurrent, predictive	The Center for Neurodevelopmental Studies. 8434 North 39th Ave. Phoenix, Arizona, USA 85051 (Miller and. Parachek 1974)	Developed for elderly inpatients Takes 3–5 min
Rapid Disability Scale—II	18 items ADL—eating, walking, mobility, bathing, dressing, toileting, grooming, adaptive tasks Four levels per item.	Reliability—inter-rater, test-etest Validity—predictive, concurrent Factor structure	Linn and Linn (1982) USA	Developed for both elderly community and institutional residents Takes 5–10 min to complete.

Table 10.2 Functional assessment instruments of performance

Test	Items	Psychometric properties	Source	Comments
Refined Activities of Daily Living Scale (RADL)	70 items 14 subtasks within 5 activities—toileting, washing, grooming, dressing, eating Six levels per task	Reliability—inter-rater, item Validity—content, concurrent.	Tappen (1994) USA	Developed for the cognitively impaired institutional residents Measured over one day
Structured Assessment of Independent Living Skills (SAILS)	50 items Fine motor skills, gross motor skills, dressing, eating, expressive language, receptive language, time and orientation, instrumental activities, social interaction Four levels of performance per task	Reliability—test-retest, inter-rater, item Validity—construct, concurrent.	Mahurin et al. (1991) USA	Developed for the cognitively impaired community residents Takes up to an hour to complete
Direct Assessment of Functional Status (DAFS)	30 items Time orientation, communication, financial skills, driving orientation, shopping, eating, dressing or grooming Two levels of performance	Reliability—inter-rater, test-retest Validity—concurrent, construct.	Loewenstien et al. (1989) USA	Developed for cognitively impaired community residents To be conducted during a day period or longer
ADL Situational Test	Four tasks, dressing (10 items), meal preparation (9 items), telephone use (11 items), purchasing (8 items). Four levels of performance.	Validity—concurrent, construct.	Skurla et al.(1988) USA	Developed for dementia clients Takes up to 30 min

functional assessments. Functional assessments are best carried out within an environment that is familiar to the individual with dementia (Geldmacher and Whitehouse, 1996; Nygard *et al.*, 1994; Park *et al.*, 1994). While direct observation in a standardized artificial environment may be preferable from one point of view, clinicians could underestimate the everyday variability of functional ability because the 'test' environment is unfamiliar. Often a caregiver is able to see and assess the individual in the less stressful and more familiar environment in which activities are usually carried out.

So it can be seen that if the clinician wishes to know whether patients with suspected dementia are able to perform functional activities, they can be assessed in the clinic. If the clinician is primarily interested in knowing whether people with suspected dementia can still manage at home, they should be assessed in their own familiar environment.

How to select an instrument for a functional assessment

The choice of a functional instrument will depend upon a number of criteria. These include the purpose for which the assessment is used, the population for which the measure was developed and upon whom the measure was tested, the theoretical and psychometric properties of the measure, whether it is meaningful to determine the performance capacity or ability, the ease of administration, the time needed to complete the test, and the economy of the instrument.

Functional assessments are used to help in establishing a diagnosis, to establish a baseline of function, to monitor change over time, to plan useful intervention strategies, to advise family caregivers, or to assess the efficacy of treatments or interventions. A measure used *to help in establishing a diagnosis* should have demonstrated sensitivity and specificity. Functional assessments used *to establish a baseline of function* (to monitor change over time or to assess efficacy of interventions) must demonstrate responsiveness to change. Functional assessments that incorporate *the process of performance* may be most appropriate for helping family caregivers and assess the efficacy of treatments or interventions.

There are potential problems in using scales that were not designed for use in dementia so it is important to select a functional assessment that has been developed for, and tested upon individuals who have dementia. The validity of a functional assessment scale is strengthened when it is developed for the population on which it is being used (McDowell and Newell, 1996). Functional assessments that have been established for the assessment of older people who have physical rehabilitation needs, or measure function in persons with affective disorders, are non-specific and of limited validity for the assessment of people with dementia. They are not sensitive to change in those people who have dementia (Tappen, 1994) and often do not reflect activities that are useful for caregivers (Bucks *et al.*, 1996).

A second caveat when selecting functional assessments is the possibility of cultural bias. As long as patients have had the opportunity to engage in activities that are assessed, functional assessments do not appear to be as subject to cultural biases relative to those that occur with measures of cognition. The saliency of the items is an important factor when considering the possibility of cultural biases. Most functional assessments were developed and tested on white populations in North America and may not be appropriate for use in assessing ethnic minority groups or people living in Europe or Australia. Functional assessments that examine the process of performing an activity may be less liable to cultural bias because they explore the process of task performance using a task that is usual for that person in that culture. The functional assessments outlined in this chapter are identified in the tables by the country in which they were developed and tested.

Psychometric properties and theoretical underpinnings of functional measures will not be described in detail here. There is an excellent discussion of these aspects in Chapters 2 and 3 of the book on rating scales and questionnaires by McDowell and Newell (1996). However, any functional assessment, whatever the purpose, should have adequate reliability, validity, responsiveness, and clinical utility.

Responsiveness of a functional assessment that is used to monitor change over time or ascertain the efficacy of treatment or interventions is increased with the number of items in an instrument and with the levels of score within each item. For example an instrument that has 25 items, each with a possible score of 1 to 5 (as in a Likert scale) is more responsive than a measure that has 5 items with a possible score of yes/ no.

Finally, the measure should be clinically practicable. Is the measure easy to use or does it have complicated instructions? Does an evaluator need to be trained? Does it require a great deal of time and thus fatigue both the patient and the evaluator? Are the results meaningful and respond to the mandate of the clinic or department? Do the results lead to meaningful and useful interventions? These questions must be answered to the satisfaction of those using the assessments.

Measures of functional assessment

There is a considerable literature detailing and examining functional assessments. Measures that appear in this section have been chosen using the above criteria and have been classified into three categories: scales of ADL and IADL capacity, scales of ADL and IADL performance, and scales of ADL and IADL process. These instruments were developed specifically for a population with dementia and are either the most frequently used, or are recent instruments. Further information on functional assessments can be found in the following references: McDowell and Newell (1996); Kane and Kane (1981); Israel (1984). Table 10.1 details instruments that use self or caregiver report, Tables 10.2 and 10.3 are comprised of instruments that use observation to assess function.

Factors which impinge upon a functional assessment in dementia

There are intrinsic and extrinsic factors that influence the assessment of functional performance. Intrinsic factors include motivation, attention, focus, ability to remember instructions, the stage of the dementia, and previous experiences with assessments. Extrinsic factors include the social, physical, and cultural environment of the individual.

Clinicians must be aware of the impact of these factors on functional performance. Depending upon the type of functional assessment used, these factors are observed informally during an assessment or are measured as part of the assessment. Awareness of these factors is helpful in guiding clinicians to the selection of appropriate management strategies. People with dementia deserve the best possible situation to enhance their performance, and the clinician may need to choose between a measure of capacity or a measure of performance as the most helpful method of data collection.

Case outlining the process

Mrs C. was brought to the clinic by her daughter who was concerned because her mother seemed depressed and unable to cope at home. Mrs C., who is 78 years old, has lived in her home since her marriage 59 years ago. She cares for her husband who has severe emphysema and diabetes. He is dependent upon Mrs C. and a considerable array of home services. Mrs C's daughter reports that her mother seems to have 'given up'. She no longer visits with friends, her usual high standard of housekeeping has declined, and she seems to be forgetful and 'uninterested in life'.

An initial interview was conducted with Mrs C. and her daughter. Mrs C. denied that she had any difficulties in caring for her husband or managing her home. She denied any health problems although she was tired, 'Who wouldn't be with all that I have to do!', and complained that her daughter 'should just mind her own business'. Mrs C's daughter reported that even though the family received many home services (including nursing and meals-on-wheels), her parents did not eat well, her mother seemed to be muddled about finances, and she had withdrawn from her usual activities at the church. During the interview Mrs C. was asked to complete a brief cognitive screen, which she

Table 10.3 Functional assessment instruments of process

Test	Items	Psychometric properties	Source	Comments
Functional Performance Measure (FPM)	39 items Motor performance, context, attention, perception, concentration, processing, planning, quality of performance Likert scale 1–10 per item.	Reliability—inter-rater, between tasks Validity—construct, concurrent, content.	Carswell et al. (1995) Canada	Observational outcome measure examining the underlying process of any ADL or IADL performance Developed for clients with dementia
Assessment of Motor and Process Skills (AMPS)	36 items Posture, mobility, co-ordination, strength, energy, using knowledge, temporal organization, space and objects, adaptation Calibrated scale using many-faceted Rasch analysis	Reliability—test-retest, inter-rater, intrarater Validity—factor structure, concurrent, construct	Fisher (1995) USA Canada	Observational tool using previously calibrated tasks examining IADL Developed for physically and cognitively impaired clients
Kitchen Task Assessment (KTA)	Initiation, organization, performance of all steps, sequencing, judgement and safety, completion Four levels per item—independent, verbal cue, physical assistance, incapable	Reliability—inter-rater Validity— construct, factor analysis, criterion-concurrent	Baum and Edwards (1993) USA	Functional measure that records the level of cognitive support needed to complete a cooking task Developed for clients with dementia

firmly refused to do saying, 'Why do you need to know that? I'm not crazy. My daughter's the one who needs her head examined!'. Based on this interview, a physical examination, a neuropsychological examination, psychiatric examination, and a functional assessment were planned.

As Mrs C. was still living at home it was decided to undertake the assessment in her home. A performance based assessment was used to examine Mrs C's functional ability. It was selected by the clinic because it helped to determine a differential diagnosis, provided a baseline of function, would be used to monitor change, and to determine future service needs. It was reliable and valid, had been developed for use in an elderly population, and provided concrete information on which to base intervention strategies.

While Mrs C. was still at the clinic, an evaluator met with her and arranged to visit with Mrs C. at home for an afternoon to observe her performing her usual daily tasks. Mrs C. accepted the visit of the evaluator as she was familiar with home services because of her husband, she was in her own environment, and she was 'in control'.

The evaluator noted how Mrs C. performed the tasks, whether there were issues of safety, and the time that it took to complete the tasks. It was clear from the score and observations that Mrs C. had a number of difficulties in IADL (meal preparation, laundry, homemaking, managing the banking, and using transportation). She was quite able in ADL, except for bathing (particularly getting in and out of the tub).There were safety issues related to stove elements (while making a cup of tea Mrs C. boiled the first kettle dry) and what to do in an emergency.

The evaluator also assessed Mr C's functional capacity, using a self-report instrument of IADL and ADL. This took about 10 minutes and was done to determine the overall service needs for the family. The data collected during this visit, together with the results from additional examinations, helped to establish a diagnosis of dementia and enabled planning for support for both Mr and Mrs C.

Conclusion

In dementia the observed loss of functional ability progresses from IADL to ADL. These IADL and ADL disabilities are often the first clinical indicators of dementia. They are recognized as an important part of the disease process and should be assessed along with assessments of cognitive and specific neuropsychological processes. Functional assessments are useful measures for establishing a diagnosis, monitoring change, planning appropriate intervention strategies, and planning future health services. A variety of approaches are used to assess function in patients with dementia including caregiver report, self-report, and direct observation. In the final analysis functional assessment tools should be chosen according to the needs of the clinic and the individual with dementia.

References

Key references recommended by the authors are marked with an *.

American Psychiatric Association (1994). *Diagnostic and Statistical Manual of Mental Disorders: DSM-IV*. (4th ed.). American Psychiatric Association, Washington, DC.

Ashford, J.W., Kumar, V., Barringer, M., Becker, M., Bice, J., Ryan, N. and Vicari, S. (1992). Assessing Alzheimer severity with a global clinical scale. *International Psychogeriatrics*, **4**, 55–74.

Auer, S.R., Sclan, S.G., Yafee, R.A. and Reisberg, B. (1994). The neglected half of Alzheimer disease: Cognitive and functional concomitants of severe dementia. *Journal of the American Geriatrics Society*, **42**, 1266–1272.

Baum, C. and Edwards, D.F. (1993). Cognitive performance in senile dementia of the Alzheimer's type: The Kitchen Task Assessment. *American Journal of Occupational Therapy*, **47**, 431–438.

Berg, K., Wood-Dauphinee, S. and Williams, J.I. (1995). The Balance Scale: Reliability assessment with elderly residents and patients with acute stroke. *Scandinavian Journal of Rehabilitation Medicine*, **27**, 37–36.

Blessed, G., Tomlinson, B.E. and Roth, M. (1968). The association between quantitative measures of dementia and of senile change in the cerebral grey matter of elderly subjects. *British Journal of Psychiatry*, **114**, 797–811.

*Bucks, R.S., Ashworth, D.A., Wilcock, G.K. and Siegfried, K.S. (1996). Assessment of activities of daily living in dementia: Development of the Bristol Activities of Daily Living Scale. *Age and Ageing*, **25**, 113–120.

Burns, T., Mortimer, J.A. and Merchak, P. (1994). Cognitive performance test: A new approach to functional assessment in Alzheimer's disease. *Journal of Geriatric Psychiatry and Neurology*, **6**, 46–54.

Carswell, A. and Eastwood, R. (1993). Activities of daily living. Cognitive impairment and social function in community residents with Alzheimer disease. *Canadian Journal of Occupational Therapy*, **60**, 130–136.

*Carswell, A., Dulberg, C., Carson, L. and Zgola, J. (1995). The Functional Performance Measure for persons with Alzheimer disease: Reliability and validity. *Canadian Journal of Occupational Therapy*, **62**, 62–69.

Cohen-Mansfield, J., Reisberg, B., Bonnema, J., Berg, L., Dastoor, D.P., Pfeffer, R.I. and Cohen, G.D. (1996). Staging methods for the assessment of dementia: Perspectives. *Journal of Clinical Psychiatry*, **57**, 190–198.

Fillenbaum, G.G., Wilkinson, W.E., Welsh, K.A. and Mohs, R.C. (1994). Discrimination between stages of Alzheimer's disease with subsets of MMSE items: An analysis of Consortium to Establish a Registry of Alzheimer's Disease data. *Archives of Neurology*, **51**, 916–921.

Fisher, A.G. (1995). *Assessment of Motor and Process Skills*. Three Star Press, Fort Collins, CO.

Fisk, J.D., Rockwood, K., Handas, B., Tripp, D.A., Stadnyk, K. and Doble, S.E. (1995). Cognitive screening in a population-based sample of community-living elderly: Effects of age and education on the construct of cognitive status. *International Journal of Geriatric Psychiatry*, **10**, 687–694.

Folstein, M. F., Folstein, S.E. and McHugh P.R. (1975). Mini-mental State Examination. A practical method for grading the cognitive status of patients for the clinician. *Journal of Psychiatric Research*, **12**, 189–198.

Geldmacher, D.S. and Whitehouse, P.J. (1996). Evaluation of dementia. *The New England Journal of Medicine*, **335**, 330–336.

*Gelinas, I. (1994). Development, content validation and testing or reliability of a disability assessment in dementia of the Alzheimer type. *Programme and abstracts for the 5th Research Colloquium in Rehabilitation*, May, Montreal, Canada,

Gill, T.M., Richardson, E.D. and Tinetti, M.E. (1995). Evaluating the risk of dependence in activities of daily living among community-living older adults with mild to moderate cognitive impairment. *Journal of Gerontology*, **47**, S245–253.

Green, C.R., Mohs, R.C., Schmeidler, J., Aryan, M. and Davis, K.L. (1993). Functional decline in Alzheimer's disease: A longitudinal study. *Journal of the American Geriatrics Society*, **41**, 654–661.

Grenier, P.A., Snowdon, D.A., and Schmitt, F.A. (1996). The loss of independence in activities of daily living: The role of low normal cognitive function in elderly nuns. *American Journal of Public Health*, **51B**, S201–208.

Hill, R.D., Backman, K. and Fratiglioni, L. (1995). Determinants of functional abilities in dementia. *Journal of the American Geriatrics Society*, **43**, 1092–1097.

Huppert, F.A., Brayne, C., Gill, C., Paykel, E.S. and Beardsall, L. (1995) CAMCOG—a concise neuropsychological test to assist dementia diagnosis: Socio-demographic determinants in an elderly population sample. *British Journal of Clinical Psychology*, **34**, 529–541.

Israel, L. (1984). *Source Book of Geriatric Assessment*. S. Karger, New York.

Jagger, C., Spiers, A. and Clarke, M. (1993). Factors associated with decline in function, institutionalization and mortality of elderly people. *Age and Ageing*, **22**, 190–197.

Johnston, B., Scott, N., Po, A.L. and Jack, D.B. (1995). Psychometric profiling of the elderly using the Cambridge Cognitive Examination. *Annals of Phramacotherapy*, **29**, 982–987.

Kane, R.A. and Kane, R.L. (1981). *Assessing the Elderly. A Practical Guide for Measurement.* Lexington Books, Toronto.

Katz, S., Ford, A.B., Moskowitz, R.W., Jackson, B.A. and Jaffe, M.W. (1963). Studies of illness in the aged. *Journal of the American Medical Association,* **185**, 914–19.

Katz, S. and Stroud, M.W. (1990). Functional assessment in geriatrics. A review of progress and directions. *Journal of the American Geriatrics Society,* **37**, 267–271.

Kittner, S.J., White, L.R., Farmer, M.E., Wolz, M., Kaplan, E., Moes, E., Brody, J.A. and Feinleib, M. (1986). Methodological issues in screening for dementia: The problem of education adjustment. *Journal of Chronic Diseases,* **39**, 163–170.

Kiyak, H.A., Teri, L. and Norson, S. (1994). Physical and functional health assessment in normal aging and in Alzheimer disease: Self-reports vs. family reports. *Gerontologist,* **34**, 324–330.

Klein, L.E., Roca, R.P., McArthur, J., Vogelsang, G., Klein, G.B., Kirby, S.M. and Folstein, M. (1985). Diagnosing dementia. Univariate and multivariate analyses of the mental status examination. *Journal of the American Geriatrics Society,* **33**, 483–488.

Lawton, M.P. and Brody, E.M. (1969). Assessment of older people: Self-maintaining and instrumental activities of daily living. *Gerontologist,* **9**, 179–186.

Lawton, M.P., Moss. M., Fulcomer, M. and Kleban, M.H. (1982). A research and service oriented multilevel assessment instrument. *Journal of Gerontology,* **37**, 91–99.

Lezak, M.D. (1996). *Neuropsychological Assessment* (3rd edn). Oxford University Press, Oxford.

Lindeboom, J., Ter Horst, R., Hooyer, C., Dinkgreve, M. and Jonker, C. (1993). Some psychometric properties of the CAMCOG. *Psychological Medicine,* **23**, 213–219.

Linn, M.W. and Linn, B.S. (1982). The Rapid Disability Scale—2. *Journal of the American Geriatrics Society,* **30**, 378–382.

Loewenstein, D.A., Amigo, E., Duara, R., Guterman, A., Hurwitz, D., Berkowitz, N., Wilkie, F., Weinberg, G., Black, B., Gittelman, B. and Eisdorfer, C. (1989). A new scale for the assessment of functional status in Alzheimer's disease and related disorders. *Journal of Gerontology,* **44**, P114–121.

Loewenstein, D.A., Ardila, A., Rosselli, M., Hayden, S., Duara, R., Berkowitz, N., Linn-Fuentes, P., Mintzer, J., Norville, M. and Eisdorfer, C. (1992). A comparative analysis of functional status among Spanish- and English-speaking patients with dementia. *Journal of Gerontology,* **47**, P389–394.

Mahurin, R.K., DeBettignies, B.H. and Pirozzolo, F.J. (1991). Structured Assessment of Independent Living Skills: Preliminary report of a performance measures of functional abilities in dementia. *Journal of Gerontology*, **46**, P58–66.

Mattis, S. (1976). Mental status examination for organic mental syndrome in the elderly patient. In *Geriatric Psychiatry* (eds L. Bellack and T.B. Karasu), pp. 77–121.Grune and Stratton, New York.

*McDowell, I. and Newell, C. (1996). *Measuring Health. A Guide to Rating Scales and Questionnaires.* Oxford University Press, Oxford.

Miller, E.R. and Parachek, J.F. (1974). Validation and standardization of a goal oriented, quick screening geriatric scale. *Journal of the American Geriatrics Society*, **22**, 278–283.

Moore, J.T., Bobula, J.A., Short, T.B. and Mischel, M. (1983). A functional dementia scale. *Journal of Family Practice*, **16**, 499–503.

Nygard, L., Bernspang, B., Fisher, A.G. and Winblad. B. (1994). Comparing motor and process ability of persons with suspected dementia in home and clinic settings. *American Journal of Occupational Therapy*, **48**, 689–696.

Oliver, R., Blathwayt, J., Brackley, C. and Tamaki, T. (1993). The Safety Assessment of Function and the Environment for Rehabilitation (SAFER) tool. *Canadian Journal of Occupational Therapy*, **60**, 78–82.

Park, S., Fisher, A.G. and Velozo, C. (1994). Using the Assessment of Motor and Process skills to compare occupational performance between home and clinic settings. *American Journal of Occupational Therapy*, **48**, 697–709.

Patterson, M.B., Mack, J.L., Neundorfer, M.M., Martin, R.J., Smyth, K.A. and Whitehouse, P.J. (1992). Assessment of functional ability in Alzheimer disease: A review and a preliminary report on the Cleveland Scale for Activities of Daily Living. *Alzheimer Disease and Associated Disorders*, **6**, 145–163.

Pfeffer, R.I., Kurosaki, T.T., Harrah, C.H., Chance, J.M. and Filos, S. (1982). Measurement of functional activities in older adults in the community. *Journal of Gerontology*, **37**, 323–329.

Podsiadlo, D. and Richardson, S. (1991). The timed 'Up & Go': A test of basic functional mobility for frail elderly persons. *Journal of the American Geriatrics Society*, **39**, 142–148.

Reisberg, B., Ferris, S.H., De Leon, M.J. and Crook, T. (1982). The global deterioration scale for assessment of primary degenerative dementia. *American Journal of Psychiatry*, **139**, 1136–1139.

Rogers, J.C., Holm, M.B., Goldstein, G., McCue, M. and Nussbaum, P.D. (1994). Stability and change in functional assessment of patients with geropsychiatric disorders. *American Journal of Occupational Therapy*, **48**, 914–918.

Roos, N.P. and Havens, B. (1993). Predictors of successful aging: A twelve-year study of Manitoba elderly. *American Journal of Public Health*, **81**, 63–68.

Roth, M., Tym, E., Mountjoy, C.Q., Huppert, F.A., Hendrie, H., Verma, S. and Goddard, R. (1986). A standardized instrument for the diagnosis of mental disorder in the elderly with special references to the early detection of dementia. *British Journal of Psychiatry,* **149**, 698–709.

Skurla, E., Rogers, J.C. and Sunderland T. (1988). Direct assessment of activities of daily living in Alzheimer's disease. A controlled study. *Journal of the American Geriatrics Society,* **36**, 97–103.

*Spiegel, R., Brunner, C., Ermini-Funfschilling, D., Monsch, A., Notter, M., Puxty, J. and Tremmel, L. (1991). A new behavioural assessment scale for geriatric out- and in-patients: The NOSGER (Nurses' Observation Scale for Geriatric Patients). *Journal of the American Geriatrics Society,* **39**, 339–347.

Tappen, R.M. (1994). Development of the refined ADL assessment scale for patients with Alzheimer's and related disorders. *Journal of Gerontological Nursing,* **20**, 36–42.

Tremmel, L and Spiegel, R. (1993). Clinical experience with the NOSGER (Nurses' Observation Scale for Geriatric Patients): Tentative normative data and sensitivity to change. *International Journal of Geriatric Psychiatry,* **8**, 311–312.

Warren, E.J., Grek, A., Conn, D., Herrmann, N., Icyk, E., Kohl, J. and Silberfeld, M. (1989). A correlation between cognitive performance and daily functioning in elderly people. *Journal of Geriatric Psychiatry and Neurology,* **2**, 96–100.

World Health Organization (1980). *International Classification of Impairments, Disabilities, and Handicaps.* WHO, Geneva.

Zimmerman, S.I. and Magaziner, J. (1994). Methodological issues in measuring the functional status of cognitively impaired nursing home residents: The use of proxies and performance-based measures. *Alzheimer Disease and Associated Disorders,* **8**, S281–290.

11 The assessment of dementia in the community setting

Laurie Herzig Mallery, Sean Page, and Alistair Burns

Introduction

Dementia is a medical syndrome with important psychosocial implications for the patient, family, and community at large. Assessment of dementia is commonly conducted in a clinic, where, in most cases, an accurate diagnosis can be made efficiently. However, the needs of the patient and/or caregiver cannot always be fully appreciated in a clinic setting. Behavioural disturbances, such as delusions and agitation, may worsen when patients leave the familiar home environment. As well, patients may not be willing to come to a clinic. In such cases, properly conducted community assessment can clarify unresolved issues and uncover specific needs. This chapter reviews the relative advantages and disadvantages of evaluating dementia in the home.

Whether performed in a clinic or in a home, evaluation of dementia requires careful observation of behaviour. Assessment begins when greeting the patient and during casual conversation. Information about ambulation, posture, language skills, praxis, and affect contributes to an understanding of the patient, which ultimately helps with diagnosis. For instance, when a patient enters a room and has difficulty deciding where to sit, problems with judgement may be present; pauses during conversation may indicate word-finding difficulties; and a slow, cautious gait may indicate that dementia has progressed to a point where mobility is affected. Formal testing of multiple cognitive domains using validated instruments and thorough functional assessment can corroborate and augment initial clinical impressions.

The degree of functional limitation can be used to predict need. While evaluation of dementia in a clinic does not allow first-hand observation of the patient's environment, the patient's needs can be approximated by evaluating the level of deterioration in function (i.e. staging the severity of dementia), though collateral history from a caregiver or informant will be necessary. In particular, the informant can support or provide reports of functional difficulties, which will help the clinician make a more accurate assessment and treatment plan.

Seven stages in the course of a dementia

The degree of functional difficulties can be used to determine the stage of dementia using the Functional Assessment Staging Scale (FAST) (Reisberg 1988; see also Chapter 10). The FAST delineates seven progressive stages of functional impairment in dementia (especially as found in Alzheimer's disease), and is meant to be concordant with the Global Deterioration Scale (GDS) (Reisberg, 1982). This diagnostic instrument assumes that as dementia worsens functional disabilities will decline, mirroring cognitive deterioration. Thus, as simple tasks become more demanding and are completed with more difficulty, the severity of dementia increases.

The first three stages of this instrument describe normal cognition and age-associated memory impairment. The fourth stage defines early dementia, at which time patients typically have difficulty with instrumental activities of daily living, such as cooking a complicated meal or shopping. It is generally assumed that patients in the fourth stage are able to live independently, although they may need help organizing their medications and completing other complex tasks of daily living.

The fifth stage occurs when patients begin to have trouble choosing the clothes they want to wear. They may wear the same clothes repeatedly or dress inappropriately for weather. Patients in the fifth stage almost always need assistance. They will need help with medication management, cooking, and often need help with housekeeping and other aspects of household management. The sixth stage begins when patients develop a dressing apraxia, so that assistance with dressing is necessary. Although there are exceptions to the rule, patients in the sixth stage of dementia will generally need constant supervision. During the seventh stage of this illness, patients lose the ability to communicate and may become bed ridden. Obviously, full-time care is necessary at this point.

Using staging to determine the necessity of a home visit

Understanding functional limitations (staging) allows the clinician to predict the level of care and supervision required and make appropriate recommendations to the family and the caregiver. At this point the health professional is equipped to target specific patients who may need to be seen at home for more specific assessment of need and recommendations for care. For example if a patient with severe dementia (GDS stage 6), who under ordinary circumstances would need constant supervision, is living alone, a home assessment may be needed to clarify issues of safety. In some cases, patients with advanced dementia may perform adequately in their home setting and, thus, intervention can be postponed. Conversely, if a family states that a patient in the fourth stage (where the patient is assumed to be able to live independently) is unsafe, a home assessment may be warranted to document that there are indeed behaviours that could jeopardize the safety of either the patient or the caregiver(s).

Community-based assessment in the home provides the opportunity for further observation and supplementary data collection. First-hand information can be obtained about how the patient with dementia interacts with his or her environment. The evaluator can gain knowledge about family relationships, environmental stimuli, and potential risks, and discover unreported needs. The home also provides clues about the abilities and preferences of the patient prior to the onset of dementia.

In addition, direct observation of function may clarify diagnoses where a person has ambiguous or confusing cognitive deficits (diagnostic criteria for dementia, such as the *Diagnostic and Statistical Manual of Mental Disorder*, revised fourth edition, dictate that functional impairment is a prerequisite for a diagnosis of dementia) (American Psychiatric Association 1994). The home is an ideal place for thorough evaluation of functional abilities. Here, rather than relying on the caregiver for reporting problems, a professional, such as an occupational therapist, can observe functional ability as the patient engages in activities of daily living, such as cooking or cleaning.

The observer can also assess safety issues. Home visits can reveal surprising situations which may not be apparent when the assessment takes place in a clinic setting. In extreme cases, evaluation in the home can reveal dangers which are clearly unacceptable and need immediate attention. The assessor can then quickly determine what action to take to secure safety.

Planning the home visit

A community-based visit should be carefully planned and conducted. Time devoted to preparation will be rewarded if the patient and caregiver perceive that this visit is efficient and well organized, resulting in increased confidence in the assessor and the formation of a therapeutic alliance. The relationship between the health professional and the patient begins during the initial contact. It is important to communicate with the patient to inform him or her that a visit will take place. In addition, the caregiver should be contacted and the family should be invited to participate. It is useful to learn as much about the patient as possible before the actual visit by either reviewing the chart or contacting the physician caring for the patient. A proactive approach to safety also begins in the preparation phase, before contact has been initiated. Risk to the assessor can be minimized if more information, particularly about the patient's previous behaviour, is available prior to the actual visit.

Preparation for community-based assessment should include the following points:

♦ If making appointments over the phone, be wary about leaving messages containing confidential information on answering machines which can be picked up by others.

♦ Obtain preliminary information about the nature and purpose of the assessment.

♦ Know as much about the patient as you can before visiting at home.

♦ Contact the caregiver as well as the patient.

The home visit

The visit should be conducted in such a way that it does not overtax or confuse the patient. In many instances the patient will have impaired concentration or attention, impaired memory, and, in addition, may be frail. The process of assessment, although rigorous, should not lead to undue anxiety or distress; therefore the assessor should break down activities into discrete segments allowing the assessor to determine the patient's level of understanding and willingness to proceed at the close of each activity. This approach provides for natural breaks, which may help alleviate fatigue or distress. One should begin by explaining the assessment process and negotiating ways in which potential interruptions can be minimized and privacy established.

If a patient has not been seen, or will not be seen in an office or clinic prior to a home visit, the assessor would need to record a history from the caregiver, complete a cognitive assessment using a validated instrument (such as the Folstein MMSE (Folstein *et al.* 1975) or Brief Cognitive Rating Scale (Reisberg and Ferris1988)), conduct a physical examination, determine the stage of dementia, and evaluate the home and social situation. Laboratory studies may be ordered, where applicable.

During a home visit the following observations can be made:

♦ Examine how the home is managed. Is it neat and clean, disorganized, or cluttered? Is more help necessary?

♦ Observe the patient's demeanour. Does the patient appear comfortable? Does he or she ask you to sit down or do they seem disoriented in their environment? Are they over or under stimulated (e.g. is there a television playing in the background)?

- Look for clues about premorbid abilities, interests, skills, and personality. Such information will allow the clinician to understand the patient's present disabilities in the context of their past and present experience.

- If appropriate, assess recent and remote memory by asking about pictures within the home.

- Assess functional abilities either directly, by observing the patient, or indirectly through a caregiver history.

- Observe social dynamics and interview members of the household. Does the caregiver appear relaxed? Does the patient follow the caregiver around? How is the caregiver coping? Studies show that consultations can focus excessively on the patient and that the needs of the caregiver may be overlooked (Twigg 1992). Thus, the evaluator should confirm that adequate support systems are available for the caregiver. The caregiver should be asked directly about the presence of behavioural disturbances such as insomnia, agitation, pacing, or wandering, which add further stress to caregiving.

- Continue to observe the patient attentively throughout the course of your stay. Is the patient anxious, agitated, or restless? Are behavioural problems, such as wandering or pacing, present?

To assess issues of safety the assessor should:

- Look for hazards within the home. As cognitive impairment and functional dependence worsen, the risk of injury increases. A recent study (Oleske *et al.* 1995) showed that a common mechanism of injury was striking against furniture and building structures. This finding suggests that a home environment which is confusing, cluttered, or dark may increase the risk of injury. Rugs, slippery floors, appliances (such as the stove), knives, swinging and rocking chairs, wall sockets, and unsecured cabinets present potential threats.

- Evaluate medications. Look for these in the medicine chest, refrigerator, night stand, and bedroom.

- Assess the level of compliance. Are there medications in the home which are not being used correctly?

- Assess the patient's nutritional intake. With permission, evaluate the contents of the refrigerator and cupboard.

- Inspect the patient's ambulation. As dementia progresses mobility declines. In addition, behavioural problems can lead to the use of neuroleptics and other sedating medications which increase the risk of falling.

- Try to notice any odours of urine or alcohol.

- Pay attention to signs of potential elder abuse.

♦ Evaluate the home to ascertain whether it will meet the requirements of future care needs, thus allowing the caregiver to provide continuity of care within the home. Will changes in the home need to be made should mobility decline? Is there a place for a caregiver to stay, should continuous supervision be necessary?

The team approach

The above dementia assessment works well when carried out by an inter-disciplinary team, which could include social workers, nurses, physicians, psychologists, occupational therapists, and/or physical therapists. Studies have shown that nurses are able to recognize cases of dementia (O'Connor *et al.* 1988) and that their care of patients with dementia is of high quality (Dick and Mandy 1989). Social workers provide counselling and support and direct families to outside resources. Occupational therapists can evaluate function and safety. Patients can be observed as they carry out tasks within the home. Physicians can complete detailed cognitive assessment, perform physical examinations, and assess behavioural disturbances. If well-trained pro-fessionals are involved and roles are allowed to blur, the team will function effectively with the goal of supporting individuals in the community and maximizing independence. In communities where a full complement of pro-fessions needed to form a multidisciplinary team is not available, it may take several visits to complete a home assessment, but in many instances a well planned visit from one member of the team may be adequate.

Recommendations and treatment

Once assessment is completed, recommendations and treatments can be tailored to the individual and his or her family. Flexibility is essential to meet the needs of the particular patient. Potential treatment recommendations include:

1. Counselling the patient. As patients are identified earlier in their disease course the likelihood that they will be aware of their deficits and wish to discuss their diagnosis will increase.

2. Counselling the caregiver. Caregivers need to understand the diagnosis, expected course, and problems that commonly occur. Caregivers should be encouraged to learn about dementia and the varied manifestations of this illness. Attention to the well being of the caregiver is an essential aspect of treating this condition.

3. Liaising with community resources such as Alzheimer's societies, day care

programmes, home care, Meals-On-Wheels, respite, and support groups for caregivers.

4. Adapting the environment to compensate for loss of function. Certain areas of the house, such as the bathroom or kitchen, can be blockaded, fuses from the stove can be removed, furniture can be moved away from the centre of the room to the periphery, and medications can be placed out of reach.

5. Treating behavioural disturbances (e.g. aggression, depression, agitation, delusions, or hallucinations) by environmental manipulation, changes in routine of care, or with medication, such as neuroleptics, as necessary.

6. Supervising medication use. If the patient has moderate to severe dementia (stage six and seven), medications should be kept out of reach and medication use should be closely monitored. With milder dementia a dosette/medidose which is filled by a caregiver on a weekly basis will simplify drug use and reduce the risk of error. Any medication that is not currently being used should be removed from the home.

7. Discussion of issues of advanced directives.

8. Recommendation of respite care.

9. Consideration of an exercise programme (which may be as simple as regular walking) to maintain mobility.

10. Increasing home supports.

11. Recommendation of nursing home placement if dangers associated with living at home are considered to be excessive.

12. Assessment and treatment of common illnesses of the frail elderly (constipation, incontinence, and vision and hearing impairment).

13. Recommendations about driving.

Cases of acute illness

Another role for the dementia multidisciplinary team or health professional caring for patients with dementia would be to care for the patient during times of acute illness. For many patients it may be appropriate to assess and treat acute medical problems within the home, thus avoiding hospitalization. Home treatment will allow the patient to remain in familiar surroundings, avoid the risk of exacerbating confusion that occurs when changing environment, increase the patient's comfort level, and avoid the risk of excessive medication use and overly aggressive medical care. Whether this practice is feasible will be determined by the patient's preferences. These may have been determined at an earlier stage in the disorder when the patient drew up an advanced directive. It will also depend on family preferences, community resources, financial status, and the willingness of health-care providers (such as nurses and physicians) to provide home care. When dementia is severe, palliative care from the home may be appropriate. Co-ordinated home care for ill patients can provide meaningful benefits to patients and their families.

Advantages and disadvantages of home assessment

Overall, home-based assessment is convenient for the patient and allows the clinician to obtain first-hand information about how the patient is managing in their home. Many patients are more relaxed in their home, which may make assessment less stressful. One study confirmed that cognitive evaluation in the home resulted in an improved MMSE score (Ward *et al.* 1990). Possible advantages and disadvantages of community assessment are outlined in Table 11.1.

However, in addition to added expense and increased travel time, home-based cognitive assessment can pose its own difficulties (see Table 11.1). In particular, driving to the patient's home may be time consuming, or the patient may view the home visit as an invasion of privacy (Packman and

Table 11.1 Advantages and disadvantages of community-based assessment

Advantages	Disadvantages
More convenient and less anxiety provoking for the patient and family (perhaps making it easier to assess patients with behavioural disturbances such as delusions or agitation)	May be regarded as an invasion of privacy
Allows the patient a greater feeling of control	May put the assessor at risk from the patient or their family
May be easier to collect information if patient and family are be relaxed	Interruptions and distractions cannot always be controlled (e.g. television, telephone, visitors)
May improve the patient/ health professional relationship and thus improve compliance	Privacy cannot be assured
More thorough assessment of social factors such as housing of and family or interpersonal relationships is possible	May reduce the availability or practicability of some tests
Observations of patient's environment may reveal information about memory, mood, or behaviour	May take more time and may not be cost effective
Questions about safety can be clarified	May create a sense of isolation in the assessor

Bickby 1996). Due to lack of a private space, it may be impossible to interview the caregiver alone; thus, the caregiver may be unable to provide an honest collateral history. Physical examination may be awkward, and interruptions in the home may make it more difficult for the patient to concentrate. It may take several visits to complete a comprehensive home assessment.

Another disadvantage to home assessment is the feeling of isolation that may occur as a consequence of working alone in the community. This is a potential risk for all health and social service staff who see patients outside the hospital setting. Although the nature of community work allows for increased independence and autonomy, heavy caseloads can lead to an isolated practice and psychological detachment from the team. The solution, of course, is to hold regular meetings which bring the team together to review patients. Such meetings can be a vehicle to discuss difficult problems and unresolved issues, providing each team member with support.

Safety issues for the assessor

Safety can be a concern for those working in the community setting. In the hospital, the presence of other professionals provides a feeling of security. In the community, where the assessor is often isolated, the experience can be dangerous. Although aggression and hostility may occur less commonly when assessing patients with dementia, it would be wrong to deny that such situations arise.

Packman and Bickby (1996) have addressed the safety of assessors working in the community. They identified a number of points which are worth highlighting. It is important to let others in the team, or team leaders, know where the assessor is going and when they are expected to return. When the expected time of return has passed, there should be a procedure in place for contacting the assessor.

The risk of managing an aggressive patient is minimal in comparison to the greater risks posed by opportunist theft of personal equipment, particularly while working in urban or inner city areas. Assessors can minimize risk by carrying little personal equipment and few valuables, always locking and alarming vehicles, and being discrete about such things as lap-top computers and mobile phones.

Conclusion

There is evidence that a home visit can reduce the number of admissions to nursing homes. In a study by Stuck et al. (1995) a programme of in-home, comprehensive geriatric assessment delayed decline in functional status and reduced nursing home admission among elderly people living at home. However, since those with 'severe' cognitive impairment were excluded from the study, it is not clear to what extent home assessment for the people with dementia will provide additional useful information that will alter relevant outcomes. Favourable outcomes that would justify routine home visits would include delaying nursing home placement, reducing caregiver stress, preventing injury, and improving quality of life for either the patient or the caregiver. Although some advocate community-based home assessments either in addition to or in place of clinic visits for all patients with cognitive deficits, in many places, time and financial constraints, in conjunction with scarce resources, dictate that home assessment be reserved for particularly difficult cases. In addition, several studies of home-based geriatric assessment and intervention suggest that outcomes improve when services are limited to patients with identified needs (Rubenstein 1996; Stuck *et al.* 1993). Home visits may be necessary when the patient is too frail to leave the home, if information about functional abilities cannot be elicited, when there are doubts about the reliability of the informant, if functional abilities are reported as better or worse than one would expect given the patient's cognitive and functional limitations (stage), or if there are concerns about safety.

Rigorous assessment of dementia should allow for an understanding of the patient's abilities within different cognitive domains. When a full understanding of a patient's limitations is not possible within a clinic, the home visit can provide a wealth of additional, first-hand information about the patient's overall status. After a home visit has been completed, one should have a comprehensive understanding of the patient, which would include information about how the patient interacts with their environment (i.e. functional limitations), problems with ambulation and safety, and social relationships. When used appropriately, community assessment of dementia should clarify diagnosis and stage, facilitate more meaningful decision making for both patients and their families, maintain safety, and potentially ease caregiver burden, thus postponing admission to nursing home and improving quality of life.

References

Key references recommended by the authors are marked with an *.

American Psychiatric Association (1994). *Diagnostic and Statistical Manual of Mental Disorders*, (4th edn.), (DSM IV). American Psychiatric Association, Washington, D.C.

Dick, D.H. and Mandy, C. (1989). Improving organization of service for the elderly mentally ill. *Geriatric Medicine*, **19**, 14–17.

Folstein, M.F., Folstein, S.E., and McHugh, P.R. (1975). Mini-Mental State: A practical method for grading the cognitive state of patients for the clinician. *Journal Psychiatric Research*, **12**, 189–98.

O'Connor, D.W., Pollitt, P.A., Hyde, J.B., *et al.* (1988). Do general practitioners miss dementia in elderly patients? *British Medical Journal*, **297**, 1107–10.

Oleske, D.M., Wilson, R.S., Bernard, B.A., Evan, D.A., and Terman, E.W. (1995). Epidemiology of injury in people with Alzheimer's disease. *Journal of the American Geriatric Society*, **43**, 741–6.

Packman, S. and Bickby, S. (1996). Community interviewing: Experiences and recommendations. *Psychiatric Bulletin*, **20**, 72–4.

Reisberg, B. (1988). Functional Assessment Staging (FAST). *Psycho - pharmacology*, **24**, 653–5.

Reisberg, B. and Ferris, S.H. (1988). The Brief Cognitive Rating Scale (BCRS). *Psychopharmacology Bulletin*, **24**, 629–36.

Reisberg, B., Ferris, S.H., de Leon, M.J. and Crook, T. (1982). The Global Deterioration Scale for assessment of primary degenerative dementia. *American Journal of Psychiatry*, **139**, 1136–9.

Rubenstein, L.Z. (1996). The Emergency Department: A useful site for CGA? *Journal of the American Geriatrics Society*, **44**, 601–2.

Stuck, A.E., Siu, A.L., Wieland, G.D., Adams, J., and Rubenstein, L.Z. (1993). Comprehensive geriatric assessment: A meta-analysis of controlled trials. *Lancet*, **342**, 1032–6.

Stuck, A.E., Aronow, H.U., Steiner, A., Allessi, C.A., Bula, C.J., Gold, M.N., *et al.* (1995). A trial of annual in-home comprehensive geriatric assessments for elderly people living in the community. *New England Journal of Medicine*, **333**, 1184–9.

Twigg, J. (1992). Carers in the service system. In J. Twigg (Ed) *Carers: Research and Practice.* pp 59–93. HMSO, London.

Ward, H.W., Ramsdell, J.W., Jackson, E., Revall, M., Swart, J., and Rockwell, E. (1990). Cognitive function testing in comprehensive geriatric assessment. A comparison of cognitive testing performance in residential and clinic settings. *Journal of the American Geriatric Society*, **38**, 1088–92.

12 Research potential

S. Gauthier, J. Byrne, and L Byrne

Introduction

Research into Alzheimer's disease has greatly advanced in the past decade (High, 1993). This has resulted in improvements in understanding the disease process, patient care, and in diagnosis. Indeed, it is now estimated that misdiagnosis of probable Alzheimer's disease is less than 10 percent (Katzman and Jackson, 1991).

The need to use humans as research participants in Alzheimer's disease is greater than in many other areas of research because there is no successful animal model of Alzheimer's disease, although the transgenic mouse model may change this. Therefore, unlike other diseases where valid animal models exist, the prospect of effective diagnosis and treatment will be greatly reduced if research using human subjects is not undertaken. If it is accepted, therefore, that there is a scientific and ethical imperative to undertake research into Alzheimer's disease and related disorders (Kapp, 1994), then the question of how best to conduct such research is raised.

Research opportunities for the multidisciplinary team

The interdisciplinary nature of memory disorders teams and the referrals they receive results in considerable potential for research. The clientele of memory disorders teams is a mixture of adults with various concerns about their cognitive abilities and their friends or family members. Each of these individuals is a potential research subject (see Table 12.1). It must be remembered that they are not necessarily representative of the population at large and, as such, form a 'convenience' rather than a representative sample, although the generalizability of findings from such studies can be enhanced by large numbers of subjects from many sites. Individuals with disorders which are difficult to diagnose are often referred to memory disorders clinics and thus the clinics present an opportunity to observe many patients with uncommon

Table 12.1 Groups attending a memory disorders team and their research potential

Group	Research potential
Individuals concerned about their genetic risk for Alzheimer's disease	Counselling strategies
Individuals with early cognitive symptoms	Early diagnosis, stabilization studies
Individuals with mild to moderate Alzheimer's disease	Natural history, symptomatic drug therapy, defining treatment effects, aetiological studies
Individuals with moderate to late Alzheimer's disease	Delay to reach clinical milestones studies, treatment emergent behaviour drug studies, day programme strategies
Individuals caring for people with dementia	Caregiver burden and quality of life studies
Individuals with depression	Therapeutic studies
Individuals with subjective memory disorder but no objective evidence of cognitive impairment or depression	Therapeutic studies

or rare disorders, who would be missed in representative samples of the dementia population. Opportunities for research exist in many different areas of the disease process, the overall effect on the patient, and the subsequent effect on others (see Table 12.2).

Aetiology of cognitive impairment

Although there are a number of suggested aetiological hypotheses for Alzheimer's disease, the most common cause of dementia in western countries, a great deal remains to be learned from observations made of patients in memory disorders clinics. Biological fluids such as blood, cerebro-spinal fluid, and urine are usually easily accessible from routine tests and scientists can, and have, made valuable discoveries from such clinic-based samples—for example ApoE 4 in sporadic Alzheimer's disease (Poirier *et al.*, 1993). Case-control studies can also be conducted in clinic settings, with a spouse as an age and environmental control, as a pilot for large city or country-wide epidemiological research.

La Rue and Markee (1995) found, for example, that the predictive value of psychological screening tools for subclinical dementia was low and the range of time over which prediction could be demonstrated was short. These findings indicate that more research is needed in this area but with caution in drawing conclusions about the positive predictive and clinical value of preclinical cognitive screening tests (La Rue and Markee, 1995).

Genetic and risk factor studies deserve special mention because of

Table 12.2 Examples of some areas of opportunity for research in memory disorders teams

Aetiology of cognitive impairment

Familial relationships in dementia, e.g. ApoE 4 in sporadic Alzheimer's disease (Poirier *et al.*, 1993)

Diagnosis of cognitive impairment

Screening for early cognitive loss

Legal and ethical issues in the early diagnosis of dementia

Brain imaging and electrophysiological techniques in diagnosis

CSF and other biological markers for dementias

Development of diagnostic tools and assessments e.g. neuropsychological measures

Research into the sensitivity, specificity, validity, etc. of current diagnostic assessment tools

Pharmacological treatment trials

Phase I and phase IIIa studies

Post-licensing studies, e.g. the development of protocols for drug administration and research into interactions with concomitant medications

Non-pharmacological treatment trials

Counselling of people with dementia—assessment of outcome

Counselling of the primary caregivers of people with dementia—assessment of outcome

Outcome measures for intervention trials

Development of behavioural and other outcome measures e.g. the BADLS for activities of daily living in dementia (Bucks *et al.*, 1996) and validation in different cultures and subgroups

Development of cognitive outcome measures e.g. the ADAS-cog and validation in different cultures and subgroups

Development of quality of life measures and validation in different cultures and subgroups

Clinical audit

Using clinical assessments already carried out, which may improve clinical practice

Caregiver effects

Development of outcome measures for the primary care givers of people with dementia e.g. Behavioural and Instrumental Stressors in Dementia (Keady and Nolan, 1996)

Disease in caregivers and possible links to the caregiver burden

the current awareness among the public about genetic predisposition to Alzheimer's disease. Some clinics elect to offer specific genetic counselling services, a rich source of research opportunities, but requiring a high index of legal and ethical sensitivity (Post *et al.*, 1997), as well as adequate resources.

Diagnosis of cognitive impairment and types of dementia

Many opportunities exist to refine the sensitivity and specificity of different types of diagnostic strategies in the early stages of dementia. The differential diagnosis of benign memory loss and various causes of dementia are discussed in the following chapters. Each of the specific diagnostic groups (see Table 12.3) requires further study. Certain scales are gaining in recognition as useful markers of disease progression, and are thus potentially useful in stabilization studies (Table 12.4). These require validation in different cultural milieu, as well as refinement and further validation generally.

Table 12.3 Common diagnostic groups found in memory disorders clinics (alphabetically)

Age-associated memory impairment
Alzheimer's disease
Alzheimer's disease with atypical features
Anxiety disorders
Depression
Frontotemporal dementias
Lewy body dementia
Mixed Alzheimer's disease and vascular dementia
'Normal'
Questionable dementia
Vascular cognitive impairment
Vascular dementia

Table 12.4 Examples of commonly used scales to assess the progression of dementia

Mini-mental state examination (MMSE) (Folstein and Folstein, 1975)
Alzheimer's Disease Assessment Scale, cognitive section (ADAS-cog) (Rosen, *et al.*, 1984)
Disability Assessment in Dementia (DAD) (Gauthier *et al.*, 1993)
Neuropsychiatric Inventory (NPI) (Cummings *et al.*, 1994)
Clinical Dementia Rating (CDR) (Hughes *et al.*, 1982)

Management of dementia

Pharmacological treatment trials

Adults referred to memory disorders teams may expect an accurate diagnosis and curative therapy. Unfortunately, therapy is still often restricted to removing medications such as sedatives and tranquillisers, correcting associated metabolic deficiencies, and prescribing antidepressants and neuroleptics. A variety of cholinesterase inhibitors, however, which are a palliative treatment, are now available for use in some countries. Research opportunities exist in the development of guidelines for the use of such medication, based on the experience gained by memory disorders teams.

These drugs have been tested in phase II and phase IIIa protocols with patients with 'probable Alzheimer's disease' without or with limited concomitant disease and medication. Careful observation of *real life* use is essential, and possible, in the memory disorders team setting. There is also a research potential in observing patterns of response to these drugs based on diagnostic groups or subgroups, for example ApoE genotypes and based on neuropsychological profile information. The efficacy profile for the patient and family may also be of interest to the researcher. There are thus opportunities for investigation with pharmacological treatments, both pre- and post-licensing.

Some teams will have the interest and resources to test new antidementia drugs, for example the newer cholinesterase inhibitors and muscarinic agonists, in early phases of development (II and IIIa). This will require dedicated study managers and raters. Potentially, other drugs having selective serotoninergic, noradrenergic, or dopaminergic activity will also have therapeutically useful effects.

Symptomatic drug studies are being followed by disease modification studies and prevention studies in people at risk or with minimal symptoms, for example oestrogens, anti-inflammatory, and cholesterol-modifying drugs (Gray and Gauthier, 1997). The use of pharmacological treatments for the dementias is discussed in detail in Chapter 17.

Non-pharmacological treatment trials

Since treatment has been typically pharmacological, there is a paucity not only of non-pharmacological treatments in use but of research evaluating such interventions. Some non-pharmacological treatments and interventions for people with dementia and their caregivers do exist, for example counselling, validation therapy, and memory management. If there is an intention, as proposed in Chapter 18, that 'the purpose of treatment is to reduce stress and improve quality of life', then opportunities exist in the assessment of non-pharmacological treatment with these variables as outcome measures. The areas in which research is necessary are the same as pharmacological treatment trials and include development of outcome measures and further development of useful interventions. The use of non-pharmacological treatment for the dementias is discussed in detail in Chapter 18.

Research practicalities

Research design

The memory disorders team setting provides a forum for a wide range of research designs. Cross-sectional studies will be possible by recruiting the family of those attending the clinic along with the clinic patients. This methodology is often used in clinical geropsychological assessment studies, but has the problem of cohort confounds (La Rue and Markee, 1995), as differences discovered may be attributable not only to age differences but also cohort differences—that is differences in environment due to being brought up in a different time period.

Longitudinal studies are made possible where follow-up appointments are routine. Ordinarily, these studies are disadvantaged by the time and economic expense of following up and maintaining links with groups of people over long periods of time. Longitudinal studies become more viable in a memory disorders clinic setting, where follow-up visits are offered to clarify diagnosis and monitor the disease process. However, some problems remain, such as a high drop out rates, due to death, migration, and sufferers becoming too severe for measurement, amongst other reasons, resulting in large amounts of missing data and possibly a biased sample.

Quantitative studies often require large numbers of participants for statistical power. Although there may be problems recruiting for such studies, a memory disorders team setting may offer opportunities for qualitative research involving interviews and discussion groups with both patients and carers. Single case design studies are useful in interventional research and case study methodology is a powerful clinical neuropsychological method. Both of these designs involve smaller numbers of patients and are potentially rich sources of research information, but as with all methods should be employed only to answer very specific research questions (Miller, 1993).

The randomized control trial, whilst suitable for pharmacological treatment trials, may not be adequate to answer more subtle questions about quality of life or life satisfaction. Qualitative research is often viewed as simpler than quantitative research. However, although qualitative research typically involves fewer participants, the wealth of data obtained from each individual may be time consuming to collect and difficult to interpret.

Outcome measures

Every research question and design will have appropriate outcome measures. The choice of appropriate outcome variables in symptomatic drug studies for dementia has often been a compromise between regulatory requirements and the investigator's best clinical judgement. Furthermore, some scales, particularly in the domains of functional autonomy and behaviour, were initially borrowed from other fields such as geriatric medicine, and thus researchers had to build and validate novel instruments specific to dementia, such as the Disability Assessment in Dementia (DAD) (Gauthier *et al.*, 1993), the Neuropsychiatric Inventory (NPI) (Cummings *et al.*, 1994), and the Bristol Activities of Daily Living Scale (BADLS) (Bucks *et al.*, 1996). Recently, with the advent of a more holistic attitude towards the measurement of health and disease, quality of life has been proposed as an important measure of therapeutic outcome. The use of quality of life measures in dementia is particularly problematic since they are preferably subjective measures and thus the language and decision making deficits which can arise in dementia will result in measurement difficulties. Indeed, the World Health Organization Quality of Life Group has outlined diseases and disorders with a communi-cational dysfunction component as an important area for the development of an accurate quality of life outcome module to complement their existing 'core' quality of life measure (WHOQOL, 1995).

Measures which focus on the effect of disease and various interventions on the primary care givers of people with dementia are being increasingly used. Some measures look at the amount of time spent caring and the consequent effect on the behaviour of the carer, whilst others focus more on the emotional burden of caring. Originally developed as objective measures, the majority now require subjective assessment. As with other measures, most have been adapted from carers of people with other diseases (e.g. the Social Behaviour Assessment Scale (Platt *et al.*, 1978) and the Caregiver Strain Index (Robinson, 1983)). Others, however, have been specifically designed for the primary care givers of people with dementia (e.g. Behavioural and Instrumental Stressors in Dementia (Keady and Nolan, 1996)).

Those evaluating non-pharmacological treatments have typically used person-centred evaluations of outcome and such outcome measures may also prove to be useful in the evaluation of licensed drug therapy among individuals.

Where could research begin?

A starting place may be in evaluation and audit of clinical services offered. This can be used to highlight areas requiring change as well as encouraging standardized practice. Small scale, inexpensive pilot projects to evaluate the viability of larger scale research can be undertaken with relatively little time and financial cost, and will increase confidence and expertise. The team can then consider larger scale research and collaborative projects.

Finding the time

Research will be viable only if supported by management. Those with an interest in research will need to negotiate time and facilities. As well as creating costs, research can benefit the clinic in terms of finance and improving clinical practice.

Where should the research be conducted?

This will depend on the nature of the research. Some research involving invasive procedures and controlled environments may be necessarily carried out in the clinic. There are pros and cons of undertaking research in either the clinic or the home. One advantage of research at home is that measurements of cognitive performance can be more reliable because people are relaxed and measurement is thus less confounded by anxiety. Additionally, participants are more likely to understand that the consultation is not clinical—an important point when considering consent to research. The disadvantages of being at home include the fact that one is not able to control the research environment to the same extent as in a clinic. Additionally, some people would rather be seen in a neutral setting, so that their privacy is not invaded. For further discussion on assessment in the community please see Chapter 11.

Sampling

The issue of sampling is germane when considering the individuals who are entered into a drug trial and the subsequent generalizability of the trial findings. Schneider *et al*. (1997) found that the selection criteria for pharmacological clinical trials in Alzheimer's disease do indeed result in unrepresentative sampling of the population of Alzheimer's disease sufferers, with inclusion criteria including community living and having a carer to supervise medication. However, exclusion criteria for clinical trials are determined by the pharmaceutical company involved and not by the individual clinic and thus, although the team may be consulted, they are not independent in deciding how generalizable the trial data will be.

Recruitment

Recruitment from a population with dementia has its own difficulties. There are ethical issues, for example consent and recruiting people for research when they are unaware that they have a dementing disorder. These issues will be discussed in more detail later in the chapter. There are also practical considerations. People may be recruited in person whilst attending the clinic or their general practice surgery. One some occasions, recruits will first be contacted by letter or telephone. Since people with dementia necessarily have a memory deficit, they will not always remember having been contacted, or the nature of the research. This creates practical difficulties for the researcher. Additionally, potential participants are not offered the same opportunity as people without memory deficits to decide whether or not to take part in research. This must be considered by the researcher and every effort made to ensure that the potential recruit is fully aware of what they are being asked to do, and when. This may be achieved by informing a relative of the research appointment, or by asking them over the telephone to make a note of your appointment in a diary.

Some researchers have budgets to enable them to pay an honorarium to research participants. If this is not the case, then it should be made clear to the potential recruit that there will be no financial reward for the research involvement. When making a funding application, funds to pay participants for their involvement should be a consideration. Although there may not be a budget to pay participants for their time, there may be funds to pay for travelling expenses, either of the researcher or of the participant. Again, this should be discussed with the participant and provision made for such expenses in grant applications.

Cross-sectional research involves study of an experimental and control sample. The researcher will need, therefore, to consider how to recruit participants from a control population. Local groups of older adults may be interested in contributing to the research programme and can be met and approached through local libraries and other members of the community. Control groups should be matched, as far as possible, to the group under study, in order that any differences found can not be attributable to factors other than the disease process. Although this is a difficult task, it may be overcome by recruitment of relatives of the participants in the experimental group, who may wish to take part in the research. It may be helpful to them to see the kind of things that their relatives experience and the researcher may be advantaged by having matched control groups, as relatives are often a close match in terms of socioeconomic group, predicted IQ, and, in the case of spouses, age.

Other issues

Funding

Research can generate important revenues in terms of salaries for staff and overheads for administrative and educational activities. Many studies will require a competent administrator, a study manager, and dedicated support staff, as well as committed researchers. Careful budget planning is an important component of such a study. Smaller research initiatives may have to be funded from within existing budgets, but will still need an identified co-ordinator.

Since the clinic's resources may be augmented by research initiatives, research can be seen to be an asset rather than a burden to the clinic. However, increasing the research productivity of the clinic may require more technical and human resource time. The issue of how to pay for transport is also pertinent, as the researcher may have their own mileage covered by grants, but may have no funding for participant transportation (please see the section on recruitment above). Chapter 3 discusses information management and Chapter 2 organizational aspects, in detail.

Multidisciplinary teams

The multidisciplinary nature of the memory disorders teams (including, for example, physicians, psychologists, nurses, speech therapists, physio-therapists, occupational therapists, and academic researchers) offers both practical and intellectual advantages. There is opportunity for intellectual interactions between its members and it provides non-clinical researchers with access to patients under the supervision of a clinician. This dissemination of knowledge and expertise should be facilitated by regular research meetings, above and beyond meetings concerning the everyday running of the clinical service.

Collaboration

Links with other memory disorders teams

Groupings of memory disorders clinics such as the Consortium of Canadian Centres for Clinical Cognitive Research (C5R, Pryse-Phillips, 1995) and the NIA-funded Alzheimer Disease Co-operative Study (ADCS, Ferris *et al.*, 1997) offer both academic and economic advantages. Additionally, multi-centre recruitment may be one solution to the difficulty in recruiting sufficiently large samples to ensure the statistical power of quantitative research.

Links with other complementary teams

In addition to collaborative projects with other memory disorders teams, a team may consider collaboration with those working in complementary services, for example neurochemistry and genetics. Such collaboration will increase the range of possible research initiatives, facilitating those projects which require different specialties from those typically found in the memory disorders team.

Links with academic researchers

For non-clinicians, being based within a memory disorders team offers an established communicational network with clinical staff. In the absence of such a network, studies conducted by non-clinical staff require establishing communication with clinical staff in order to gain access to patients. This can be time consuming and will thus slow down the research programme. Memory disorders teams may consider establishing firm links with academic re-searchers in order to facilitate continuing collaboration. Concurrently, clinical researchers can benefit from the academic input of the non-clinical staff.

Facilitating collaboration

To facilitate collaboration with other teams, networks may be established through conferences, group meetings, and now through the World Wide Web. There are an increasing number of electronic journals, many of which can be accessed with no charge. Additionally, researchers can contact others through email lists and news group discussion lists, such as 'candid-dementia'. Such groups can be invaluable for the instantaneous discussion of research ideas and agendas.

Ethics

Capacity to consent

The assumption that as a person begins to dement he or she loses their ability to consent to medical and other procedures raises the issue of whether it is ethical to carry out research in the absence of such consent. How to establish that someone is legally incapacitated is also important, since it is not true to say that every person with a diagnosis of dementia has lost their legal capacity. Indeed, individuals with dementia are often able to make legal wills and set up enduring powers of attorney. In these cases it is the imperative of their legal representative to decide if the person has legal capacity.

There are important considerations in research which exist above and beyond those in legal situations. Firstly, there is the potential for a conflict of interest when the researcher requires participants for their study. This is not true for individuals in a therapeutic situation, where there is no gain by the practitioner (Kapp, 1994). However, research is often conducted which will be of no direct benefit to the subject taking part, but which will benefit the researcher. Many participants do, however, gain pleasure and a feeling of worth from having contributed to the research process. Additionally, in the case of therapeutic research, participants may benefit from receiving therapy which is possibly as yet unavailable to other disease sufferers.

In the early stages of a dementing illness, an individual may have legal capacity and may understand their decision to consent but may not be able to remember his or her decisions. If this is the case, it is imperative that they are reminded of their decision and perhaps asked to reaffirm it.

If, at least in some cases, an individual with dementia is legally incapacitated, the question arises as to how justifiable it is for them to participate in research studies, since it can be inferred from their legal incapacitation that they will be unable to give informed consent. The Declaration of Helsinki (Kennedy and Grubb, 1994) and the Nuremberg Code (Kennedy and Grubb, 1994) both state that it is absolutely necessary to obtain an individual's consent to research procedures.

Non-therapeutic and therapeutic research

A useful distinction when considering issues of consent is that between therapeutic and non-therapeutic research. There seems to be little disagreement that research for and with people who are mentally incapacitated, for *therapeutic* purposes, is acceptable. The Committee of Ministers of the Council of Europe stated that 'a legally incapacitated person may not undergo medical research unless it is expected to produce a direct and significant benefit to his health' (Working Party on Research on the Mentally Incapacitated, 1991). The legal position in England and Wales is that a doctor can give treatment to an individual who is unable to consent (with the court endorsing the good practice of consultation both of the patient and the relatives of that patient). This principle holds in therapeutic research (Working Party on Research on the Mentally Incapacitated, 1991).

Patients may make 'living wills' to indicate their decisions about treatment they may receive when they are no longer able to consent. These could conceivably include decisions about research involvement, particularly in therapeutic research. In England and Wales these have no legal force, although they may influence clinicians and provide insight for researchers. In Canada, they have legal standing in a number of provinces (Singer *et al.*, 1996).

Non-therapeutic research is more problematic. A doctor's obligations to patients include beneficence, non-maleficence, and respect for the autonomy of the individual. In non-therapeutic research the obligation of beneficence is not upheld and it is possible that the other two obligations may be violated if the research has risk involved, or if the patient would not have consented to the research if he or she had been able. However, if there is a belief that the individual would have consented to the research but was excluded because of a dementing illness then the principle of respect for autonomy is equally breached.

A conflict arises from the need to consider societal good along with the principles of beneficence, non-maleficence, and autonomy (Berghmans and Ter Meulen, 1995). The Committee of Ministers of the Council of Europe state that 'national law may authorise research involving a legally incapacitated person which is not of direct benefit to his health when that person offers no objection provided that the research is to benefit persons in the same category and that the same scientific results can not be obtained by persons who do not belong to this category' (Working Party on Research on the Mentally Incapacitated, 1991). Thus it can be seen to be acceptable to conduct non-therapeutic research when the person is assumed to consent and when the research is necessarily carried out on a person who is unable to consent.

Further to this, the Royal College of Psychiatrists propose that it is unethical not to undertake research as this deprives future and present patients of better treatment and the prospect of prevention (Working Party on Research on the Mentally Incapacitated, 1991). Procter (1995) proposes that it is unethical not to research on people with dementia as this is a breach of trust of those people who have already contributed to research. Berghmans and Ter Meulen (1995) ask whether it is morally wrong to expect a person with dementia to help medical researchers in return for their care by society. Kitwood (1995), although he is not totally disagreeing with non-therapeutic research, replies that this argument is without merit as it is not society as a whole which generally cares for the dementing individual but rather an individual's family, and that society has a moral duty to care for its weaker members without expecting mutualism.

The general conclusion is that non-therapeutic research should not be vetoed *per se* but that there is a need for guidelines for and monitoring of research of this nature.

Proxy consent

An adult can give legal consent on behalf of another adult when a power of attorney exists. A power of attorney is a legal document enabling one person to act on behalf of another person. In England and Wales an ordinary power of attorney ceases to be valid if the person granting the power of attorney becomes legally incapacitated (Power of Attorney Act, 1971). An enduring power of attorney enables a named person to make decisions on behalf of a mentally incapacitated individual and is agreed by the patient before he or she becomes legally incapacitated. This legal power is evident in many parts of the world, including the British Isles, United States of America, Australia, and Canada (Power of Attorney Act, 1971). However, the power of attorney can be exercised over material goods only and not to decide on treatment or research involvement. Proxy consent may be sought for treatment and research participation, but it has no legal standing in England and Wales. Indeed, the Law Commission of England and Wales have rejected the introduction of a general authority to make decisions for an individual purely on the basis of a family relationship (Kennedy and Grubb, 1994). Additionally, a discrepancy has been observed between proxy decisions and decisions made by individuals, especially in research settings (Warren *et al.*, 1986 and Cassel, 1990 as cited in Kapp, 1994). Despite this, in Scotland there is a way that an adult can give consent on behalf of another adult. A 'tutor-dative' who has the power to consent for the 'patient' may be appointed through a court procedure and the patient is then in the legal position of a child (Working Party on Research on the Mentally Incapacitated, 1991). Although in the majority of countries this power does not exist, it is useful for the researcher, if they are to embark on non-therapeutic research with a legally incapacitated individual, to have an idea of whether that individual would consent if they were able. In essence, the proxy should try to make the decision on behalf of the incapacitated individual, by making a cost-benefit analysis of what is involved in the research. In addition to this, the patient should be seen to be consenting to the research. If there are any verbal or non-verbal indications that the patient is not consenting then the research should be discontinued—even if proxy consent has been obtained (Procter, 1995).

Most research, however, in the field of dementia is necessarily carried out on people in the mild to moderate stage of disease progression, as this is often when research is most viable and also necessary in the case of researching possible therapeutic and preventative measures and diagnosis. Given that in these early stages individuals with dementia will possibly retain capacity to consent, most research conducted in this area is no more ethically problematic than research *per se.*

Recruitment of people unaware of their diagnosis

The issue of telling the diagnosis is discussed in Chapters 18 and 19. The policy on telling the diagnosis will have implications for the research programme. Recruitment for research when the potential participants do not know their diagnosis has ethical and practical implications. Ethically, a participant can not make informed consent if they are unaware of why they are being recruited into a study. Practically, the participant can not be shown literature which mentions why they are being recruited into the study. Therefore, research with people who do not know their diagnosis should be avoided but often is not because this would include most people with moderate and severe dementia and many with mild dementia.

Predictive genetic testing

Another ethical issue in the field of dementia research is that of genotyping, for example for ApoE, as this could be open to abuse. There is a consensus in the literature that since having the ApoE 4 genotype is not a predictive test of Alzheimer's disease, genotyping should be restricted solely to research use and not used as a early diagnostic marker in a clinical setting (Roses, 1996; American College of Medical Genetics/American Society of Human Genetics Working Group on ApoE and Alzheimer's disease, 1995; Post *et al.*, 1997; Mayeux and Schupf, 1995).

Other issues

The effect of the licensing of acetylcholinesterase inhibitors on research into Alzheimer's disease

The recent licensing of anticholinesterases for use in mild to moderate Alzheimer's disease is expected to have a marked effect on research into the illness. Although it is expected that the availability of medicines will increase the profile and expand the spectrum of research, the effect on research may not be wholly positive. Neuropsychological or cognitive research often must be conducted on individuals not taking cognitive enhancing medication. The window of opportunity for research with individuals with Alzheimer's disease, therefore, will be decreased. Patients may only be recruited into research in the period between diagnosis of probable Alzheimer's disease and prescription of the medication, or after they have ceased to respond to the medication. Consequently, more research may necessarily be conducted on individuals unsuitable for the medication, those who fail to respond to the medication, or those who are more severely demented. Thus the research sample will become biased. Additionally, once these medications become more widely available, they will limit placebo controlled trials of new preparations.

The conflict between clinical and research aims

The ideal in research is to have full, clean data sets by reducing missing data. In a clinical environment this is not always possible. It may not be appropriate for the patient to complete a full psychological battery of tests at a particular time. The team must state explicitly that in such situations the needs of the patient must override the research imperative.

Minimizing distress

Maximizing a person's sense of well being and comfort during assessment will result in the assessments being more representative of true ability. Thus, although the research and clinical aims of the team may conflict in other areas, making sure that the patient is comfortable and is not over anxious is both a clinical and a research priority (see Chapter 7).

Safeguards in research with people with dementia

There are a number of ways of safeguarding people involved in research, including research ethics committee approval. It is important to consider *how* research is conducted rather than simply *what* research is conducted, as procedure as well as content can often have ethical significance. It is preferable, for example, that the researcher should not be medically responsible for the patient as this may induce a conflict of interests between medical practice and the research objectives.

Monitoring research involvement—gate keeping

The team must consider how the research involvement of each individual is to be monitored. An individual's request not to be approached for research purposes should be adhered to and a willing individual should not be constantly approached for multiple projects. A way of pooling research information could be implemented to facilitate this. As the team grows, it is imperative that such information is available to all researchers. Additionally, by pooling such information, judgements can be made about whether to approach an individual for entry to a certain project (see Chapter 3 on information management). Team managers should also consider how to restrict and facilitate access to the patients under their care. This 'gate-keeping' provides a good back-up to the local research ethics committees, as each proposed research project will be scrutinized by the team prior to access to patients being granted.

Dissemination of research findings

Conferences and symposia are important for information dissemination, avoiding the time lag between research completion and publication in journals, which is typically 12 to 18 months, but may extend up to 2 years. Meetings in the immediate locality will be a good place to begin, either a local or a hospital group. Once the team increases in expertise and confidence they can begin presenting at national and then international meetings.

Selection of journals is also important. Journals are very specific in what they aim to publish and who they aim to attract as readers. A good rule of thumb is to submit to journals which publish similar work. Information about the targeted readership of a journal and the format they accept for publication are often available from the journal editors. The World Wide Web is increasing in importance as a way of dissemination of findings, as discussed earlier in this chapter.

Conclusion

There are important opportunities for research to be built into the operations of memory disorders teams, whose role should increase greatly as new therapeutic strategies become widely available. An enhanced educational role for memory disorders clinics is also likely, since most of the individuals seeking medical help will be first screened by their family physician, who must be well aware of the state of the art in the diagnosis and treatment of memory disorders. The multidisciplinary nature of memory disorders teams, however, whether in a clinic or a community setting, is also an asset in research. Research can also be an important component of the funding structure of the clinic in terms of salaries for raters and study overheads being reinvested in pilot projects and educational activities.

References

Key references recommended by the authors are marked with an *.

American College of Medical Genetics/ American Society of Human Genetics Working Group on ApoE and Alzheimer's disease (1995). Anonymous statement on use of apolipoprotein E testing for Alzheimer disease. *Journal of the American Medical Association* **274**: 1627–1629.

*Berghmans, R.L.P. and Ter Meulen, R.H.J.T. (1995). Ethical issues in research with dementia patients. *International Journal of Geriatric Psychiatry* **10**: 647–651.

Bucks, R.S., Ashworth, D.L., Wilcock, G.K. and Siegfried, K. (1996). Assessment of activities of daily living in dementia: development of the Bristol Activities of Daily Living Scale. *Age and Ageing* **25**: 113–120.

Cassel (1990). (As cited in Kapp, M.B. (1994). Proxy decision making in Alzheimer's disease research: durable powers of attorney, guardianship, and other alternatives. *Alzheimer's Disease and Associated Disorders* **8**: 28–37.

Cummings, J.L., Mega, M., Gray, K. *et al.* (1994). Neuropsychiatric inventory—comprehensive assessment of psychopathology in dementia. *Neurology* **44**: 2308–2314.

Ferris, S.H., Mackell, J.A., Mohs, R., Schneider, L.S., Galasko, D., Whitehouse, P.J., Schmitt, F.A., Sano, M., Thomas, R.G., Ernesto, C., Grundman, M., Schafer, K., and Thal, L.J. (1997). A multicentre evaluation of new treatment efficacy instruments for Alzheimer's disease clinical trials: an overview and general results. The Alzheimer's Disease Co-operative Study. *Alzheimer's Disease and Associated Disorders* **11** (Suppl 2): S1–12.

Folstein, M., Folstein, S, and McHugh, P. (1975) Mini-Mental State: A practical method for grading cognitive state of patients for the clinician. *Journal of Psychiatric Research* **12**: 189–198.

Gauthier, L., Gauthier, S., Gelinas, I., *et al.* (1993). Assessment of functioning and ADL. *Abstract of the 6th Congress of the International Psychogeriatric Association*, Berlin, September 5–10: 9.

Gray, J.A. and Gauthier, S. (1997) Stabilization Approaches to Alzheimer's Disease. In Gauthier, S. (ed) *Clinical Diagnosis and Management of Alzheimer's Disease*. Martin Dunitz, London.

High, D.M. (1993). Advancing research with Alzheimer disease subjects: investigators' perceptions and ethical issues. *Alzheimer Disease and Associated Disorders* **7**: 165–178.

Hughes, C.P., Berg, L., Danziger, W.L., *et al.* (1982). A new clinical scale for the staging of dementia. *British Journal of Psychiatry* **140**: 566–572.

Kapp, M.B. (1994). Proxy decision making in Alzheimer's disease research: durable powers of attorney, guardianship and other alternatives. *Alzheimer's Disease and Associated Disorders* **8**: 28–37.

Katzman, R. and Jackson, J.E. (1991). Alzheimer's disease: Basic and clinical advances. *Journal of the American Geriatric Association* **39**: 516–525.

Keady, J. and Nolan, M. (1996). Behavioural and instrumental stressors in dementia (BISID): refocussing the assessment of caregiver need in dementia. *Journal of Psychiatric and Mental Health Nursing* **3**: 163–172.

*Kennedy, I. and Grubb, A. (1994). *Medical Law: text with materials* (2nd edn). Butterworths, London.

*Kitwood T. (1995). Exploring the ethics of dementia research: A response to Berghmans and Ter Meulen: A psychosocial perspective. *International Journal of Geriatric Psychiatry* **10**: 655–657.

La Rue, A. and Markee, T. (1995). Clinical assessment research with older adults. *Psychological Assessment* **7**: 376–386.

Mayeux, R. and Schupf, N. (1995). Apolipoprotein E and Alzheimer's disease: The implications of progress in molecular medicine. *American Journal of Public Health* **85**: 1280–1284.

Miller, E. (1993). Dissociating single cases in neuropsychology. *British Journal of Clinical Psychology* **32**: 155–167.

Platt, S., Weyman, A., and Hirsch, S. (1978). *Social Behaviour Assessment Schedule (SBAS)* (2nd edn, revised). Department of Psychiatry, Charing Cross Hospital: London..

Poirier, J., Davignion, J., Bouthillier, D, *et al.* (1993). Apolipoprotein E polymorphism and Alzheimer's disease. *Lancet* **342**: 697–699.

Post, S.G., Whitehouse, P.J., Binstock, R.H., Bird, T.D., Eckert, S.K., Farrer, L.A., *et al.* (1997) The clinical introduction of genetic testing for Alzheimer disease. An ethical perspective. *Journal of the American Medical Association* **227**: 832–836.

Powers of Attorney Act (1971).

*Procter, A.W. (1995). Ethical issues in research with dementia patients: A neuroscience perspective—a response to Berghmans and Ter Meulen. *International Journal of Geriatric Psychiatry* **10**: 653–654.

Pryse-Phillips, W. (1995). New Canadian initiatives in dementia research. *Canadian Journal of Neurological Science* **22**: 3–4.

Robinson, B.C. (1983). Validation of a caregiver strain index. *Journal of Gerontology* **38**: 344–348.

Rosen, W.G., Mohs, R.C., and Davis, K.L. (1984). A new rating scale for Alzheimer's disease. *American Journal of Psychiatry* **141**: 1356–1364.

Roses, A.D (1996). Apoliprotein E and Alzheimer's disease. A rapidly expanding field with medical and epidemiological consequences. *Annals of the New York Academy of Sciences* **802**: 50–57.

Schneider, L.S., Olin, J.T., Lyness, S.A., and Chui, H.C. (1997). Eligibility of

Alzheimer's disease clinic patients for clinical trials. *Journal of the American Geriatrics Society* **45**: 923–928.

Singer P. *et al.* (1996) Bio-ethics for clinicians: 6. Advance care planning. *Canadian Medical Association Journal* **155**: 1689–1692.

Warren *et al.* (1986). (As cited in Kapp (1994) *Alzheimer's Disease and Associated Disorders* **8**: 28–37.

World Health Organization Quality of Life Assessment (WHOQOL) (1995). Position paper from the World Health Organization. *Social Science and Medicine* **41**: 1403–1409.

Working Party on Research on the Mentally Incapacitated (1991). *The Ethical Conduct of Research on the Mentally Incapacitated*. MRC Ethics Series, MRC Headquarters Office, London.

2   Diagnostic process

13 Age-related memory and cognitive decline

R. W. Jones and S. H. Ferris

Introduction

Memory and cognitive decline in normal ageing have been well documented. It is, however, extremely difficult to define what can be considered normal decline. The distinction between severe dementia and normal ageing is obvious but establishing the difference between, for example, early, mild Alzheimer's disease and age-related cognitive loss is a much more difficult task. This is also complicated by those who suggest, with some—mainly clinical—evidence, that Alzheimer's disease is on a continuum with normality and that, if we lived long enough, we would all eventually succumb. What is less clear is whether a disease entity exists which lies between dementing disorders on the one hand and normal age-related changes on the other.

A conceptual problem arises if these issues are only considered in the context of the traditional disease model. Some of the changes are undoubtedly a direct consequence of normal brain ageing and will represent a decline that will be relative to an individual's previous cognitive performance, not relative to norms for age. On the other hand there is an overall shift in the performance distributions between the young and elderly populations, at least in some age-sensitive aspects of cognition such as memory function (Ferris and Kluger 1996). Another difficulty is in the assessment of an individual's decline in the absence of longitudinal data.

Unfortunately there is a plethora of terminology describing these changes; this is illustrated by our own difficulty in selecting a title for this chapter. No term is entirely satisfactory. Studies often vary in the criteria chosen, making direct comparison difficult. Finally, the diagnosis and definition of mild dementia itself is not easy. In the context of the memory clinic and other community dementia assessment services, patients falling into this broad area represent a real challenge. Some undoubtedly do go on to develop a dementia while others clearly do not. At present, time may be the only clear-cut way of separating these two extremes. This chapter will review the current situation and terminology in an attempt to provide information of practical relevance to those working in memory disorder or dementia assessment teams.

Normal memory functioning and changes with age

The term memory covers the registration, retention, and retrieval of information. It is one part of cognition—thinking processes through which knowledge is gained, stored, manipulated, and expressed. Cognition includes a variety of functions in addition to memory including language, praxis, visuospatial and perceptual function, and conceptualization/ flexibility (Rabins 1992). Human memory is not a single unitary function. It comprises a series of complex interconnected systems that serve different purposes and behave in a variety of ways so that we should think in terms of memories rather than memory. Classification is complex and the terminology confusing. Declarative memory (Squire 1987) is concerned with our abilities to learn about and remember information, objects, and events; it is the 'memory' of common parlance (Deutsch Lezak 1995). Within this, it is reasonable to consider three major and interacting systems—sensory memory, short-term memory, and long-term memory.

Sensory memory

Sensory memory enables us to make use of stimuli entering our nervous system. Information is held at a subconscious level long enough to recognize patterns and to select the information that needs to be further processed as short-term memory (Greene and Hicks 1984).

Short-term memory (primary, immediate, or working memory)

Short term memory is the temporary storage of events and information perceived in the very immediate past, no more than a few minutes ago and usually a much shorter period. A classical test for this would be reading out a series of numbers (digit span) or words (word span) with the subject immediately repeating them back. An explanation of the need for a short-term store has been provided by Baddeley and Hitch's (1974) working memory model. Working memory is the temporary storage of information that is essential for activities such as comprehension, learning, and reasoning. The concept proposes a collection of temporary storage subsystems co-ordinated by a central executive. There are subsystems for verbal material (the phonological loop), and pictures and spatial position (the visuospatial scratch pad). The central executive controls the depositing and receiving of memories to and from the subsystems but in the main has a supervisory role in attention control, particularly when concurrent processing is required (e.g. maintaining a memory whilst dealing with another attention-demanding task at the same time).

Long-term memory (secondary or recent and tertiary or remote)

Long-term memory seeks to be a permanent store of information that will be needed for future retrieval. Whether it has a finite capacity and how much information is lost from it are unanswerable questions. Long-term memory is also known as secondary memory, although some authors refer to secondary memory as recent memory by contrast to tertiary or remote memory (Kazniak *et al.* 1986).

Yet another distinction can be made between procedural and propositional memory (Tulving 1983). Procedural memory involves abilities such as walking, dressing, and eating. It is usually implicit, not subject to conscious awareness, and well retained in patients who may remember nothing of recent events and little from their past history. Propositional memory refers to learning of factual knowledge and can be subdivided into episodic and semantic memory.

Episodic memory refers to memories of one's own experience (e.g. where you went on holiday) and is localizable in time and space. Semantic memory refers to knowledge of the world that is unrelated to a person's life (e.g. the capital of France, historical dates) and generally consists of words and concepts. Information that has been semantically rather than episodically coded is subsequently more accurately retrieved (Tulving 1983).

Methodological problems

There is considerable difficulty in dissociating different memory systems. Other problems also complicate research that attempts to measure changes in memory and cognitive abilities across the lifespan (Rabins 1992).

The cohort effect

Most studies examining changes in memory and cognition with age have been cross sectional, comparing young and old subjects. Obviously, people of varying ages at a given time will have had different psychological, educational, and other experiences, which may affect their performance on psychometric tests. Changes seen may reflect these differences rather than a difference due to ageing. Also, the older the study cohort the more selective the group becomes ('survivor effect'). Longitudinal studies are practically and financially demanding and by the time the results are available they may be out of date. The death of some elderly subjects may mean that the subjects continuing in the study were well above 'normal' at the outset, again giving a bias to the results obtained.

The effects of physical and mental illness

With age there is an increasing prevalence of illness and abnormality affecting the organs through which cognition is expressed. For example arthritis, hearing difficulties, and deteriorating eyesight may all affect relevant skills upon which successful testing depends. Whilst some studies have excluded subjects with obvious problems in these areas (and this may introduce bias), subjects with milder difficulties are rarely identified.

Complaints of memory loss and cognitive dysfunction can be symptoms of depression. Around 40 per cent of people over the age of 60 report depressive symptoms such as weight or appetite changes, loss of interest, and dysphoria (desRosiers *et al*. 1995). Up to 5 per cent will meet psychiatric criteria for a diagnosis of clinical depression (Paykel 1989). In 20 per cent of these people, there is also a feeling that there have been changes in their ability to reason or judge properly, pay attention, and remember things as they used to (desRosiers *et al*. 1995).

There may be a loss of motivation and this may be reflected in poor test scores on mnemonic and other intellectual functions. The pattern of impairment associated with adult depression is somewhat different from that associated with ageing and dementia. For example tests of attention and concentration may be somewhat impaired (Larrabee and Levin 1986) and responses may be slowed (Hart and Kwentus 1987); there is also less impairment on delayed recall tasks in comparison with non-depressed Alzheimer's disease patients.

The effects of medication

Many relatively healthy elderly people receive medications that may affect sensory, primary and secondary memory, and interfere with a subject's ability to perform memory and cognitive tests. Although subjects taking particular medications can be excluded from studies, there is again the possibility of bias. If medically feasible, subjects can be withdrawn from psychoactive medication several weeks prior to cognitive evaluation.

Inclusion of subjects with early disease

In any study of ageing-related changes in memory, there is a likelihood that at least some of the subjects included will be in the very early stages of a dementing process. The diagnosis of mild dementia is notoriously difficult and such patients may therefore bias the interpretation of the data obtained.

Memory and age

The impression that ageing affects some systems, processes, or performance characteristics more than others mirrors the reports that older people commonly volunteer about their subjective experience of memory and cognitive change (Rabbitt 1992). They infrequently complain that they are losing all of their cognitive faculties but usually make more specific complaints about loss of memory. In particular, they complain specifically about loss of memory for events in their recent past whilst they claim that they have no problems with events from their remote past such as their childhood. The implication is that different cognitive systems may age at different rates both within and between individuals (Rabbitt 1992).

Subjective reports of memory changes with ageing

Clinicians frequently encounter healthy, non-demented older patients who complain that their memory abilities have declined from what they once were. How accurate are such complaints and do they signify the earliest evidence of a dementing illness? Evidence for an association between self-rating of memory and cognition and actual performance on memory and cognitive tests is conflicting. Some studies have reported a positive association that is usually small whilst others have reported mixed results or no association. (Wilson and Evans 1996). This variation probably reflects differences in study design and study populations. Cross-sectional studies have observed, at best, a weak relationship between self-reports and actual performance on laboratory-based memory tests (Taylor *et al.* 1992).

Few longitudinal studies have been carried out although they would be better and could observe objective changes in memory performance over time whilst assessing whether subjects perceive and report such changes. In a small, 4-year longitudinal study of 30 older adults with memory complaints (who had initially been recruited for a clinical trial), a significant decline in word-recall scores was found, and this was accompanied at the group level by significant self-reported decline in everyday memory and non-significant decline in the WAIS Digit Symbol Substitution Score (Taylor *et al.* 1992). At the individual level, memory change did not significantly correlate with change in self-report or change in Digit Symbol score.

Relevant variables such as depression have not always been measured or considered in the same way, complicating comparisons between different studies. Certainly some studies on depressed patients suggest that complaints are related to the level of depression and not to the performance on cognitive tests (Jonker *et al.* 1996). However people with early dementia do have an increased tendency to complain about their memory in comparison with non-demented subjects (O'Connor *et al.* 1990).

Most studies have been conducted on selected samples of patients, for example those seeking advice from a memory clinic or healthy volunteer samples. Barker *et al.* (1994) compared memory performance, reports of memory loss, and depressive symptoms in attenders at a general practice-referral and a self-referral memory clinic, with age- and sex-matched community controls. The general practice-referred patients were older, had lower Mini-Mental State Examination (MMSE) scores, and had levels of memory complaint and depression between the control and self-referred subjects. The self-referrers had cognitive test performance similar to community controls but complained more of memory loss, were more depressed, and more frequently reported a past history of treated depression.

More recently, a cross-sectional study on a population-based sample of 2537 non-demented and non-depressed individuals from Amsterdam has suggested that subjective memory complaints may be a potential indicator of significant memory impairment (Jonker *et al.* 1996). Within this sample, 34.3 per cent reported memory complaints and 37.3 per cent memory-related problems in daily functioning. Whilst this prevalence is higher than the 23 per cent found in an older UK community sample (Livingston *et al.* 1990), it is much lower than the 80 per cent reported in one healthy volunteer sample (Bolla *et al.* 1991).

Objective measures of memory changes with ageing

Sensory memory, primary (short term), and tertiary (remote) memory decline little with age but tests of secondary (recent) memory show notable differences between young and old subjects (e.g. Crook *et al.* 1986; Rabbitt 1992). In particular, the retrieval process in secondary memory appears to be affected (Bowles *et al.* 1989) even when cohort effects have been accounted for (Arenberg 1990). A number of interpretations have been placed on what is a large amount of data. One involves the concepts of 'crystallized' and 'fluid' intelligence to describe abilities that hold up with increasing age from those that decline (Rabbitt 1992). Overlearned, well practised familiar abilities and knowledge are 'crystallized' and remain essentially unchanged whilst 'fluid' activities, involving reasoning, problem solving, and the efficient processing of rapid information, decline with increasing age. Others have suggested that psychomotor slowing can account for most if not all of the measured changes in performance that deteriorate with age (e.g. Van Gorp *et al.* 1990).

Neurobiological changes with ageing

Many changes in brain structure and neurochemistry accompany ageing. Material is usually only available at autopsy and changes that occur with age may be subtle, varied, and require special techniques. Results are still often controversial (Esiri 1994). There have been no large autopsy studies of the brains of prospectively assessed, cognitively well preserved, elderly subjects.

Macroscopic changes

The weight and volume of the brain diminish gradually and unremittingly in healthy older people. The evidence is mainly from autopsy data but volume changes have also been assessed using computed tomography. Brain weight and volume remain more or less constant up to about 50 years of age after which there is a loss of about 2 to 3 per cent per decade over the following four decades (Esiri 1994). There is slight narrowing of the cortical gyri and widening of the sulci together with some atrophy of the hippocampus and amygdala. Cortical atrophy is maximal in the frontal and temporal association cortex (Morris and McManus 1991). As the brain shrinks, the volume of the ventricular system and the subarachnoid space enlarges. There are regional variations in loss of weight and volume and the loss of brain substance with ageing may not be inevitable. For example the volume loss of white matter after 70 is greater than that of grey. Anderson *et al.* (1983) found a volume loss in neocortex of only 2 to 3 per cent between 70 and 85 years but a decrease of 11 per cent in cerebral white matter, whilst atrophy in the subiculum of the hippocampus was greater at 28 per cent.

Microscopic changes

Alterations with normal ageing in the number and size of nerve cells are still controversial with variations that are not easy to account for in the results from different studies. There is probably definite, but not very severe, nerve cell loss in the brain in normal ageing and rather more shrinkage of nerve cells, for example in cortical and hippocampal pyramidal neurones (Morris and McManus 1991). These changes also continue, apparently steadily, into extreme old age but do not occur in all nerve cell populations

Plaques and tangles, the two main pathological features of Alzheimer's disease, are found in normal ageing increasing progressively from 60 to 90 years of age (although the number of very old subjects studied is limited). For example in one study (Miller *et al.* 1984), 9 per cent of brains of subjects under 55 and 90 per cent of brains of those over 85 contained tangles whilst for plaques the figures were zero and 72 per cent. The critical difference is that in Alzheimer's disease there are much larger numbers of plaques and especially tangles. There is also a tendency for the densities of plaques and tangles to be greater in younger Alzheimer's disease patients (Mann *et al.* 1985). It seems that the numbers of plaques and tangles in Alzheimer's disease and normal ageing show a bimodal distribution rather than a continuum. Tangle distribution is also more widespread in Alzheimer's disease.

An important related issue concerns age and Alzheimer's disease related synaptic loss preceding neuronal death. There is undoubtedly an age-related reduction of about 15 to 20 per cent in synapses in frontal cortex (Masliah *et al.* 1993). In Alzheimer's disease, the degree of synaptic loss is greater than that found in normal ageing and shows a strong correlation with cognitive impairment (Terry *et al.* 1991).

From a pathological viewpoint, it seems clear that ageing and dementia, particularly Alzheimer's disease, do not form a continuum. What is not clear is whether what changes that do occur are an inevitable consequence of ageing or how these changes relate to patients that appear to have age-related cognitive decline.

There are cellular changes in the nucleus basalis of Meynert that are of interest because of the cholinergic output of the nucleus and because of the profound loss of cells that occurs here in Alzheimer's disease (Bartus *et al.* 1982). De Lacalle *et al.* (1991) studied neurologically intact, pathologically normal patients and estimated that compared to young adults, 26 per cent of nucleus basalis neurones are lost by the age of 60 and 50 per cent by the age of 100. This reduction in numbers was accompanied by an increase in cell size up to the age of 60 but thereafter cell size also decreased. The authors suggested that neuronal plasticity was lost at around 60 years of age and that benign memory impairment is seen because the brain cannot then compensate for any further ageing-related cell loss.

Neurochemistry

A range of neurochemical properties can be assessed in tissue sections and many appear to be altered by age in brain areas thought to be important for memory. Reductions have been noted for cholinergic, noradrenergic, serotoninergic, dopaminergic, and several neuropeptidergic systems (for references see Crook *et al.* 1986).

The cholinergic system has received the most attention because of its importance in memory dysfunction and Alzheimer's disease (Bartus *et al.* 1982). However, few recent published reports on the cholinergic system of the ageing mammalian brain have included man. This reflects the difficulty of obtaining clinically and pathologically assessed normal brain tissue over the lifespan. Also, Decker's 1987 review highlighted the controversy between reports on human brain published previously, with equal numbers of authors claiming a significant decrease or no change in choline acetyltransferase in the neocortex or hippocampus (Decker 1987). A fresh appraisal has been made including mainly animal studies to the beginning of 1991 (Perry *et al.* 1994). If proper account is taken of species and regional variations and to the possible existence of behaviourally impaired subgroups within the aged population, then normal ageing is characterized by disruption of cholinergic input to the hippocampus and to the cortex. For example the enzyme choline acetyl-transferase is reported as being decreased in eight of ten independent investigations.

Age-related cholinergic dysfunction will interact with changes in other neurotransmitters (Decker and McGaugh 1991). Neuronal cells become less sensitive to acetylcholine but not to glutamic acid, suggesting that there may not be a generalized reduction in neurotransmitter system activity with increasing age.

At present. no direct link can be proved between, for example, a decline in hippocampal cholinergic activity and the mild deficits in memory experienced by many older people. However, it is not unreasonable to expect that such changes may be connected to age-related memory and cognitive impairment (see also next section).

Neuroimaging

Demented individuals as a group have more atrophy than age-matched control subjects. The overlap between normal and abnormal is too great to expect any one-off measure of atrophy reliably to separate dementia from normal ageing in an individual, although comparing serial magnetic resonance images may be helpful (Fox *et al.* 1996).

Hippocampal atrophy appears to be a common accompaniment of normal ageing and is associated with significant reductions in delayed verbal recall (Golomb *et al.* 1993). A more recent report (Golomb *et al.* 1996) suggests that hippocampal atrophy may be a risk factor for accelerated memory dysfunction in normal ageing.

Electroencephalography frequency also declines in later life but remains above 8.5Hz in healthy people (Obrist 1980). Recent data (Prichep *et al.* 1994) using quantitative electroencephalography analysis shows a progressive slowing with greater cognitive decline, and this was sensitive to the earliest presence of subjective dysfunction. For a more detailed discussion of neuroimaging see Chapter 6.

Review of terminology

Benign senescent forgetfulness (BSF)

BSF is a term that has been widely used to describe elderly people with poor memories who are not thought to be suffering from dementia. The term originally described a form of intermittent impairment of memory retrieval in elderly residents in a retirement home (Kral 1958, 1962). Benign forgetfulness was characterized by poor or inconsistent retrieval of relatively minor details of an episode in the recent past, but with no memory loss for the episode itself. The residents with BSF were generally aware of their memory troubles and tried to compensate for them.

It differed from a 'malignant' form in terms of the quality of symptoms, the milder severity and the relatively non-progressive nature. Kral also described a 'normal' group but did not produce objective criteria to distinguish BSF from normality and also described BSF as an expression of a 'senium naturale'. The senescent forgetfulness groups were defined by comparison with the unimpaired peer group but the subjects were not assessed by formal cognitive testing.

The initial study assessed residents of an old people's home (Kral 1958), many of whom had neurological signs (37.5 per cent of those aged 60–80 years). A further study followed chronically institutionalized psychiatric patients (Kral *et al.* 1964). Clearly neither groups were representative of the general population nor was any distinction made between those with long-standing problems and those with problems of recent onset.

Age-associated memory impairment (AAMI)

The term 'age-associated memory impairment' was proposed with specific research diagnostic criteria by a National Institute of Mental Health work group in the United States 'to describe the memory loss that may occur in healthy, elderly individuals in the later decades of life' (Crook *et al.* 1986). The group noted that there was neither a generally accepted diagnostic term to describe individuals who experience such loss nor any precise diagnostic criteria to distinguish these individuals from subjects who have experienced no such loss or those who experience memory loss that is likely to be associated with specific disease states.

The group felt that terms such as benign senescent forgetfulness were semantically inappropriate, imprecisely defined (with little psychometric assessment included), and intended to describe a particular subset of older people with memory impairment. They commented that, although some elderly people accept AAMI as they accept age-related physical limitations, for many people the impairment was distressing and was not relieved by assurances that the impairment is 'normal', that they were 'just getting older', or that they were not becoming demented.

The work group's paper highlighted research into ageing-related changes. It concluded that while memory decline may be more widely recognized, there are similar changes in other cognitive functions that together make up fluid intelligence. Despite this, it is memory rather than cognitive loss that is focused on in both the diagnostic criteria and the term AAMI.

The diagnosis of AAMI was limited to people at least 50 years old although this did not imply that such impairment was qualitatively different from that occasionally seen in younger adults. Equally, the term did not imply that the disorder was necessarily non-progressive although marked progression would exclude individuals. Detailed diagnostic criteria for selecting research participants were proposed including subjective complaints of everyday memory loss supported by a memory test performance at least one standard deviation below the mean established for young adults on a standardized test of recent memory for which there are adequate normative data. Other criteria included evidence of adequate intellectual ability and absence of specific medical and psychiatric causes of memory impairment. The work group expected that both the diagnostic terminology and criteria would be revised as further research was conducted and the views of researchers and clinicians expressed.

The original description of AAMI led to some confusion regarding both the construct and the inclusion criteria (Barker and Jones 1993). One misconception is that AAMI is describing a disease. Whilst diagnosis and treatment of AAMI is frequently mentioned, and the criteria are described as diagnostic criteria, AAMI is never referred to as a disease because it is intended to describe a consequence of normal ageing. Psychometric scores that distinguish AAMI from pathological memory loss have since been published (Crook 1989); this is consistent with the notion that AAMI is not pathological. Thus it was not adequately clarified that AAMI is intended to define the subgroup of elderly people with memory changes who are concerned by memory changes which are frequently seen in normal ageing.

Memory complaint has been a particular problem. It is not clear whether the work group really meant 'complaint' or 'report' (Barker and Jones 1993). A questionnaire (Larrabee *et al.* 1992) to select people with AAMI for drug studies asks subjects to record how their memory performance has changed since high school or college days. Whether this constitutes a complaint or demonstrates that the subject is distressed by the change is doubtful. On the other hand, it might be inappropriate to treat individuals who are not aware of the problem. If complaint is an important element, then this may create problems because memory complaint is more closely correlated with depression than performance (e.g. Barker *et al.* 1994). Although depression as evidenced by a Hamilton Depression Rating Scale score of 13 or more is an exclusion criterion for AAMI, even milder depression may affect a person's perception of their own performance (Bolla *et al.* 1991).

The choice of memory performance more than one standard deviation below the mean for young adults as the criterion for inclusion is arbitrary. Whilst this can be considered as a less than ideal surrogate for 'decline' in the absence of longitudinal data, it does mean that 16 per cent of normal young subjects would themselves satisfy this part of the criteria. When trying to describe an individual who shows a decline in memory with age, it would obviously be more appropriate to compare their present memory with an internal and retrospective measure of their original cognitive functioning. Tests such as the National Adult Reading Test are available for estimating pre-existing IQ and these have been evaluated in organic conditions (Crawford *et al.* 1988) but there are no tests which accurately estimate earlier memory performance.

In the original AAMI publication, cut-off scores for specific memory tests have been given and these are one standard deviation below the mean for young adults, yet these scores have been altered in a subsequent publication (Crook 1989) without explanation. It is not clear what the significance is if one test result is below the cut-off but the other tests are above this level. Equally, there is no discussion as to why adequate intellectual function is required for the diagnosis. There is a danger that people of lesser original intelligence can never be described as having AAMI despite memory complaints and memory decline; on the other hand, subjects with well above average original intellectual function whose memory has declined may still perform above the cut-off point for memory and not qualify for inclusion despite potentially even greater distress at their age-related decline.

Age-related cognitive decline (ARCD)

More recently, the broader construct, Age-Related Cognitive Decline (ARCD), has been included in the fourth edition of the DSM-IV (American Psychiatric Association 1994) and essentially replaces the previous AAMI terminology. This is not necessarily a rejection of the AAMI construct but merely a generalization and simplification.

The original AAMI criteria were presented with the expectation that modifications would occur as a result of further research and the views of clinicians and researchers. Unlike AAMI, no specific operational criteria have been included in DSM-IV for identifying cases with ARCD. Despite this, ARCD is a helpful step forward because it broadens the concept beyond memory but continues to represent the same basic phenomenon of declining cognitive performance with age.

People with ARCD may report problems remembering names or appointments or may experience difficulty in solving complex problems. The focus of clinical attention is an objectively identified decline in cognitive functioning consequent to the ageing process which is within normal limits for the given age.

There are two important issues concerning ARCD which remain to be addressed (Ferris and Kluger 1996). First is the difficulty of subject selection criteria. How do we know if an individual has really experienced significant decline in the absence of data documenting previous cognitive performance? The second is the important suggestion that we must accept that ARCD is an appropriate and desirable target for treatment. Individuals who subjectively experience and are concerned about ARCD, who show objective evidence of decline and are not depressed, should be candidates for receiving putative cognitive-enhancing compounds in well-controlled clinical trials.

Mild cognitive impairment (MCI)

Over the past few years there has also been considerable work on MCI which is an intermediate 'at risk' category between ARCD/ AAMI and Alzheimer's disease. The further study of MCI is an important current research topic which will help clarify similarities and differences between normal ageing and Alzheimer's disease as well as for identifying the earliest clinical signs of Alzheimer's disease.

Patients with MCI can be identified because they have a Global Deterioration Scale (GDS) of 3 (Reisberg *et al.* 1988) or a Clinical Dementia Rating (CDR) of 0.5 (Hughes *et al.* 1982). These individuals also appear to be at high risk for further decline and conversion to Alzheimer's disease (Flicker *et al.* 1991). However, further work is also needed to understand the differences between those MCI cases who appear to have 'preclinical' Alzheimer's disease and those who do not show significant further decline and who may represent the more severe end of the ARCD spectrum (Ferris and Kluger 1996).

Other terms

A number of other terms have been described which attempt to define the area between mild dementia and normality. These include very mild cognitive decline (Reisberg *et al.* 1982) and age-consistent memory impairment (Blackford and La Rue 1989).

Evaluation

There are numerous neuropsychological tests which can be used to evaluate patients for memory and cognitive impairment. There should be adequate documentation clearly stating the aims of the test, the theoretical basis of the test, and its recommended range of use. Techniques of administration and scoring should be clear. Tests should be reliable (and caution exercised in reducing the number of test items for elderly subjects because this reduces reliability) and valid. Face validity is especially relevant when dealing with elderly subjects (Cunningham 1986). In addition, sensitivity to change is important and tests with marked ceiling or floor effects may be limited in their value.

'The diminished sensory acuity, motor strength and speed, and particularly flexibility and adaptability that accompany advancing age can affect the elderly person's test performance adversely' (Deutsch Lezak 1995, p135). This can give spuriously low scores and incorrect conclusions about the cognitive functioning of older people. It is important to check that auditory and visual acuity are adequate and written materials should use large print and high contrast. The general slowing associated with advanced age requires age norms for all timed tests. It is also essential to obtain the subject's co-operation and consent to assessment.

With growing evidence from longitudinal studies that the earliest signs of more rapid cognitive decline may be clinically detectable, memory clinics offer the ideal situation for identifying subjects with MCI. For example greater impairment of verbal list learning predicted, with more than 90 per cent accuracy, which MCI subjects subsequently declined to dementia (Flicker *et al.* 1991). Delayed paragraph recall was also 92 per cent accurate in predicting which MCI cases declined to Alzheimer's disease (Ferris *et al.* 1993). It would appear that mild decline in delayed memory, psychomotor performance (e.g. digit symbol substitution), and language function (e.g. WAIS vocabulary) may indicate individuals with a greater risk of developing Alzheimer's disease (Ferris and Kluger 1996).

There are little if any longitudinal changes in cognitive performance in ARCD subjects over 2 to 3 years and it is still difficult to predict future Alzheimer's disease in such cases. Early hippocampal atrophy may be important as previously discussed.

Management and treatment

Pharmacological and non-pharmacological treatments may be considered for alleviating or improving age-related cognitive changes.

Non-pharmacological methods

Yesavage (1985) observed that the memory decline which occurs in normal ageing can be, at least temporarily, reversed by mnemonic and other cognitive training techniques in some subjects. This may not be effective for many subjects, particularly those of advanced age. In addition, the effects may not last unless other pretraining behavioural treatments are given as well. For example the performance on a visual-based mnemonic was improved by pretraining elderly subjects in visual imagery. For a fuller discussion of current approaches to non-pharmacological methods, please see Chapter 18.

Pharmacological methods

Part of the driving force behind the concept of AAMI appears to be the rationale that it would be useful to focus clinical studies of drugs for memory and dementia on a healthy population of older people who have experienced memory loss yet appear not to be suffering from dementia. The original AAMI working party report comments that many of the neurochemical changes seen with age are similar, although less severe, to those in Alzheimer's disease and related conditions and 'it may be argued that compounds that reverse these deficits may be of therapeutic value in both AAMI and dementing disorders' (Crook *et al.* 1986).

A few positive treatment studies have now been published. For example 149 subjects meeting criteria for AAMI participated in a 12-week, double-blind parallel study comparing 300 mg of phosphatidylserine with placebo (Crook *et al.* 1991). There was an improvement relative to placebo on performance tests related to learning and everyday memory tasks. It also appeared that the subgroup of people who performed at a relatively low level before treatment were most likely to respond with improvement on both computerized and standard neuropsychological performance tests, and also on clinical global performance ratings of improvement.

This area has been controversial and led to fears that large numbers of 'normal' elderly people will be offered such drugs and that this may be inappropriate and potentially hazardous. Establishing the clinical relevance of improvements on computerized and other neuropsychological tests is not easy. However, for individuals with cognitive decline, treatment with very safe compounds might improve their quality of life since many, whilst neither disabled nor demented, are distressed by their cognitive deficiency.

Conclusions

Memory disorders services encourage early referral of people with mild memory or cognitive impairment. With the increasing availability of treatments for Alzheimer's disease, patients and their families will be increasingly willing to seek expert advice at an earlier stage. Even if initially seen by a community team outside a clinic setting, people with mild impairment are best referred to a memory clinic, where this is available, for further assessment and diagnosis.

The distinction between age-related changes and early dementia is still a difficult and challenging problem and time may be the only clear-cut way to separate the two. We should be seeking to identify patients with MCI since the majority appear to be in a 'preclinical' stage of Alzheimer's disease. Such patients would also seem to be potential recipients of drugs which improve cognition and memory or delay progression to Alzheimer's disease and clinical trials are undoubtedly needed.

The situation with ARCD is more complicated and further longitudinal studies are required to determine what percentage of patients do go on to develop dementia and whether a prognostic factor such as early hippocampal atrophy is helpful. People with ARCD might still benefit from drug therapy but this is still controversial. Such therapies may bring an improved quality of life to elderly people but will need careful clinical evaluation and a high benefit to risk ratio.

References

Key references recommended by the authors are marked with an *.

American Psychiatric Association (1994). *Diagnostic and Statistical Manual of Mental Disorders* (4th Ed.) Washington, DC: Author.

Anderson, J.M., Hubbard, B.M., Coghill, G.R., and Slidders, W. (1983). The effect of advanced old age on the neurone content of the cerebral cortex. *Journal of the Neurological Sciences,* **58**, 233–44.

Arenberg, D. (1990). Longitudinal changes in cognitive performance. In *Advances in Neurology*, Volume 51: Alzheimer's disease (ed R.J. Wurtman). Raven Press, New York.

Baddeley, A.D. and Hitch G.J. (1974). Working memory. In *The Psychology of Learning and Motivation*, Volume 8 (ed. G.A. Bower), pp. 47–90. Academic Press, New York.

Barker, A. and Jones, R. (1993). Age-associated memory impairment: diagnostic and treatment issues. *International Journal of Geriatric Psychiatry*, **8**, 305–10.

Barker, A., Carter, C., and Jones, R. (1994). Memory performance, self-reported memory loss and depressive symptoms in attenders at a GP-referral and a self-referral memory clinic. *International Journal of Geriatric Psychiatry*, **9**, 305–11.

Bartus, R.T., Dean, R.L., Beer, B., and Lippa, A.S. (1982). The cholinergic hypothesis of geriatric memory dysfunction. *Science*, **217**, 408–17.

Blackford, R.C. and La Rue, A. (1989). Criterion for diagnosing age associated memory impairment; proposed improvements from the field. *Developmental Neuropsychology*, **5**, 298–300.

Bolla, K.I., Lindgren, K.N., Bonaccorsy, C., and Bleecker, M.L. (1991). Memory complaints in older adults. Fact or fiction? *Archives of Neurology*, **48**, 61–4.

Bowles, N., Obler, L., and Poon, L. (1989). Aging and word retrieval: naturalistic, clinical and laboratory data. In *Everyday Cognition in Adult and Late Life* (ed. L. Poon, D. Rubin, and B. Wilson). Cambridge University Press, Cambridge.

Crawford, J.R., Parker, D.M., and Besson, J.A. (1988). Estimation of premorbid intelligence in organic conditions. *British Journal of Psychiatry*, **153**, 178–81.

Crook, T.H. (1989). Diagnosis and treatment of normal and pathologic memory impairment in later life. *Seminars in Neurology*, **9**, 20–30.

Crook, T., Bartus, R.T., Ferris, S.H., Whitehouse, P., Cohen, G.D., and Gershon, S. (1986). Age-associated memory impairment: proposed diagnostic criteria and measures of clinical change—report of a National Institute of Mental Health work group. *Developmental Neuropsychology*, **2**, 261–76.

Crook, T.H., Tinklenberg, J., Yesavage, J., Petrie, W., Nunzi, M.G., and Massari, D.C. (1991). Effects of phosphatidylserine in age-associated memory impairment. *Neurology*, **41**, 644–9.

Cunningham, W.R. (1986). Psychometric perspectives: validity and reliability. In *Handbook for Clinical Memory Assessment of Older Adults* (ed. L.W. Poon). American Psychological Association, Washington D.C.

Decker, M.W. (1987). The effects of aging on hippocampal and cortical projections of the forebrain cholinergic system. *Brain Research Reviews,***12**, 423–38.

Decker, M.W. and McGaugh, J.L. (1991). The role of interactions between the cholinergic system and other neuromodulatory systems in learning and memory. *Synapse*, **7**, 151–68.

De Lacalle, S., Iraizoz, I., and Ma Gonzalo, L. (1991). Differential changes in cell size and number in topographic subdivisions of human basal nucleus in normal ageing. *Neuroscience*, **43**, 445–56.

desRosiers, G., Hodges, J.R., and Berrios, G. (1995). The neuropsychological differentiation of patients with very mild Alzheimer's disease and/or major depression. *Journal of the American Geriatric Society*, **43**, 1256–63.

Deutsch Lezak, M. (1995). *Neuropsychological Assessment* (3rd edn). Oxford University Press, New York.

Esiri, M. (1994). Dementia and normal aging: neuropathology. In *Dementia and Normal Aging* (ed F.A. Huppert, C.Brayne, and D.W. O'Connor), pp. 385–436. Cambridge University Press, Cambridge.

Ferris, S.H. and Kluger, A. (1996). Commentary on age-associated memory impairment, age-related cognitive decline and mild cognitive impairment. *Aging, Neuropsychology, and Cognition*, **3**, 1–5.

Ferris, S.H., Kluger, A., Golomb, J., de Leon, M.J., Flicker, C., and Reisberg, B. (1993). Assessment in early detection of age-associated cognitive decline (Abstract). In *Proceedings of the Sixth Congress of the International*

Psychogeriatric Association, p46. International Psychogeriatric Association, Berlin.

Flicker, C., Ferris, S.H., and Reisberg, B. (1991). Mild cognitive impairment in the elderly: predictors of dementia. *Neurology*, **41**, 1006–9.

Fox, N.C., Freeborough, P.A., and Rossor, M.N. (1996). Visualisation and quantification of rates of atrophy in Alzheimer's disease. *Lancet*, **348**, 94–7.

Golomb, J., de Leon, M.J., Kluger, A., George, A.E., Tarshish, C., and Ferris, S.H. (1993). Hippocampal atrophy in normal aging. An association with recent memory impairment. *Archives of Neurology*, **50**, 967–73.

Golomb, J., Kluger, A., de Leon, M.J., Ferris, S.H., Mittelman, M., Cohen, J., and George, A.E. (1996). Hippocampal formation size predicts declining memory performance in normal aging. *Neurology*, **47**, 810–3.

Greene, J. and Hicks, C. (1984). *Basic Cognitive Processes*. Open University Press, Milton Keynes.

Hart, R.P. and Kwentus, J.A. (1987). Psychomotor slowing and subcortical-type dysfunction in depression. *Journal of Neurology, Neurosurgery and Psychiatry*, **50**, 1263–66.

Hughes, C.P., Berg, L., Danziger, W.L., Coben, L.A., and Martin, R.L. (1982). A new clinical scale for the staging of dementia. *British Journal of Psychiatry*, **140**, 566–72.

Jonker, C., Launer, L.J., Hooijer, C., and Lindeboom, J. (1996). Memory complaints and memory impairment in older individuals. *Journal of the American Geriatric Society*, **44**, 44–9.

Kazniak, A.W., Poon, L.W., and Riege, W. (1986). Assessing memory deficits: an information-processing approach. In *Handbook for Clinical Memory Assessment of Older Adults*. American Psychological Association, Washington D.C.

Kral, V.A. (1958). Neuro-psychiatric observations in an old people's home. *Journal of Gerontology*, **13**, 169–76.

Kral, V.A. (1962). Senescent forgetfulness: benign and malignant. *Canadian Medical Association Journal*, **86**, 257–60.

Kral, V.A., Cahn, C., and Mueller, H. (1964). Senescent memory impairment and its relation to the general health of the aging individual. *Journal of the American Geriatric Society*, **12**, 101–13.

Larrabee, G.J. and Levin, H.S. (1986). Memory self-ratings and objective test performance in a normal elderly sample. *Journal of Clinical and Experimental Neuropsychology*, **8**, 275–84.

Larrabee, G.J., McEntee, W.J., and Crook, T. (1992). Age-associated memory impairment. In *Cognitive Disorders: Pathophysiology and Treatment* (ed. L.J.Thal, W.H.Moos, and E.R.Gamzu). Marcel Dekker, New York.

Livingston, G., Hawkins, A., Graham, N., Blizard, B., and Mann, A.H. (1990). The Gospel Oak study: prevalence rates of dementia, depression and activity limitation among elderly residents in Inner London. *Psychological Medicine*, **20**, 137–46.

Mann, D.M.A., Yates, P.O., and Marcyniuk, B. (1985). Some morphometric observations on the cerebral cortex and hippocampus in Alzheimer's presenile dementia, senile dementia of Alzheimer type and Down's syndrome in middle age. *Journal of the Neurological Sciences*, **69**, 139–59.

Masliah, E., Mallory, M., Lansen, L., DeTeresa, R., and Terry, R.D. (1993). Quantitative synaptic alterations in the human neocortex during normal aging. *Neurology*, **43**, 192–7.

Miller, F. de W., Hicks, S.P., D'Amato, C.J., and Landis, J.R. (1984). A descriptive study of neuritic plaques and neurofibrillary tangles in an autopsy population. *American Journal of Epidemiology*, **120**, 331–41.

Morris, J.C. and McManus, D.Q. (1991). The neurology of aging. Normal versus pathologic change. *Geriatrics*, **46**, 47–54.

Obrist, W.D. (1980). The electroencephalogram of healthy aged males. In *Human Aging* (ed. J.E. Birren, R.N. Butler, S.W. Greenhouse, L. Sokoloff, and M.R. Yarrow). Arno Press, New York.

O'Connor, D.W., Pollitt, P.A., Roth, M., Brook, P.B., and Reiss, B.B. (1990). Memory complaints and impairment in normal, depressed, and demented elderly persons in a community survey. *Archives of General Psychiatry*, **47**, 224–7.

Paykel, E. (1989). The background, extent and nature of the disorder. In *Depression: an Integrative Approach* (ed. K. Herbst and E. Paykel). Heinemann Medical Books, New York.

Perry, E.K., Court, J.A., Piggott, M.A., and Perry, R.H. (1994). Cholinergic component of dementia and aging. In *Dementia and Normal Aging* (ed F.A. Huppert, C.Brayne, and D.W. O'Connor), pp. 437–69. Cambridge University Press, Cambridge.

Prichep, L.S., John, E.R., Ferris, S.H., Reisberg, B., Almas, M., Alper, K., and Cancro, R. (1994). Quantitative EEG correlates of cognitive deterioration in the elderly. *Neurobiology of Aging*, **15**, 85–90.

Rabbitt, P. (1992). Memory. In *Oxford Textbook of Geriatric Medicine* (ed. J. Grimley Evans and T. Franklin Williams), pp. 463–79. Oxford University Press, Oxford.

Rabins, P.V. (1992). Cognition. In *Oxford Textbook of Geriatric Medicine* (ed. J. Grimley Evans and T. Franklin Williams), pp. 479–83. Oxford University Press, Oxford.

Reisberg, B., Ferris, S.H., de Leon, M.J., and Crook, T. (1982). The global deterioration scale for assessment of primary degenerative dementia. *American Journal of Psychiatry*, **139**, 1136–9.

Reisberg, B., Ferris, S.H., de Leon, M.J., and Crook, T. (1988). The Global Deterioration Scale (GDS). *Psychopharmacology Bulletin*, **24**, 661–3.

Squire, L.R. (1987). *Memory and Brain.* Oxford University Press, New York.

Taylor, J.L., Miller, T.P., and Tinklenberg, J.R. (1992). Correlates of memory decline: a 4-year longitudinal study of older adults with memory complaints. *Psychology and Aging*, **7**, 185–93.

Terry, R.D., Masliah, E., Salmon, D.P., Butters, N., DeTeresa, R., Hill, R., Hansen, L.A., and Katzman, R. (1991). Physical basis of cognitive alterations in Alzheimer's disease: synapse loss is the major correlate of cognitive impairment. *Annals of Neurology*, **30**, 572–80.

Tulving, E. (1983). *Elements of Episodic Memory*. Oxford Psychology Series No. 2, Clarendon Press, Oxford.

Van Gorp, W.G., Satz, P., and Mitrushina, M. (1990). Neuropsychological processes associated with normal aging. *Developmental Neuropsychology*, **6**, 279–90.

Wilson, R.S. and Evans, D.A. (1996). How clearly do we see our memories? *Journal of the American Geriatric Society*, **44**, 93–4.

Yesavage, J.A. (1985). Nonpharmacologic treatment for memory losses with normal aging. *American Journal of Psychiatry*, **142**, 600–5.

14 Differentiation of the common dementias

Howard H. Feldman and John T. O'Brien

The conceptual basis of dementia

With the greying of society, diseases causing dementia are now recognized as being one of the most important challenges facing western medicine in the 21st century. The term 'dementia' describes a syndrome of acquired loss of cognitive function, behavioural changes, and loss of social function. There is no implied aetiology for dementia and most broadly it represents a neuro-behavioural syndrome that occurs in a large number of diseases. Most dementias occur on the basis of primary degenerative disorders of the central nervous system, though some occur with multisystem inflammatory diseases, infectious diseases, or metabolic/endocrine disorders. Surgically treatable dementias account for a very small percentage of all cases. The potential reversibility of dementia has been emphasized, though longitudinal studies from dementia clinics have demonstrated that in practice this is seen in only 3 to 8 per cent of cases (Clarfield 1988). In patients with dementia associated features such as depression, toxicity related to medications and metabolic disorders are the most frequently modifiable/ reversible problems (Clarfield 1988). The course of dementia is quite variable, though most typically a progressive declining disorder is seen. However, with careful workup and management of treatable components of dementia patients may live with an optimal level of function through their illnesses. The broadest goal for each dementia clinic, community based team, and individual practitioner should be to diagnose and manage each individual to their best level of cognition, behaviour, and function.

This chapter will focus on the three most common causes of dementia and their diagnostic differentiation; Alzheimer's disease (AD), vascular dementia (VaD), and dementia with Lewy bodies (DLB). Not only are these the most common individual causes of dementia but additionally they frequently occur together. Post-mortem studies have reported that up to 15 to 30 per cent of clinically diagnosed AD have significant Lewy body pathology (Hansen *et al.*

231

1990), while 20 to 30 per cent of AD subjects have comorbid cerebrovascular lesions (Gearing *et al.* 1995) which appear to worsen cognitive function (Snowdon *et al.* 1997). How these comorbid pathologies are identified and assigned a place in the diagnosis is evolving with the advent of operational diagnostic criteria for each of these disorders. There may also be significant regional variations in frequency distributions of these disorders. In North American epidemiological studies, the prevalence of AD rises to 35 to 48 per cent in the population over the age of 85 (Evans *et al.* 1989; Canadian Study of Health and Aging Working Group 1994) whereas in Scandinavia, vascular dementia has been estimated to account for 46.9 per cent of dementia cases over the age of 85 (Skoog *et al.* 1993). In specialized dementia clinics, the triad of AD, VaD, and DLB will generally account for 65 to 80 per cent of all referrals.

Alzheimer's disease

Alzheimer's disease (AD) is the most common cause of referral for community assessment or to a specialized dementia clinic and typically will account for 50 to 70 per cent of referrals. Most epidemiological studies have suggested that the community based prevalence is similar (Canadian Study of Health and Aging Working Group 1994). AD has marked clinical, neurochemical, and neuropsychological heterogeneity and it has been speculated that it represents a syndrome rather than a unitary disease (Blass 1993). Though some linearity of decline can be seen on disease staging scales through the mild and moderate disease phases (Koss *et al.* 1996), there is considerable variability in the rates of decline. Many of the commonly used cognitive assessments such as the Mini Mental State Exam (MMSE) (Folstein *et al.* 1975) do not have linear rates of decline but rather are better characterized as following a sigmoidal function (Feldman and Gracon 1996). Some clinical subgroups of 'fast' versus 'slow' decliners have been proposed (Mann *et al.* 1992), where the early involvement of language (Snowdon *et al.* 1996), early age of onset, extrapyramidal signs, and psychosis may predict a more rapid decline. However, the predictability of course in an individual referred case is limited (Koss *et al.* 1996).

The genetics of AD are heterogeneous and evolving rapidly. Familial AD has been reported to affect 5.3 per cent of patients referred to specialized dementia clinics (Sadovnick *et al.* 1989). In familial AD several mutations have been characterized including those on chromosome 21 of the amyloid precursor protein gene (Goate *et al.* 1991), chromosome 14 of the presenilin 1 gene, and chromosome 1 presenilin 2 gene (Sherrington *et al.* 1995). A strong association has also been identified between the E4 allele of the Apolipoprotein E gene on chromosome 19 and late onset AD. The presence of the E4 allele is associated with an increased odds ratio for AD of 10 to 17.9 for homozygosity and 3 to 5 for heterozygosity (Mayeux *et al.* 1993). However, at the present time apoE genotyping cannot be routinely advised for either clinical or predictive testing until additional population risk information is available (Bird 1995).

Clinical diagnosis

The use of standardized criteria

The NINCDS-ADRDA criteria (McKhann *et al.* 1984) continue to provide the clinical diagnostic standard in research studies with applicability to clinical practice. These criteria have been validated both clinically and pathologically (Morris *et al.* 1988) and with their rigorous use the error rate of diagnosis has been lowered to 10 to 15 per cent (Tierney *et al.* 1988). Within the framework of these criteria (see Table 14.1) there are features which are consistent with the disease and those that should alert the clinician that an AD diagnosis is unlikely.

An apoplectic onset, the occurrence of early seizures, and the presence of focal neurological signs are considered to be 'unlikely AD'. By contrast 'clinically probable AD', which is the highest clinical likelihood, is diagnosed when the presentation of cognitive decline is gradual in onset, progressive in course, and without rapid or stroke-like declines. When the course of and presentation of AD are typical, but there is a comorbid identified disorder capable of, but not causing, the dementia, the diagnosis of 'clinically possible' AD is applied. This grouping includes some variations in presentation though the clinical impression remains that AD is the best diagnosis. The diagnosis of 'clinically definite' AD requires that there is histopathological evidence of AD obtained either post-mortem or by biopsy tissue examination. Other diagnostic criteria currently used include those of the DSM-IV (APA 1994) and ICD-10 (WHO 1989) which have not had the same scrutiny of neuropathological correlation. A comparison of the criteria is shown in Table 14.2.

Each of these sets of diagnostic criteria are dependent on clinical expertise with application that is subjective (Cummings and Khachaturian 1996). The anchor points for diagnosis and the determination of the extent of deficit required to fulfil criteria are not specified. There is an explicit need to exclude other brain disorders capable of causing the dementia syndrome such as Parkinson's disease, frontotemporal degenerations, and VaD, though the diagnostic criteria for these groups are less well operationalized. The group of mixed dementias which is pathologically common is not well handled within the framework of the NINCDS-ADRDA criteria and still requires further operationalization.

Table 14.1 NINCDS-ADRDA criteria for clinical diagnosis of Alzheimer's disease

I. Criteria for clinical diagnosis of PROBABLE Alzheimer's disease include:
  - dementia established by clinical examination and documented by the Mini-Mental Test, Blessed Dementia Scale, or some similar examination, and confirmed by neuropsychological tests:
  - deficits in two or more areas of cognition;
  - progressive worsening of memory and other cognitive functions;
  - no disturbance of consciousness;
  - onset between ages 40 and 90, most often after age 65; and
  - absence of systemic disorders or other brain diseases that in and of themselves could account for the progressive deficits in memory and cognition.

II. The diagnosis of PROBABLE Alzheimer's disease is supported by:
  - progressive deterioration of specific cognitive functions such as language (aphasia), motor skills (apraxia), and perception (agnosia);
  - impaired activities of daily living and altered patterns of behaviour;
  - family history of similar disorders, particularly if confirmed neuropathologically; and
  - laboratory results of
    - normal lumbar puncture as evaluated by standard techniques,
    - normal pattern or nonspecific changes in EEG, such as increased slow-wave activity, and
    - evidence of cerebral atrophy on CT with progression documented by serial observation.

III. Other clinical features consistent with the diagnosis of PROBABLE Alzheimer's disease, after exclusion of causes of dementia other than Alzheimer's disease, include:
  - plateaus in the course of progression of the illness;
  - associated symptoms of depression, insomnia, incontinence, delusions, illusions, hallucinations, catastrophic verbal, emotional, or physical outbursts, sexual disorder, weight loss;
  - other neurologic abnormalities in some patients especially with more advanced disease and including motor signs such as increased muscle tone, myoclonus, or gait disorder;
  - seizures in advance disease; and
  - CT normal for age.

IV. Features that make the diagnosis of PROBABLE Alzheimer's disease uncertain or unlikely include:
  - sudden, apoplectic onset;
  - focal neurologic findings such as hemiparesis, sensory loss, visual field deficits, and inco-ordination early in the course of the illness; and
  - seizures or gait disturbances at the onset or very early in the course of the illness.

V. Clinical diagnosis of POSSIBLE Alzheimer's disease:
  - may be made on the basis of the dementia syndrome, in the absence of other neurologic, psychiatric, or systemic disorders sufficient to cause dementia, and in the presence of variations in the onset, in the presentation or in the clinical course;
  - may be made in the presence of a second systemic or brain disorder sufficient to produce dementia, which is not considered to be the cause of the dementia; and
  - should be used in research studies when a single gradually progressive severe cognitive deficit is identified in the absence of other identifiable cause.

VI. Criteria for diagnosis of DEFINITE Alzheimer's disease are:
  - the clinical criteria for probable Alzheimer's disease and
  - histopathologic evidence obtained from a biopsy or autopsy.

VII. Classification of Alzheimer's disease for research purposes should specify features that may differentiate subtypes of the disorder, such as:
  - familial occurrence;
  - onset before age of 65;
  - presence of trisomy-21; and
  - coexistence of other relevant conditions such as Parkinson's disease.

Reprinted from G. McKhann et al. Clinical diagnosis of Alzheimer's disease—Report of the NINCDS-ADRDA Work Group under the auspices of the Department of Health and Human Services Task Force on Alzheimer's Disease. Neurology 1984; 34: 939–44 by permission of Lippincott-Raven Publishers.

Table 14.2 Comparison of three commonly used criteria for the diagnosis of Alzheimer's disease

Characteristics	ICD-10	DSM-IV	NINCDS-ADRDA Probable AD
Memory decline	+	+	+
Thinking impairment	+	–	–
Aphasia, apraxia, agnosia, or disturbed executive function	–	+	–
Impairment of at least one non-memory intellectual function	+	+	+
Dementia established by questionnaire	–	–	+
Dementia confirmed by neuropsychological testing	–	–	+
ADL impairment	+	–	–
Social or occupational impairment	-	+	–
Decline from previous level	+	+	+
Onset between age 40 and 90	–	–	+
Insidious onset	+	+	–
Slow deterioration	+	–	–
Continuing deterioration	–	+	+
Absence of clinical or laboratory evidence of another dementing disorder	+	+	+
Absence of sudden onset	+	–	U
Absence of focal neurological signs	+	–	U
Absence of substance abuse	–	+	–
Deficits not limited to delirious period	+	+	+
Absence of another major mental disorder	–	+	–

ICD -10 - *International Classification of Diseases*, 10th revision; DSM-IV - *Diagnostic and Statistical Manual of Mental Disorders*, 4th edition; NINCDS-ADRDA - National Institute of Neurological and Communicative Disorders and Stroke-Alzheimer's Disease and Related Disorders Association; AD- Alzheimer's Disease; ADL - activities of daily living; U - criteria that make the diagnosis of probable AD but do not specifically exclude the diagnosis.

Reprinted from J. Cummings and Z. Khachaturian, Definitions and diagnostic criteria. In Clinical Diagnosis and Management of Alzheimer's Disease. Ed. S Gauthier, Martin Dunitz, London, 1996, by permission of Martin Dunitz Ltd.

Clinical features and the assessment of early, suspected dementia

A particularly common reason for referral is the need for assessment of early-stage, suspected AD. Referral of this type may be received from the primary care physician, the community mental health team, but (in North America) commonly comes directly from the patient/ family. It may be driven by genetic concerns when there is a positive family history, or by subtle changes noted at home or in the workplace. At this early point an individual may be presenting with either cognitive symptoms or behavioural features and diagnosis is often not straightforward. Both detailed cognitive and behavioural assessment are mandatory at this stage to identify a patient as being either at high risk for, or in the incipient stages of, AD. The formal diagnostic criteria may not be met at this point yet very early disease can be recognized. This stage is becoming particularly important as very early intervention research studies are currently in planning to try and delay the onset and progression of disease. Patterns of cognitive deficit in both incipient and early AD can be identified with psychometric tests which fractionate memory and new learning as well as language and mental control. Screening measures such as the MMSE (Folstein *et al.* 1975) and the Modified Mini-Mental State (3MS) (Teng 1987) lack diagnostic sensitivity for early diagnosis where by contrast, delayed recall on verbal learning tests has been a distinguishing feature of early disease as has an impaired acquisition of new information with failure to improve with semantic cues (Petersen *et al.* 1994; Tierney *et al.* 1996). Reported impairment in visuospatial problem solving as tested through the 'clock test' has also been shown to have good diagnostic sensitivity and specificity for AD (Freedman *et al.* 1994). For community mental health teams and primary care physicians referral for neuropsychological testing is an important adjunct to identify early disease. The utility of early diagnosis apart from the evident need for early therapeutic intervention, includes the opportunity to address vocational issues, financial decision making, caregiver education, and advanced directives.

Depression

Often the question of depression will be an active one during this early disease stage and this should be addressed with review of pertinent symptoms and with diagnostic assessment. Formal rating on instruments such as the Hamilton Depression Scale (Hamilton 1960), Beck Depression Inventory (Beck *et al.* 1961), Cornell Depression Scale (Alexopoulous *et al.* 1988), or the Neuropsychiatric Inventory (Cummings *et al.* 1994) can be very helpful in identifying depression and allowing a treatment plan to be instituted. Tenacious pharmacological treatment of depression may be required with reassessment of cognitive function following treatment to clarify the diagnostic issues. Up to 50 per cent of AD patients will develop depression during the course of their dementia. (Lazarus *et al.* 1987). The interested reader can review Chapter 5 on 'Psychiatric assessment' in this text for a more in-depth discussion of depression and other psychiatric symptoms in dementia. Other more subtle changes in personality and executive functions can be identified early on as well and should be investigated.

Investigations

Both functional and structural brain imaging have contributed significantly to our understanding of the pathophysiology of AD (see also Chapter 6). Their place in establishing a positive diagnosis of AD, however, continues to be limited. Structural imaging with CT or MR imaging allows the assessment of comorbid brain pathologies as well as a qualitative assessment of regional brain atrophy (Mattman *et al.* 1996). Overlapping findings, both with cognitively normal subjects as well as those with non-Alzheimer dementias, limits its utility for positive AD identification. There has been recent interest in measurement of hippocampal volumes with MRI and it remains to be established whether this will have sufficient diagnostic utility for AD. Functional imaging studies with positron emission tomography (PET) and single photon emission computed tomography (SPECT) have demonstrated that there are characteristic regional patterns of impaired cerebral metabolism and blood flow with temporoparietal hypoperfusion/hypometabolism (Foster *et al.* 1983). The cost and technical complexity of PET has limited its application to research settings and the diagnostic sensitivity and specificity of SPECT for AD is debated and has yet to be established. SPECT outside research centres is not recommended at this time for routine clinical practice (Mattman *et al.* 1996).

From the laboratory perspective, biological markers such as Apolipo-protein E4 (Corder *et al.* 1993; Petersen *et al.* 1995), cerebrospinal fluid Tau levels (Arai *et al.* 1995), and β-amyloid fragments in blood and cerebrospinal fluid (Nitsch *et al.* 1995) have been proposed as diagnostic tests for AD. None can be endorsed for routine clinical care at the present time as there is a lack of proven diagnostic sensitivity and specificity with significantly enhanced post-test probability. As a dynamic area of research there will continually be new claims for specific diagnostic tests for Alzheimer's disease that will require careful study and further validation (de la Monte *et al.* 1992; Kennard *et al.* 1996).

Summary

Though there are emerging paraclinical supportive diagnostic tests in development, at present the diagnosis continues to be clinically based with emphasis on neurobehavioural symptoms and cognitive assessment with the careful exclusion of other causes of the dementia syndrome.

Vascular dementia

Vascular dementia (VaD) generally accounts for 10 to 30 per cent of referrals for dementia assessment either in the community or to specialized clinics. There are a range of ischaemic/ heamorrhagic disorders which can produce vascular cognitive impairment and dementia including both cortical and subcortical infarctions, congophilic angiopathy, subacute arteriosclerotic encephalopathy, granular cortical atrophy, and anoxic/hypoxic encephalopathy. The current conceptual framework is that the site in concert with the volume of infarction determines whether dementia will result. In the original neuro-pathological correlative studies, a volume of 100 cc of infarcted tissue was associated with dementia (Blessed *et al.* 1968), though more recently it has been proposed that infarctions as small as 10 cc strategically located can contribute to or cause dementia (del Ser *et al.* 1990).

Clinical diagnosis

Clinical features

The clinical presentations of VaD reflect the diversity of stroke mechanisms and it has been difficult consequently to set diagnostic rules. Vascular risk factors including hypertension, smoking, diabetes mellitus, hyperlipidaemia, and family history of stroke are frequently present. Clinical features will often include a sudden onset, a course that has stepwise decline, or fluctuation with transient or residual focal neurological signs on examination. Bilateral upper motor neurone signs and pseudobulbar palsy support the multifocal nature of the vascular infarcts, particularly those related to lacunas as well as subacute arteriosclerotic encephalopathy (Binswanger's disease). Multifocal sub-cortical infarctions can produce gait disorders including parkinsonism or apraxia, urine incontinence, paratonic rigidity, and bradyphrenia. The cogni-tive deficits are often patchy with relative preservation of some higher cortical functions typically involved in AD, such as new learning. Neuropsychological referral of patients with such atypical patterns of cognitive impairment should be considered and neuroimaging studies carefully reviewed for clinical radiological correlations.

The use of standardized criteria

There have been numerous proposed clinically based criteria for VaD which date back to the early 1970s (Hachinski *et al.* 1974). For vascular dementias, traditional classification protocols have included the Hachinski Ischaemic Score and its modified versions (Rosen *et al.* 1980). Further updated diagnostic proposals including the State of California Alzheimer's Disease Diagnostic and Treatment Centers (ADDTC), the NINDS-AIREN, DSM IV, and ICD-10 have been proposed and are being evaluated (Chui *et al.* 1992; Roman *et al.* 1993; APA 1994; WHO 1989). They integrate CT/ MRI imaging findings addressing the need for clinical radiological correlations. Criteria incorporating imaging increase the reliability of diagnosis from 40 to 70 per cent (Erkinjuntti *et al.* 1988; Pullicino and Benedict 1996). These current criteria have been evaluated concurrently in small studies and it has been recognized that they are not equivalent scales (Verhey *et al.* 1996). It is apparent from Table 14.3 that the definition of dementia differs across criteria as does the need for focal examination findings and/or neuroimaging findings.

Table 14.3 Summary of the main ADDTC and NINDS-AIREN criteria

	The ADDTC Criteria	The NINDS-AIREN Criteria
Dementia Definition	Deterioration from a known level of intellectual function sufficient to interfere with the patient's customary affairs of life, and which is not isolated to a single category of intellectual performance.	Impairment of memory plus at least two other areas of cognitive domains, which should be severe enough to interfere with activities of daily living and not due to physical effects of stroke alone.
Probable VaD	Requires all the following: 1. Dementia 2. Evidence of two or more strokes by history, neurological signs, and/or neuroimaging, or a single stroke with a clear temporal relationship to the onset of dementia 3. Evidence of at least one infarct outside the cerebellum by CT or T1-weighted MRI	Requires all the following: 1. Dementia 2. Cerebrovascular disease: focal signs on examination + evidence of relevant CVD by brain imaging (CT/MRI). 3. A relationship between the above two disorders, manifested by one or more of the following: (a) dementia onset within 3 months of a stroke (b) abrupt deterioration in cognitive functions, or fluctuating stepwise course
Possible VaD	1. Dementia and one or more of the following: 2(a). History or evidence of a single stroke without a clear temporal relationship to dementia onset or 2(b). Binswanger's disease that includes all the following: (i) early onset of urinary incontinence or gait disturbance; (ii) vascular risk factors; (iii) extensive white matter changes on neuroimaging	May be made in the presence of dementia and focal neurological signs in patients with: 1. No evidence of CVD on neuroimaging; or 2. In the absence of clear temporal relationship between stroke and dementia; or 3. In patients with subtle onset and variable course of cognitive deficit and evidence of CVD

CVD-Cerebrovascular Disease.

Reprinted from K Amar, GK Wilcock, M Scott. The Diagnosis of Vascular Dementia in the Light of the New Criteria. Age Ageing 1996;25:51-55, by permission of Oxford University Press.

Investigations

Structural brain imaging is increasingly recognized as essential for the accurate clinical diagnosis of VaD and is required for the application of some proposed diagnostic criteria for VaD. For example the absence of vascular lesions on CT or MRI excludes the possibility of VaD according to the NINDS-AIREN criteria (Table 14.4) (Roman *et al.* 1993). A variety of imaging changes may be seen, reflecting the many different vascular pathologies that can lead to dementia, including single infarcts, hypotension, leukoaraiosis, multiple infarcts, incomplete stroke, and haemorrhage. One major difficulty is deciding which imaging changes represent significant cerebrovascular disease and which may be incidental findings, unrelated to cognitive impairments. As noted, currently two dimensions are deemed important—the first is the location of the lesion, the second its size. Strategically placed infarcts (e.g. in the thalamus) may cause significant cognitive impairment even if small, while diffuse white matter change (leukoaraiosis) or cortical infarcts may sometimes be insignificant (Table 14.4). Not all proposed criteria agree on the imaging changes which are required for accurate clinical diagnosis of VaD, reducing the reliability of these criteria (Lopez *et al.* 1994). In the California criteria (Chui *et al.* 1992), much less weight is placed on the presence of leukoaraiosis than in the NINDS-AIREN criteria, considering it more of interest for research unless accompanied by clinical features suggestive of Binswanger's disease (Table 14.3).

It is important to note that CT has lower sensitivity for detecting vascular lesions, though when they are seen they are more often clinically significant.

Table 14.4 Radiological features considered consistent with vascular dementia according to the NINDS-AIREN criteria.

1. Site

    A. Large-vessel strokes in the following territories:

        (a) Bilateral anterior cerebral artery
        (b) Posterior cerebral artery
        (c) Parietotemporal and temporo-occipital association areas
        (d) The superior frontal and parietal watershed territories

    B. Small-vessel disease:

        (a) Basal ganglia and frontal white matter lacunes
        (b) Extensive periventricular white matter lesions
        (c) Bilateral thalamic lesions

2. Size

        (a) Large-vessel lesions of the dominant hemisphere
        (b) Bilateral large-vessel hemispheric strokes
        (c) Leukoencephalopathy involving at least 25% of total white

Reprinted from GC Roman *et al.* Vascular dementia: Diagnostic criteria for research studies. *Neurology* 1993; 43: 250–260 by permission of Lippincott-Raven Publishers.

MRI has greater sensitivity for detecting vascular lesions, but so much so that periventricular changes and mild/ moderate white matter lesions are seen in over 50 per cent of non-demented elderly subjects (O'Brien *et al.* 1996). While the classic studies of Tomlinson *et al.* (1970) suggested that between 50 and 100 mls of infarcted tissue was needed to develop dementia, imaging studies do support the current notion that both severity and location of lesions are important (Liu *et al.* 1992), though much work still needs to be undertaken to establish the value of imaging changes. Until then, neuroimaging changes should be interpreted in conjunction with clinical history and cognitive and neurological examination. A common mistake is the overinterpretation of small and insignificant cerebrovascular lesions in patients with otherwise typical features of AD or other dementias.

SPECT scanning may be diagnostically useful in VaD, showing a patchy, asymmetric distribution of cerebral blood flow instead of the bilateral, symmetric changes suggestive of AD or DLB (if temporoparietal) or frontal lobe dementia (if frontal). Confirmation of this SPECT utility is still required. The usefulness of other imaging techniques, such as functional MRI, remains to be established.

Summary

The diagnosis of VaD or mixed dementia requires the synthesis of clinical assessment with correlation of neuroimaging vascular lesions. Which of the currently proposed diagnostic criteria will achieve the most widespread use and have the most accurate clinical pathological correlations is not yet clear. Similarly how to integrate neuropathological findings for final diagnosis is not yet settled. With up to 30 per cent of dementia having mixed pathologies of AD and vascular disease, resolution of some of these issues is mandatory to further our clinical approach and to set the way for appropriate patient selection for emerging VaD pharmacological treatments. Whether there will be a differential response of AD, VaD, and mixed dementias to cholinesterase inhibitors or muscarinic agonists remains to be established.

Dementia with Lewy bodies

It has been increasingly recognized that a primary progressive disorder with the clinical profile of fluctuating cognitive impairment, parkinsonism, and psychotic features, characterized neuropathologically by the presence of Lewy bodies in the cortex, is an important cause of dementia. A variety of diagnostic labels have been attached to this condition, including the Lewy body variant of Alzheimer's disease (Hansen *et al.* 1990), dementia associated with cortical Lewy bodies (Byrne *et al.* 1991), diffuse Lewy body disease (Dickson *et al.* 1991), and senile dementia of Lewy body type (Perry *et al.* 1990). A recent consensus meeting advocated use of the term dementia with Lewy bodies (DLB) (McKeith *et al.* 1996), which will be adopted here.

The prevalence of DLB in the community is unknown, but recent neuropathological autopsy studies have found DLB in 15 to 25 per cent of all cases, suggesting it may be the largest pathological subgroup after pure AD. Accurate antemortem diagnosis of DLB is important as such patients have a characteristic and often rapidly progressive clinical syndrome, respond adversely to neuroleptic (antipsychotic) medication, which may hasten their decline, and may possibly be the best responders to cholinesterase inhibitors (McKeith *et al.* 1996).

Clinical diagnosis

The use of standardized criteria

At present, there are no internationally agreed criteria for diagnosing DLB, which does not feature in either ICD-10 or DSM IV. However, shortly after detailed clinical descriptions of case series were reported, two sets of operationalized criteria were proposed (Byrne *et al.* 1991; McKeith *et al.* 1992). These were broadly similar, although the criteria of Byrne *et al.* specified parkinsonism as mandatory for diagnosis. Subsequently, both groups and others agreed on consensus criteria at an international workshop held at Newcastle in 1995. These are shown in Table 14.5 (McKeith *et al.* 1996), though it is important to note that neither the two original sets of criteria nor the current consensus criteria have as yet been prospectively validated by clinical pathological study.

Clinical features

DLB may initially present with dementia, parkinsonism, or both together— the order of onset of mental and motor symptoms being highly variable, particularly in elderly people. Sometimes patients with classic Parkinson's disease develop a dementia characteristic of DLB. As with AD, onset of DLB is insidious and the disorder progressive. Some cases progress rapidly to an end stage of profound dementia and parkinsonism after 1 to 5 years, although in other cases the course may more closely resemble that of AD. The prevalence and demographic features of DLB still have to be accurately defined, though some evidence suggests that men may be more susceptible than women and also have poorer prognosis (Kosaka 1990).

Fluctuation in cognitive function is common and regarded by some as the hallmark of DLB. In the early stages, patients may show global deficits in cognitive function which alternate with periods of normal or near-normal performance. No typical diurnal pattern to this fluctuation has been identified and the periodicity and amplitude of fluctuations are variable, occurring

Table 14.5 Proposed Consensus Criteria For the Clinical Diagnosis Of Probable And Possible Dementia With Lewy Bodies (DLB)

1. The central feature required for a diagnosis of DLB is progressive cognitive decline of sufficient magnitude to interfere with normal social or occupational function. Prominent or persistent memory impairment may not necessarily occur in the early stages but is usually evident with progress. Deficits on tests of attention and of frontal-subcortical skills and visuospatial ability may be especially prominent.

2. Two of the following core features are essential for a diagnosis of probable DLB, one is essential for possible DLB.

   (a) Fluctuating cognition with pronounced variations in attention and alertness.

   (b) Recurrent visual hallucinations which are typically well formed and detailed.

   (c) Spontaneous motor features of parkinsonism.

3. Features supportive of the diagnosis are

   (a) Repeated falls

   (b) Syncope

   (c) Transient loss of consciousness

   (d) Neuroleptic sensitivity

   (e) Systematized delusions

   (f) Hallucinations in other modalities.

4. A diagnosis of DLB is less likely in the presence of

   (a) Stroke disease, evident as focal neurological signs or on brain imaging.

   (b) Evidence on physical examination and investigation of any physical illness, or other brain disorder, sufficient to account for the clinical picture.

Reprinted from IG McKeith *et al.* Consensus guidelines for the clinical and pathological diagnosis of dementia with Lewy bodies (DLB). *Neurology* 1996; 47: 1113–24 by permission of Lippincott-Raven Publishers.

rapidly (lasting minutes or hours), slowly (weekly or monthly), or both. In many cases fluctuation is so severe as to resemble episodes of delirium. As such, before making the diagnosis of DLB, it is important to exclude several conditions including medication toxicity, intercurrent illness, and vascular events as possible causes for the clinical picture. Fluctuation is often a difficult symptom to elicit and quantify but it is helpful to ask carers for detailed descriptions of the patient's mental abilities and functioning at their best compared to their worst. Caregivers frequently report that patients with DLB are somnolent, show reduced awareness, and have episodes of going blank or switching off.

Visual hallucinations are reported in over 90 per cent of cases of DLB. They are typically recurrent, well formed, and detailed and appear to be the only psychotic symptom which reliably distinguishes DLB from AD or VaD (McShane *et al.* 1995). Themes are often of people and animals intruding into the patient's home though inanimate objects and abstract perceptions such as writing on walls and ceilings are not unusual. Some degree of insight into their unreality is often present. It is the persistence (over several months) of visual hallucinations in DLB which helps to distinguish them from episodic perceptual disturbances which may occur transiently in other dementias or during a delirium.

Spontaneous motor features of parkinsonism, typically mild, are frequently present. Rigidity and bradykinesia are the usual symptoms while hypophonic speech, masked faces, stooped posture, and a slow shuffling gait may also be seen. Resting tremor is less common. As parkinsonian signs may be found in advanced AD and other dementias, parkinsonism appearing for the first time late in the course of the dementia is consistent with a diagnosis of DLB, but not specific for it. An adverse and extreme reaction to neuroleptics is suggestive of DLB and has been found in up to 50 per cent cases in some series.

Personal and social function, as well as performance in daily living skills, may be markedly impaired, even in the early stages of the illness by a combination of cognitive and neurological disability. Other features which would support the diagnosis of DLB include a history of repeated falls, syncope, and transient loss of consciousness with no other definable cause as well as systematized delusions and hallucinations in other modalities (see Table 14.5).

Neurological signs consistent with parkinsonism, as described above, may be found but are not essential for the diagnosis. Focal neurological signs are absent. Their presence, with a history of fluctuating cognitive impairment, should raise the suspicion of a VaD. As with AD, a variety of non-localizing neurological signs may be present in DLB patients with advanced dementia.

Fluctuation in cognition should, where possible, be demonstrated by documenting variability in cognitive performance over time using standard-ized cognitive tests such as the MMSE. It may be possible during mental status examination to observe attentional impairments and infer the presence of hallucinations from a patient's behaviour. This is most likely if the patient is observed passively, as both will diminish during a conversational interview. Cognitive testing either performed in the office or with the assistance of a neuropsychologist should include tests of memory, attention, visuospatial ability, and executive function (see also Chapter 7). While DLB patients have global impairments or dementia (by definition), they exhibit a profile of impairment quite distinct from those seen in AD. There are prominent deficits on tests of executive function and problem solving such as the Wisconsin Card Sorting Test, the Trail-Making Test, and verbal fluency. There may also be disproportionate impairments on tests of visuospatial performance such as block design, clock drawing, or copying figures. Memory may be less impaired (McKeith *et al.* 1996). However, with the progression of dementia, this selectivity may be lost, making differential diagnosis based upon clinical examination difficult in the later stages when deficits in memory, language, and other cognitive skills overlap those seen with Alzheimer's disease.

Investigations

There are no definitive data about specific abnormalities or special investigations which confirm a diagnosis of DLB. Structural brain imaging may show generalized cortical atrophy in the absence of vascular lesions, as with AD. Prominent frontal lobe changes have been suggestive in a small number of cases (Forstl *et al.* 1993) but further work is needed to confirm this and determine whether such changes may be helpful diagnostically. Abnormalities on functional imaging show reduced cerebral blood flow with a similar pattern to that seen in AD, while electroencephalography shows early generalized background slowing with abnormal transients in the temporal lobes or frontally dominant burst patterns. No specific genetic markers have been identified, although both apolipoprotein E4 (Schneider *et al.* 1995) and debrisoquine oxidase CYP2D6B (Saitoh *et al.* 1995) appear with increased frequency in DLB.

Particular problems of differential diagnosis

The importance of excluding other systemic and brain disorders sufficient to account for dementia, as outlined in the NINCDS-ADRDA criteria discussed above, also applies to the diagnosis of DLB. Otherwise, accurate clinical diagnosis consists of recognition of the characteristic clinical triad of fluctuating cognition, visual hallucinations, and motor parkinsonism along with the exclusion of alternative causes for these symptoms. Main problems in differential diagnosis would be between DBL and AD, VaD, uncomplicated Parkinson's disease, and other conditions with parkinsonism and dementia such as progressive supranuclear palsy . Dementia, fluctuation, and psychosis are frequent in VaD but a history of gradual onset, fluctuating (rather than stepwise) progression, and the absence of vascular risk factors, stroke, focal neurology, and vascular lesions on neuroimaging would suggest DLB. Differentiation from AD is perhaps most difficult, particularly in those DLB subjects without motor parkinsonism. In these cases fluctuation, adverse reaction to neuroleptics, persistent visual hallucinations, a more rapid course, and associated features of falls and syncopal attacks may help identify those with DLB. Of these, recurrent and persistent visual hallucinations may be the most helpful. As yet, the role of genetic tests such as apolipoprotein E4 measurement are unclear, though the increased rate of E4 in DLB as well as Alzheimer's disease suggest this marker is unlikely to be helpful in differentiating AD from DLB. To determine whether other biological markers such as neuroimaging or electroencephalography are helpful in diagnosis, the results of ongoing prospective studies of DLB must be awaited.

Conclusions

While the gold standard for diagnosis of all dementia remains neuro-pathological examination, this chapter has described how the three most common dementias, AD, VaD and DLB, may be clinically diagnosed. In all cases a full history, general examination, and neurological evaluation to include the assessment of mental states are essential.

Selective neuropsychological assessment and neuroimaging studies can assist the diagnostic process, particularly for VaD. The results of further prospective clinicopathological studies will be needed to revise and improve further the clinical diagnostic criteria outlined in this chapter. Specialized dementia clinics have a unique opportunity to impact favourably on the diagnosis and care of patients with dementia in the realms of behaviour, cognition, and function. Increasingly community care teams will be charged with providing a closer to home assessment and management approach. In this setting selective referral for neuroimaging, neuropsychological assessment, and psychiatric assessment/ intervention will be required and indications for such will continue to evolve beyond the current approach. Further discussion of the non-Alzheimer dementias and diagnostic issues is covered in the following chapter.

Acknowledgement

We thank Agnes Sauter for her helpful assistance in the preparation of this work.

References

Key references recommended by the authors are marked with an *.

Alexopoulous, G.S., Abrams, R.C., Young, R.C. and Shamoian, C.A. (1988). Cornell Scale for depression in dementia. *Biological Psychiatry*, **23**, 271–284.

APA (American Psychiatric Association) (1994). *Diagnostic and statistical manual of mental disorders (DSM IV)* (4th edn). American Psychiatric Association, Washington DC.

Arai, H., Terajima, M., Miura, M., Higuchi, S., Muramatsu, T., Machida, N., *et al.* (1995). Tau in cerebrospinal fluid: A potential diagnostic marker in Alzheimer's disease. *Annals of Neurology*, **38**, 649–652.

Beck, A.T., Ward, C.H., Mendelson, M., Mock, J. and Erbaugh, J. (1961). An inventory for measuring depression. *Archives of General Psychiatry*, **4**, 561–571.

Bird, T.D. (1995). Apolipoprotein E genotyping in the diagnosis of Alzheimer's disease: A cautionary view. *Annals of Neurology*, **38**, 2–4.

Blass, J.P. (1993). Pathophysiology of the Alzheimer's syndrome. *Neurology*, **43** (Suppl), S25–S38.

Blessed, G., Tomlinson, B.E. and Roth, M. (1968). The association between quantitative measures of dementia and of senile change in the cerebral gray matter of elderly subjects. *British Journal of Psychiatry*, **114**, 797–811.

Byrne, E.J., Lennox, G., Godwin Austen, R.B., *et al.* (Nottingham Group for the study of Neurodegenerative Disorders) (1991). Diagnostic criteria for dementia associated with cortical Lewy bodies. *Dementia*, **2**, 283–284.

Canadian Study of Health and Aging Working Group (1994). Canadian Study of Health and Aging: study methods and prevalence of dementia. *Journal of the Canadian Medical Association*, **150**, 899–913.

Chui, H.C., Victoroff, J.I., Margolin, D., Jagust, W.J., Shankle, R. and Katzman, R. (1992). Criteria for the diagnosis of ischemic vascular dementia proposed by the State of California Alzheimer's Disease Diagnostic and Treatment Centers. *Neurology*, **42**, 473–480.

Clarfield, A.M. (1988). The reversible dementias: do they reverse? *Annals of Internal Medicine*, **109**, 476–486.

Corder, E.H., Saunders, A.M., Strittmatter, W.J., Schmechel, D.E., Gaskell, P.C., Small, G.W., *et al.* (1993). Gene dose of apoliprotein E type 4 allele and the risk of Alzheimer's disease in late onset families. *Science*, **261**, 921–923.

Cummings, J. and Khachaturian, Z. (1996). Definitions and diagnostic criteria. In *Clinical Diagnosis and Management of Alzheimer's Disease* (ed. S. Gauthier) pp. 3–15. Martin Dunitz, London, UK.

Cummings, J.L., Mega, M., Gray, K., Rosenberg-Thompson, S., Carusi, D.A. and Gornbein, J. (1994). The Neuropsychiatric Inventory. *Neurology*, **44**, 2308–2314.

de la Monte, S.M., Volicer, L., Hauser, S.L. and Wands, J.R. (1992). Increased levels of neuronal thread protein in cerebrospinal fluid of patients with Alzheimer's disease. *Annals of Neurology*, **32**, 733–742.

del Ser, T., Bermejo, F., Portera, A., Arredondo, J.M., Bouras, C. and Constantinidis, J. (1990). Vascular dementia. A clinicopathological study. *Journal of the Neurological Sciences*, **96**, 1–17.

Dickson, D.W., Ruan, D., Crystal, H., Mark, M.H., Davies, P., Kress, Y., *et al.* (1991). Hippocampal degeneration differentiates diffuse Lewy body disease (DLBD) from Alzheimer's disease: light and electron microscopic immunocytochemistry of CA2–3 neurites specific to DLBD. *Neurology*, **41**, 1402–1409.

Erkinjuntti, T., Haltia, M., Palo, J., Sulkava, R. and Paetau, A. (1988). Accuracy of the clinical diagnosis of vascular dementia: A prospective clinical and post-mortem neuropathological study. *Journal of Neurology, Neurosurgery,and Psychiatry*, **51**, 1037–1044.

Evans, D.A., Funkenstein, H.H., Albert, M.S., Scherr, P.A., Cook, N.R., *et al.* (1989). Prevalence of AD in a Community Population of Older Persons. *Journal of the American Medical Association*, **262**, 2551–2556.

Feldman, H. and Gracon, S. (1996). Alzheimer's disease: symptomatic drugs under development. In *Clinical Diagnosis and Management of Alzheimer's Disease*, (ed. S. Gauthier) pp. 239–259. Martin Dunitz, London UK.

Folstein, M.F., Folstein, S. and McHugh, P.R. (1975). Mini-mental state: A practical method for grading the cognitive state of patients for the clinician. *Journal of Psychiatric Research*, **12**, 189–198.

Forstl, H., Burns, A. and Levy, R. (1993). The Lewy-body variant of Alzheimer's disease. Clinical and pathological findings. *British Journal of Psychiatry*, **162**, 385–392.

Foster, N.L., Chase, T.N., Fedio, P., Patronas, N.J. and Brooks, R.A. (1983). Alzheimer's disease: Focal cortical changes shown by positron emission tomography. *Neurology*, **33**, 961–965.

Freedman, M., Leach, L., Kaplan, E., Winnocker, G., Schulman, K.I. and Dalis, D.C. (1994). *Clock Drawing and Neuropsychology Analysis*, Oxford University Press, New York.

Gearing, M., Mirra, S.S., Hedreen, J.C., Sumi, S.M., Hansen, L.A. and Heyman, A. (1995). The Consortium to Establish a Registry for Alzheimer's Disease (CERAD) Part X. Neuropathology confirmation of the clinical diagnosis of Alzheimer's disease. *Neurology*, **45**, 461–466.

Goate, A., Chartier-Harlin, M.C. and Mullan, M. (1991). Segregation of a missense mutation in the amyloid precursor protein gene with familial Alzheimer's disease. *Nature*, **349**, 704–706.

Hachinski, V.C., Lassen, N.A. and Marshal, J. (1974). Multi-infarct dementia: A cause of mental deterioration in the elderly. *Lancet*, **2**, 207–210.

Hamilton, M. (1960). A rating scale for depression. *Journal of Neurology, Neurosurgery, and Psychiatry*, **23**, 56–62.

Hansen, L., Salmon, D., Galasko, D., Masliah, E., Katzman, R., DeTeresa, R., *et al.* (1990). The Lewy body variant of Alzheimer's disease: A clinical and pathological entity. *Neurology*, **40**, 1–8.

Kennard, M.L., Feldman, H., Yamada, T. and Jefferies, W.A. (1996). Serum levels of the iron binding protein, p97 are elevated in Alzheimer's disease. *Nature Medicine*, **2**, 1230–1235.

Kosaka, K. (1990). Diffuse Lewy body disease in Japan. *Journal of Neurology*, **237**, 197–204.

Koss, E., Edland, S., Fillenbaum, G., Mohs, R.C., Clark, C., Galasko, D., *et al.* (1996). Clinical and neuropsychological differences between patients with earlier and later onset of Alzheimer's disease. Part XII. A CERAD analysis. *Neurology*, **46**, 136–141.

Lazarus, L.W., Newton, N., Cohler, B., Lesser, J. and Schweon, C. (1987). Frequency and presentation of depressive symptoms in patients with primary degenerative dementia. *American Journal of Psychiatry*, **144**, 41–45.

Liu, C.K., Miller, B.L., Cummings, J.L., Mehringer, C.M., Goldberg, M.A., Howng, S.L., *et al.* (1992). A quantitative MRI study of vascular dementia. *Neurology*, **42**, 138–143.

Lopez, O.L., Larumbe, M.R., Becker, J.T., Rezek, D., Rosen, J., Klunk, W., *et al.* (1994). Reliability of NINDS-AIREN clinical criteria for the diagnosis of vascular dementia. *Neurology*, **44**, 1240–1245.

Mann, U.M., Mohr, E., Gearing, M. and Chase, T.N. (1992). Heterogeneity in Alzheimer's disease: Progression rate segregated by distinct neuropsychological and cerebral metabolic profiles. *Journal of Neurology, Neurosurgery,and Psychiatry*, **55**, 956–959.

Mattman, A., Feldman, H., Forster, B., Li, D., Szasz, I., Beattie, B.L., *et al.* (1996). Regional HmPAO SPECT and CT measurements in the diagnosis of Alzheimer's disease. *Canadian Journal of Neurological Sciences*, **24**, 22–28.

Mayeux, R., Stern, Y., Ottman, R., Tatemichi, T.K., Tang, M.X., Maestre, G., *et al.* (1993). The apolipoprotein epsilon 4 allele in patients with Alzheimer's disease. *Annals of Neurology*, **34**, 752–754.

McKeith, I.G., Perry, R.H., Fairburn, A.F., Jabeen, S. and Perry, E.K. (1992). Operational criteria for senile dementia of Lewy body type. *Psychological Medicine*, **22**, 911–922.

*McKeith, I.G., Galasko, D., Kosaka, K., Perry, E.K., Dickson, D.W., Hansen, L.A., *et al.* (1996). Consensus guidelines for the clinical and pathological diagnosis of dementia with Lewy bodies (DLB): report of the consortium on DLB international workshop. *Neurology*, **47**, 1113–1124.

*McKhann, G., Drachman, D.A., Folstein, M., Katzman, R., Price, D.L. and Stadlan, E.M. (1984). Clinical diagnosis of Alzheimer's disease—Report of the NINCDS-ADRDA Work Group under the auspices of Department of Health and Human Services Task Force on Alzheimer's disease. *Neurology*, **34**, 939–944.

McShane, R., Gedling, K., Reading, M., *et al.* (1995). Prospective study of relations between cortical Lewy bodies, poor eyesight and hallucinations in Alzheimer's disease. *Journal of Neurology, Neurosurgery,and Psychiatry*, **59**, 185–188.

Morris, J.C., McKeel, D.W., Fulling, K., Torack, R.M. and Berg, L. (1988). Validation of clinical diagnostic criteria for Alzheimer's disease. *Annals of Neurology*, **24**, 17–22.

Nitsch, R.M., Rebeck, G.W., Deng, M., Richardson, U.I., Tennis, M., Schenk, D.B., *et al.* (1995). Cerebrospinal fluid levels of amyloid beta-protein in Alzheimer's disease: inverse correlation with severity of dementia and effect of apolipoprotein E genotype. *Annals of Neurology*, **37**, 512–518.

O'Brien, J.T., Desmond, P., Ames, D., Harrigan, S., Schweitzer, I. and Tress, B. (1996). A magnetic resonance imaging study of white matter lesions in depression and Alzheimer's disease. *British Journal of Psychiatry*, **168**, 477–485.

Perry, R.H., Irving, D., Blessed, G., Fairbairn, A. and Perry, E.K. (1990). Senile dementia of Lewy body type. A clinically and neuropathologically distinct form of Lewy body dementia in the elderly. *Journal of the Neurological Sciences*, **95**, 119–139.

Petersen, R.C., Smith, G.E., Ivnik, R.J., Kokmen, E. and Tangalos, E.G. (1994). Memory function in very early Alzheimer's disease. *Neurology*, **44**, 867–872.

*Petersen, R.C., Smith, G.E., Ivnik, R.J., Tangalos, E.G., Schaid, D.J., Thibodeau, S.N., *et al.* (1995). Apolipoprotein E status as a predictor of the development of Alzheimer's disease in memory-impaired individuals. *Journal of the American Medical Association*, **273**, 1274–1278.

Pullicino, P. and Benedict, R. (1996). Structural imaging in vascular dementia. In *Vascular Dementia* (ed.I. Prohovnik, J. Wade, S. Knezevic, T. Tatemichi and T. Erkinjuntti) pp. 247–292. Wiley Press, Cichester, UK.

*Roman, G.C., Tatemichi, T.K., Erkinjuntti, T., Cummings, J.L., Masdeu, J.C., Garcia, J.H., *et al*. (1993). Vascular dementia: diagnostic criteria for research studies. Report of the NINDS-AIREN International Workshop. *Neurology*, **43**, 250–260.

Rosen, W.G., Terry, R.G., Fuld, P.A., Katzman, R. and Peck, A. (1980). Pathological verification of ischemic score in differentiation of dementias. *Annals of Neurology*, **7**, 486–488.

Sadovnick, A.D., Irwin, M.E., Baird, P.A. and Beattie, B.L. (1989). Genetic studies on an Alzheimer clinic population. *Genetic Epidemiology*, **6**, 633–643.

Saitoh, T., Xia, Y., Chen, X., Masliah, E., Galasko, D., Shults, *et al*. (1995). The CYP2D6B mutant allele is overrepresented in the Lewy body variant of Alzheimer's disease. *Annals of Neurology*, **37**, 110–112.

Schneider, J.A., Gearing, M., Robbins, R.S., de L'Aune, W. and Mirra, S.S. (1995). Apolipoprotein E genotype in diverse neurodegenerative disorders. *Annals of Neurology*, **38**, 131–135.

Sherrington, R., Rogaev, E.I., Liang, Y., Rogaeva, E.A., Levesque, G., Ikeda, *et al*. (1995). Cloning of a gene bearing missense mutations in early-onset familial Alzheimer's disease. *Nature*, **375**, 754–760.

Skoog, I., Nilsson, L., Palmertz, B., Andreasson, L.A. and Svanborg, A. (1993). A population-based study of dementia in 85-year-olds. *New England Journal of Medicine*, **328**, 153–158.

Snowdon, D.A., Kemper, S.J., Mortimer, J.A., Greiner, L.H., Wekstein, D.R. and Markesbery, W.R. (1996). Linguistic ability in early life and cognitive function and Alzheimer's disease in late life. *Journal of the American Medical Association*, **275**, 528–532.

Snowdon, D.A., Greiner, L.H., Mortimer, J.A., Riley, K.P., Greiner, P.A., and Markesbery, W.R. (1997). Brain infarction and the clinical expression of Alzheimer disease. The Nun Study. *Journal of the American Medical Association,* **277**, 813–817.

Teng, E.L. (1987). The Modified Mini-Mental State (3MS) Examination. *Journal of Clinical Psychiatry,* **48**, 314–318.

Tierney, M.C., Fisher, R.H., Lewis, A.J., Zorzitto, M.L., Snow, W.G., Reid, *et al.* (1988). The NINCDS-ADRDA Work Group criteria for the clinical diagnosis of probable Alzheimer's disease: a clinicopathologic study of 57 cases. *Neurology,* **38**, 359–364.

Tierney, M.C., Szalai, J.P., Snow, W.G., Fisher, R.H., Nores, A., Nadon, *et al.* (1996). Prediction of probable Alzheimer's disease in memory-impaired patients: A prospective longitudinal study. *Neurology,* **46**, 661–665.

Tomlinson, B.E., Blessed, G. and Roth, M. (1970). Observations on the brains of demented old people. *Journal of the Neurological Sciences,* **11**, 205–242.

*Verhey, F.R.J., Lodder, J., Rozendaal, N. and Jolles, J. (1996). Comparison of seven sets of criteria used for the diagnosis of vascular dementia. *Neuroepidemiology,* **15**, 166–172.

WHO (World Health Organization) (1989). *ICD-10 Manual of the International Statistical Classification of Diseases, Injuries and Causes of Death* (10th edn). World Health Organization, Geneva.

15 Other dementias

William Pryse-Phillips and Lars-Olof Wahlund

Introduction

Cognition is the action or faculty of knowing—knowledge—implying consciousness. The complex faculty is taken to include orientation, attention, memory, language functions, gnosis, visual perception, comprehension, abstraction, reasoning, constructional praxis, judgement, and new learning.

Definitions of dementia emphasize memory loss, the presence of other cognitive disturbances, a progressive course, and the presence of diffuse brain disease. Thus the DSM-IIIR criteria for probable Alzheimer's disease require the presence of dementia; deficits in two or more areas of cognition; progression; normal consciousness; and the absence of other diagnosable pathologies. The diagnosis is supported by progressive deterioration of specific cognitive skills; impaired Activities of Daily Living and inappropriate behaviour; positive family history; normal cerebrospinal fluid; normal electroencephalography (EEG) or non-specific changes only; and CT evidence of cerebral atrophy. But to require the absence of other pathologies begs the question as to the diagnosis and makes the diagnosis of Alzheimer's disease one of exclusion. In this chapter, we will survey briefly those conditions which fulfil many of the criteria for Alzheimer's disease but exhibit physical signs or other clinical features which disallow that diagnosis. As there are so many of them, those occurring less frequently are included in an appendix at the end of this chapter.

The first consideration of a clinician on encountering a possibly dementing patient is to determine whether the patient is in fact demented or not, and if so, how badly? The answer comes from the clinical history (including the history from a caregiver); the family and medical history and the social history; the clinical examination of mental state; a neuropsychological examination and often the use of rating scales. Questions must target the personal, social, medical, and medication history of the subject—over-medication, depression, pseudodementia, hypothyroidism, and malnutrition are representative conditions giving rise to the appearances of a dementing state.

The next question concerns the pathology of the (true) dementia. Again, this may be answered from the clinical history (including the history from a caregiver); from the clinical examination of the central nervous system and the support systems; and from the results of investigations. However, no test result profile reliably predicts dementia pathology.

Physical signs are only a feature of Alzheimer's disease in the most advanced cases or in patients with, for example, superimposed vascular dementia. Evidence of diffuse cortical dysfunction is best assessed using the Dartmouth Battery which examines perseveration; the nuchocephalic reflex; pursuit eye movements; the glabellar tap sign; upgaze, downgaze, and gaze maintenance; gegenhalten (or paratonia, in both the arms and the legs); and limb position maintenance (Jenkyn *et al.*, 1977). In addition, the clinician must search for signs of basal ganglia disease, such as bradykinesia, dystonia, axial rigidity, tremor, chorea, and slowed responses; for other motor signs such as pyramidal, cerebellar, or lower motor neurone lesions; for abulia; and for cortical sensory deficits, including extinction. The presence of any of these makes the diagnosis of Alzheimer's disease questionable, and the same is true if seizures, myoclonus, early impairment of speech and language, autonomic features such as incontinence, gait disturbance, or any asymmetry of neurological findings are detected. The presence of any evidence of systemic vasculopathy or of other systemic disease must also raise serious question about the diagnosis of Alzheimer's disease.

Subcortical dementia

The term 'subcortical dementia' indicates that dementias occurring in degenerative disorders involving subcortical structures differ from those with mainly cortical atrophy. Clinically, the dementia in such cases is accompanied by prominent motor disturbances, especially slowing of motor responses, but also by apathy, depression, dysarthria, inappropriate emotional display (irritability or euphoria), and by impaired ability to retrieve and manipulate abstract knowledge. Other intellectual deficits include forgetfulness, apathy, and depression; very slow thought processes; altered personality with irritability, euphoria, and often inappropriate emotional display; and impaired manipulation of abstract knowledge (e.g. comprehension and calculation) (Brown and Marsden, 1988; Cummings, 1990). However, language-dependent skills and perceptual-motor abilities are relatively well preserved if the subject is not pressed for time and other such typical 'cortical' signs as aphasias, apraxias, agnosias, visual field deficits, etc. are not evident. Although criticisms of this clinical differentiation have been made and its validity is disputed, the differentiation represents a useful clinical insight which allows an initial step in diagnosis to be expedited.

These changes are thought to be based upon the primary problem of excessive delay in motor performance as in Parkinson disease and its variants, such as progressive supranuclear palsy, both multisystem degenerations in which the slowness in performance of intellectual tasks is considered as due to disturbances in the brain's activating, alerting, or timing mechanisms. Paramedian thalamic infarctions, normal pressure hydrocephalus, Binswanger and Huntington's diseases are other diseases placed in this category.

Atypical features of dementias apart from the above-mentioned neurological signs include an early age of onset, rapid course, early seizures or myoclonus, early change in personality, previous stroke, fever, and the coexistence of cancer or rheumatological disorders. In general, it may be stated that in the presence of any neurological symptoms (headache, myoclonus or seizures, cramps, sensory losses, etc.) or of localizing physical signs, then the diagnosis of Alzheimer's disease must be treated with scepticism.

A listing of the more important dementing or dementia-like syndromes other than Alzheimer's disease is provided in Table 15.1. A listing of commonly used laboratory and radiological tests is provided in Table 15.2.

Clinical syndromes of dementia

Conditions simulating dementia

Age-related cognitive decline

The unique existence of this condition or conditions is disputed, but it is described as the occurrence of mild and isolated memory changes involving recall rather than registration or retention, or other isolated cognitive change, during normal ageing. That the disorder is different from early Alzheimer's disease is still not generally accepted (see Chapter 13 for a more detailed discussion).

Pseudodementia

The term 'pseudodementia' refers to a clinical syndrome characterized by apparent dementia which, however, is not caused by organic mental dysfunction but rather is most often seen in the setting of depression (Kaplan and Sadock, 1991). The main varieties include 'Ganser syndrome', hysterical dementia, simulated dementia, and depression (Lishman 1988); the last of these is the most common cause of a pseudodementing syndrome and the other forms are extremely rare.

In one large study in England and Wales from 1974, it was found that 8 per cent of the diagnoses of dementia were later changed to depression, which implies that depression in the elderly is one of the most important differential diagnoses from dementia (Nott and Fleminger, 1975). This is of special

Table 15.1 Dementing or dementia-like syndromes other than Alzheimer's disease

A. Conditions that simulate dementia	
Delirium	Pseudodementia of depression
Depression	Paraphrenia
Drug effects	Amnestic syndrome
Age-related cognitive decline	
B. Systemic disease with cognitive deficits	
Severe nutritional disturbance	Pellagra
Wernicke–Korsakoff syndrome	Disorders of thyroid and parathyroid glands
Vitamin B_{12} deficiency	Cushing, Addison, Wilson disease
Organ failure	Dialysis encephalopathy
Hypoxic, hypoglycaemic brain damage	Collagen-vascular diseases
Metal or other toxins	Whipple disease
C. Vascular disease of the brain (see Chapter 14)	
D. Other primary degenerative diseases of the brain	
Dementia of Lewy body type (see Chapter 14)	
Progressive supranuclear palsy	
Other conditions listed in Table 15.3	
E. Neurological disease incurring cognitive deficits	
Cerebral trauma	Epilepsy
Syphilis	Normal pressure hydrocephalus
Cerebral tumour	Chronic subdural haematoma
Progressive Multifocal leukoencephalopathy	Amyotrophic lateral sclerosis
Multiple sclerosis	Muscular dystrophy
Parkinsonism-plus	Primary CNS lymphoma
Granulomatous angiitis	Fungal meningitis
AIDS	Postencephalitis or -abscess
F. Genetic diseases sometimes presenting in adult life	
Adrenoleukodystrophy	Mucolipidosis
Alexander disease	Fabry disease
Glucosylceramide lipidosis	GM1 gangliosidosis
Krabbe disease	Metachromatic leukodystroiphy
Neuronal ceroid lipofuscinosis	Niemann–Pick disease

importance since the disorder is treatable. The reason for seeming cognitive dysfunctions in patients with depression is likely to be the general psycho-motor retardation which accompanies depression, accompanied by a withdrawal of interest and attention from the environment. Events fail to register due to lack of ability to attend and concentrate. In consequence the patients show disorientation, impairment of recent memory and defective knowledge of current events. In neuropsychological tests—Mini Mental State Examination (MMSE)—and similar, the depressed patients often achieve low scores due to lack of endurance. These patients often answer 'I don't know' or 'This is too difficult for me' before truly trying to solve the problems. Of note clinically in such cases is the absence of any evidence of defects of higher cortical function such as dysphasia or apraxia.

Table 15.2 Commonly used laboratory and radiological tests in dementia

Commonly used tests	
Full/ complete blood count	
Erythrocyte sedimentation rate	Liver function tests
Urea and electrolytes	Drug levels
Syphilis serology	Thyroid function tests
Vitamin B_{12} and folate levels	
EEG	CT scan
Evoked potential studies	MRI scan
CSF studies	SPECT scanning
Other relevant investigations, when clinically appropriate include	
Collagen-vascular screen, arteriogram	
Blood sugars	
Biochemical markers of porphyria, e.g. PBG Porphobrilinogen	
Serum calcium	
Hg, As, thallium, Pb, phosphate	
Cortisols	
Cu, ceruloplasmin	
C26:22 ratio; V. Long Chain fatty acids	
HIV antibody studies	
RISA scan	
Rectal biopsy	
Specific enzyme studies (see text)	
Brain biopsy	

To differentiate depression from dementia, it is important to gather information from many sources; to demonstrate the essential normality of the neurological examination; and to record a normal EEG and CT or MRI. The absence of any blood flow reduction on SPECT images, as typically seen in Alzheimer's disease or vascular dementias, would support the diagnosis of depression. Ultimately, the effectiveness of antidepressant treatment clinches the diagnosis in a number of cases, but sometimes the picture is complicated by the fact that in early Alzheimer's disease the presence of depressive symptoms is common. Chapter 5 considers depression in dementia in more detail.

Systemic disease with cognitive features

Dementia symptoms accompanying vitamin B_{12} deficiency

Vitamin B_{12} deficiency may sometimes induce mental disturbances. Apart from clear psychiatric symptoms, signs of cognitive impairment, confusion, and psychomotor retardation may occur (Lishman, 1988). In one study of subjects with low serum vitamin B_{12} levels (Shulman, 1967), 30 per cent were found to have memory disturbances that reverted after appropriate treatment. Nevertheless, the relationship between vitamin B_{12} deficiency and mental and cognitive dysfunctions is unclear and is mainly based on single case reports.

It should be noted that despite the fact that low concentrations of vitamin B_{12} are common in elderly patients with symptoms of dementia, very few respond positively to replacement therapy. Vitamin B_{12} deficiency in many demented subjects may be due to dietary factors or pernicious anaemia; because replacement is convenient, simple, and cheap, it should be undertaken on wide indications. To assess deficiency, serum levels of vitamin B_{12} are actually insensitive; the levels of the vitamin B_{12}-dependent products homocysteine and methylmalonic acid give a more accurate measure of true vitamin B_{12} deficiency.

Folic acid deficiency

Deficiency of folic acid damages the nervous system even less often that vitamin B_{12} deficiency; but when it occurs, the clinical picture is indistinguishable (Rossor, 1990).

Hypothyroidism

Apathy and cognitive slowing are often seen in connection with hypothyroidism. The picture resembles that seen in the subcortical dementias. The process is insidious and may have reached an advanced stage by the time the diagnosis is made. It is easily overlooked. The diagnosis is most easily made by measuring the serum level of thyroid-stimulating hormone and the patient should recover completely if treated early enough (Rossor, 1990).

Other metabolic and deficiency diseases

Other vitamin deficiencies, especially of the B-vitamin complex, may produce cognitive impairment. The Wernicke–Korsakoff syndrome caused by thiamine deficiency, for instance, is characterized by a severe impairment of new learning, and nicotinamide deficiency may also cause cognitive deficits although the typical presentation is with delirium.

Abnormalities of parathyroid function, corticosteroid homeostasis, and chronic hypoglycaemia are other conditions that should be considered. Renal and hepatic failure may also cause confusional states in their acute stages, and portosystemic encephalopathy can be associated with a reversible dementia with pyramidal and extrapyramidal signs (Rossor, 1990).

Infectious or granulomatous processes such as neurosyphilis, sarcoidosis, fungal disease of the CNS, HIV-1 related disorders, (Price and Brew, 1988).

Lyme disease, paraneoplastic syndromes such as limbic encephalitis (Gascon and Gilles, 1973; Corsellis *et al.* 1968), toxicity (e.g. lead and mercury), and cerebral angiitis may need exclusion.

Some patients with epilepsy exhibit intellectual deterioration during the course of the disease, usually as a result of the neurological disorder causing the syndrome in the first place (such as Lafora body disease, cranio-cerebral trauma or mitochondrial disorders) or as side-effects of the drugs used to control seizures. The rare Landau-Kleffner and Lennox-Gastaut syndromes are associated with intrinsic cognitive deterioration.

In addition to those described above, there are a number of other conditions which can be associated with impaired cognition or dementia. Some of the more important of these are included in the appendix to this chapter.

Vascular disease of the brain

Vascular disease is considered in detail elsewhere (see Chapter 14) and is an important cause of both dementia and cognitive impairment.

Neurodegenerative conditions presenting with dementia

Frontotemporal dementias (FTD)

Frontotemporal lobe dementias account for up to 10 per cent of all dementing disorders, and may represent the second largest degenerative dementia group in younger people, after Alzheimer's disease. The group is dominated by frontal lobe degeneration of non-Alzheimer's type (FLD), which is a progressive disease predominately of the frontal lobes but also to some extent of the anterior temporal cortical areas (Fig. 15.1). Pick's disease is a histological variant of frontotemporal atrophy differing from FLD by the presence of intraneuronal inclusion bodies, but clinically FLD and Pick's disease are indistinguishable. A few cases of frontotemporal atrophy associated with the amyotrophic form of motor neurone disease have also been described (Brun and Passant, 1996).

Although the frontotemporal dementias usually exhibit bilateral and symmetrical pathology in the frontal and temporal lobes, asymmetrical distribution sometimes influences the clinical picture (Fig. 15.2). One example of this is the condition known as primary progressive aphasia (see below). The common clinical features of frontotemporal dementias comprise behavioural and affective symptoms and speech disturbances.

The typical behavioural symptoms include:

♦ insidious onset and slow progression;

♦ early loss of social awareness (lack of social tact, misdemeanours such as shoplifting);

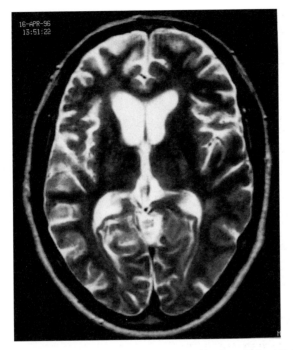

Fig. 15.1 Magnetic resonance image of the brain from a 56-year-old patient with frontal lobe degeneration. A transaxial, T_2 weighted slice through the basal ganglia is shown. The frontal horns of the lateral ventricles and the cerebrospinal fluid spaces around the frontal lobes are enlarged, reflecting an atrophy of the frontal lobes.

♦ early signs of disinhibition such as unrestrained sexuality, violent behaviour, and restless pacing;

♦ mental rigidity and inflexibility;

♦ stereotyped and perseverative behaviour;

♦ distractibility, impulsivity, and impersistence;

♦ early loss of insight into the change of the subject's mental state.

Common affective symptoms are:

♦ depression, anxiety, excessive sentimentality, delusions;

♦ hypochondriasis;

♦ emotional unconcern;

♦ amimia (with lack of spontaneity).

Typical speech disturbances include:

♦ progressive reduction of speech (with lack of spontaneity and economy of utterance);

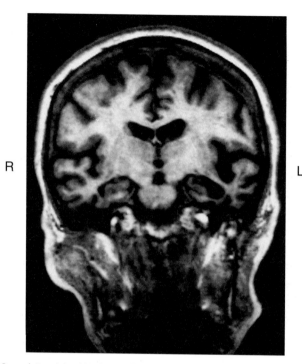

R   L

Fig. 15.2 Coronal, T_1 weighted MRI image of a patient with primary progressive aphasia. The volume of the left (dominant) temporal lobe is markedly reduced.

♦ stereotypy of speech;

♦ echolalia and perseveration;

♦ mutism (late in the process).

Other features supporting the diagnosis include normal EEG recordings, reduced blood flow in the frontal and temporal lobes on SPECT or PET scans and frontotemporal lobe atrophy on CT or MRI. Physically, early primitive reflexes and early incontinence are common (Mendez *et al.*, 1993; Pick, 1892; Brun *et al.*, 1994a).

Frontal lobe degeneration

Frontal lobe degeneration is a slowly progressive dementia with personality changes, affective symptoms, and linguistic disturbances as described above. The onset is usually in the presenium and there is strong evidence of genetic factors. The family history is positive in up to 50 per cent of cases. The mean duration of the disease is 7 years with a range of 3 to 17 years (Brun *et al.*, 1994a, 1994b; Rebeiz *et al.*, 1968).

Pick's disease

Although Pick's disease is the best known of all frontotemporal dementias, it accounts for only 1 to 2 per cent of all cases of organic dementia. Clinically it is almost indistinguishable from frontal lobe degeneration. Histopathologically, Pick's disease differs from FLD mainly by the presence of Pick's inclusion bodies (Brun *et al.*, 1994a,1994b; Mendez *et al.*, 1993; Pick, 1892).

Amyotrophic lateral sclerosis dementia

Rarely, frontal lobe dementia symptoms present in the setting of motor neurone disease such as amyotrophic lateral sclerosis (ALS). Clinically, symptoms of dementia may precede or accompany the evidence of motor neurone pathology (Brun *et al.*, 1994a, 1994b; Rebeiz *et al.*, 1968).

Primary progressive aphasia

As discussed above, speech disturbances may be the first symptoms in fronto-temporal degeneration. In such cases, the pathological process starts asymmetrically in the temporal and frontal lobes on the dominant side, resulting in early linguistic problems such as either fluent or non-fluent speech disturbances. Sometimes a Wernicke's type aphasia dominates but transcortical aphasias are also common (Tyrell *et al.*, 1990; Snowden *et al.*, 1992). None of the progressive aphasia patients express motor disorders. Eventually these patients show cognitive disturbances and personality changes, but this may take a long time and a typical dementing syndrome may not be obvious until after 8 to 10 years (Mesulam, 1982). In such cases, asymmetrical atrophy of the dominant frontotemporal lobes is shown on CT or MRI. The EEG is usually normal (Anderson *et al.*, 1997).

Other diseases with frontal lobe symptoms

Frontal lobe dementia symptoms may also be present in other diseases such as Huntington's disease and neurosyphilis.

Dementia associated with extrapyramidal features

Progressive supranuclear palsy

Progressive supranuclear palsy is a slowly-progressive dementing syndrome of later adult life characterized by the presence of ocular and other neurological signs. The cardinal clinical features include 'subcortical' dementia, parkinsonian rigidity, axial dystonia in extension, pseudobulbar palsy, vertical (later horizontal) gaze pareses, and a poor response to levadopa therapy. Defects in fixation, saccades, pursuit, convergence, and vestibulo-ocular reflexes are also notable. The cause is unknown.

Diagnostic criteria (Hauw *et al.*, 1994; Albert *et al.*, 1974) require:

All of:

♦ onset over 40;

♦ progressive course;

♦ bradykinesia;

♦ supranuclear gaze palsy.

And any three of:

♦ dysarthria;

♦ dysphagia;

♦ extended neck posture;

♦ minimal or no tremor;

♦ pyramidal tract signs;

♦ early gait disturbance;

♦ frequent falls;

♦ more axial than limb rigidity (dystonia).

Without:

♦ early or progressive cerebellar signs;

♦ unexplained polyneuropathy;

♦ dysautonomia other than isolated postural hypotension (not iatrogenic).

The combination of some features of parkinsonism and dementia is also seen in conditions listed in Table 15.3. Most of these are referred to elsewhere in this chapter, including the appendix, or are the subject of separate chapters.

Table 15.3 The combination of features of parkinsonism and dementia

Late Alzheimer's disease	Hallervorden–Spatz disease
Corticobasal degeneration	Vascular dementias
Communicating hydrocephalus (NPH)	Multisystem degenerations
Variants of Pick's disease	Lytico–Bodig (Kuru)
Sporadic ALS	Progressive subcortical glial dystrophy
Familial Parkinson-dementia (Lewy body disease)	

Huntington's disease

Huntington's disease is a progressive neurodegenerative disorder inherited as an autosomal dominant trait as a result of a mutation of a gene on chromosome 4. The clinical evidence is usually first displayed in the third to fifth decades and includes abnormal movements (chorea), deterioration in personality and in cognitive abilities, and psychiatric disturbances. The most typical neuropsychological deficits include slowness of thought, learning failures, and inability to shift mental set or attention. Behavioural changes may antedate the movement disorder by 10 years or more (Moss *et al.*, 1986; Wexler, 1988).

Criteria for the diagnosis have been defined (Folstein *et al.*, 1986):

Definite

(1) chorea or the characteristic impairment of voluntary movement which was not present at birth, was insidious in onset, and which had become gradually worse;

(2) a family history of at least one other member with these typical symptoms of the disease.

Early cases; impairment of movements requiring rhythm and speed, slow voluntary (saccadic) eye movements, mild speech abnormalities, impaired balance on tandem walking, bradykinesia.

Advanced cases; severe slowing or absence of both saccades and pursuit eye movements, severe dysarthria or mutism, inability to walk, long tract motor signs and extreme slowing of all movements.

Dementia and emotional symptoms are usually present but are not required and are not alone sufficient for the diagnosis.

Probable

The clinical features as above but with a family history that was unobtainable because of adoption or unknown parentage.

Creutzfeldt–Jakob disease

This progressive and fatal spongiform encephalopathy is due to prions and it should be considered in any patient with a rapidly progressive course, as other more characteristic features may not occur until the dementia is well established. Criteria for the diagnosis have been suggested (Masters *et al.*, 1979):

1. *Definite*

Neuropathologically confirmed spongiform encephalopathy in a case of progressive dementia with at least one of the following features:

♦ myoclonus;

♦ pyramidal and extrapyramidal signs;

♦ cerebellar signs;

♦ characteristic EEG showing a burst–suppression pattern.

2. *Probable*

As above, without pathological verification.

3. *Possible*

A history of progressive dementia with:

♦ myoclonus and a course of less than 3 years;
♦ a member of the family having transmissible definite or probable disease;
♦ at least two of the features listed under Definite above, together with the appearance of early and prominent signs of a lower motor neurone lesion (amyotrophic form).

Normal pressure hydrocephalus (NPH)

This condition, also known as adult occult hydrocephalus, is an uncommon chronic progressive dementing syndrome of adult life, characterized also by the presence of grossly enlarged cerebral ventricles under normal pressure, urinary incontinence, gait apraxia, and pyramidal signs. Radioimmunosorbent assay scans typically demonstrate reflux of the isotope into the ventricles after lumbar intrathecal injection, and ventricular decompression leads to significant improvement in the physical signs. The severity of the dementia varies from mild apathy to severe psychomotor retardation.

NPH has been claimed to constitute 1 to 6 per cent of all cases of dementia; 80 per cent of patients so diagnosed are over the age of 70 years. The root cause is the impairment of the outflow and resorption of the cerebrospinal fluid into the venous system at the arachnoid villi, which leads to increased intraventricular pressure, relieved only when the ventricles expand.

The primary or idiopathic form accounts for about a third of cases, while NPH is considered secondary to previous subarachnoid haemorrhage in about a quarter, to trauma in a fifth, and to previous strokes in a sixth of cases. Other preceding conditions reported have included intracranial surgery, meningo-encephalitis, lupus erythematosus, arthritis, and various structural causes of partial obstruction to cerebrospinal fluid circulation. Pressure gradients are formed between sites of cerebrospinal fluid production and absorption; the trans-mantle pressure is responsible for the ventricular dilatation. Changes in villi seen after meningitis are absent in idiopathic NPH. Periventricular oedema impairs microcirculation and causes loss of autoregulation. Any added vascular disease present augments the symptoms.

The manifestations of the disease may occur as a result of both mechanical stretching of periventricular fibre pathways and microcirculatory compression or periventricular oedema resulting from transependymal cerebrospinal fluid flow or hypometabolism, leading to globally-impaired cerebral blood flow (misery perfusion) resulting in parenchymal (cortical and thalamic) brain disturbance.

Features

The usual features of the condition include marked apathy, emotional indifference, lack of insight, hostility, aggressiveness, anxiety, delusions, ideas of reference, visual hallucinations, and personality change. Memory impairment is progressive, with fluctuations; a Korsakoff-like picture may supervene, but speech functions and arithmetic ability tend to be retained. Urinary (and bowel) incontinence is a classical feature (Graff-Radford *et al.*, 1989; Adams *et al.*, 1965). The disorder usually progresses over months at most. In one series of patients, 96 per cent displayed mental signs, 95 per cent gait disturbances, and 75 per cent incontinence.

Gait disturbance may precede everything else, including disorders of mentation, and is manifest by the occurrence of falls, retropulsion, and sometimes gait apraxia. Pyramidal signs in the legs, frontal release signs, impairment of postural control, bradykinesia, variable paratonia, and rigidity may be present, so that the syndrome resembles the parkinsonism dementia complex. Patients may become helpless and dependent, up to akinetic mutism. Clinical associations include diabetes, hypertension, heart disease, and cerebrovascular disease.

No single laboratory test is a reliable diagnostic indicator but the following have been employed:

Cerebrospinal fluid pressure monitoring—a single measurement is useless and 24-h monitoring is preferable. It may show:

♦ active hydrocephalus with mean intracranial pressure (ICP) >15 mm Hg and mean resistance to outflow >38 mmHg;

♦ compensated unstable, with lower pressures but with B waves >25 per cent total recording time: (#1 and 2 form about 70 per cent of cases);

♦ compensated stable, pressures< 15 mmHg and with B waves for <25 per cent total recording time.

The predictive value of this test is disputed.

Repeated lumbar puncture (LP) with cerebrospinal fluid withdrawal—30 ml can be removed at 2 to 3-day intervals. Visual reaction times and movement times may improve in patients with NPH. In another study, bladder function improved, both with removal of 50 ml cerebrospinal fluid and after shunting.

Continuous lumbar cerebrospinal fluid drainage of 15 ml/h with controlled resistance in mobile patients predicted the response to a subsequent shunting procedure. Non-responders to such drainage did not do well with shunting. A 3-day period with drainage of <200 ml cerebrospinal fluid may actually be sufficient. However, the response to cerebrospinal fluid removal does not predict the effect of shunting adequately.

Cerebrospinal fluid tap test—this composite measure of psychological and motor responses on the day before and then again within 30 min of removing 40ml of cerebrospinal fluid may have predictive value.

CT—findings include periventricular lucencies, narrow cortical sulci, ballooned ventricles. Frontal and temporal horn indices may predict the shunting response. However, reduction of ventricular size after shunting is not correlated with clinical improvement. High brain elasticity (reflected by pressure volume index) is the best predictor of rapid and marked reduction of ventricular size, but reduction may take months.

Radionucleide cisternography (RISA scan)—typically, the isotope spreads over the convexity is at The Superior Sagittal Sinus (SSS) by 24 hours, and none goes to the ventricles. In NPH, penetration into the ventricles is seen between 8 and 48 h, persisting <3 days; and collection over the surface and at the SSS is markedly reduced or absent, but these findings are not specific for NPH. The standard test is a poor predictor of response to shunting, but late ventricular stasis, as shown by a ratio of ventricular to total intracranial activity (V/T ratio) of over 32 per cent, is a useful marker.

HMPAO-SPECT studies show that regional blood flow is reduced in frontal, temporal, hippocampal, and basal ganglion regions and in the white matter, asymmetrically; but global cerebral blood flow (CBF) is normal. Values improve when ventricular pressure and volume are reduced and increased flow in frontal and hippocampal regions correlates with psychiatric improvement. Low flow rates in parietal and posterior temporal areas are associated with a poor result from shunting, perhaps because this is a pattern which is typical of Alzheimer's disease.

MRI estimation of hippocampal size (but not of ventricular cerebrospinal fluid volume) correlates well with MMSE scores in patients with NPH, but these patients probably have Alzheimer's disease as well. The T_1 and T_2 of the periventricular white matter were significantly prolonged in shunt-responsive NPH patients compared with controls; both values shortened after shunting and both T_1 and T_2 of white matter were longer than those of grey matter in this group of responders, while normals showed longer times in the grey matter. Non-responders had significant prolongation of T_1 in periventricular white matter only.

Periventricular hyperintensity also occurs with older age, encephalomalacia, ischaemia, haemorrhage, oedema, gliosis, neoplasm, axonal loss, degeneration, necrosis, de- and dysmyelination, and lipid change in the periventricular white matter.

Treatment

The usual treatment employed is diversion of the cerebrospinal fluid, using low pressure valve systems. Current criteria for the operation include:

♦ symptoms consistent with NPH;

♦ enlarged ventricles on cranial CT scans;

♦ lumbar cerebrospinal fluid pressure <200mm cerebrospinal fluid;

♦ ventricular filling and convexity block on RIA scan.

However, complications are recorded in about a third (9–50 per cent) and include subdural haematoma (<17 per cent); subdural effusion (<30 per cent); shunt infection; seizures; shunt malfunction requiring revision (13 per cent); intracerebral haemorrhage; infections; and VI palsy in 3 to 4 per cent. Death has been described as occurring in 7 to 25 per cent.

Shunting leads to improvement in 10 to 85 per cent of primary NPH, depending on selection, and in 60 to 75 per cent of secondary NPH. Poor results are reported in patients with severe dementia, even if cerebrospinal fluid outflow resistance is high or the temporal horns enlarged. Any improvement that occurs does so within 3 months of shunting and is independent of valve pressures. The best surgical results are found when there is a full triad of symptoms and signs; there is a short history and progressive features; an initiating cause can be identified; cortical atrophy is not present; there are present frontal periventricular lucencies and gait disturbance precedes cognitive failure.

Genetic diseases which may present with dementia in adult life

In addition to the conditions described above, some other primarily genetic neurological diseases present (uncommonly) for the first time during adult life with evidence of cognitive dysfunction, though almost never without accompanying neurological signs. Most of these however are usually encountered in childhood or infancy (Coker, 1991). Conditions representative of this group are included in the appendix.

Conclusion

In conclusion, although most dementias are caused by one of a relatively small number of conditions, the differential diagnosis of dementia is extensive. Many of the less common conditions are described in this chapter. Differentiating between them is the province of many of the other chapters in this manual. It is important to bear these less common diagnoses in mind as it will influence the treatment and management of the condition. Fortunately, our increased understanding of the pathological background of some of the most commonly occurring conditions is increasingly, resulting in the development of meaningful therapeutic strategies, and this knowledge may eventually be helpful in the treatment of the less common conditions described here.

Appendix

Additional systemic diseases associated with cognitve impairment or dementia

Limbic dementia

Limbic dementia is the term applied to a syndrome of amnesia and behavioural change (including denial of illness, distractibility, and an affective disorder) caused by extensive and selective destruction of the limbic system, as by the herpes simplex virus or in the Wernicke–Korsakoff syndrome (Gascon *et al.*, 1973).

Limbic encephalitis

This condition is a paraneoplastic syndrome of the adult brain characterized by inflammatory or degenerative changes in the temporal parts of the limbic system grey matter, resembling those of a viral encephalitis. Clinical manifestations include seizures, followed within weeks by an abrupt, permanent impairment of recent memory, personality changes, variable focal neurological signs, and subsequently dementia and altered consciousness (Corsellis *et al.*, 1968).

Whipple's disease

Whipple's disease is a chronic, multisystem antibiotic-responsive bacterial infection, usually affecting elderly males who manifest a malabsorption syndrome and occasionally neurological features such as gaze pareses, nystagmus, myoclonus, and hypothalamic symptoms. Brain biopsy shows sickle-particle cells and jejunal biopsy is also often positive (Halperin *et al.*, 1982).

Neoplastic angioendotheliosis

This rare, fatal condition of adults is characterized by intravascular malignant metastasis or lymphomatous spread, or diffuse malignant proliferation of endothelial cells, within the lumina of small vessels in many organs. Clinically, a subacute progressive dementing syndrome is the most typical presentation; cortical blindness and various focal or multifocal features have also been described (Knight *et al.*, 1987; Beal and Fisher, 1982).

Mitochondrial encephalopathy

The mitochondrial encephalopathies form a clinically and biochemically heterogeneous group of complex, sporadic, inborn errors of metabolism affecting the energy pathways of mitochondrial metabolism in many systems, and producing *inter alia*, central nervous system syndromes in adults such as seizures, dementia, deafness, headache, somnolence, vomiting, pigmentary retinopathy, optic atrophy, ataxia, myoclonus and/or involuntary movements, psychomotor retardation, myopathy, neuropathy,and sometimes involvement of other organ systems.

Porphyria

Delirium rather than dementia is a more common feature of this genetic disorder of haemoglobin metabolism.

Additional neurological disorders associated with cognitive impairment or dementia

Thalamic dementia

Thalamic dementia is a syndrome of global psychological defects seen rarely in adult patients with paramedian diencephalic lesions. The syndrome is characterized clinically by optic atrophy, ophthalmoplegias, myoclonic seizures, dystonias, spasticity, apathy and slow responses (as is the case of other 'subcortical dementias'), and autonomic disturbances. Mental signs include impairment of attention and of mental control with apathy, poor motivation, slowness in response, amnesia, and emotional lability.

Familial myoclonic dementia (Stern–Garcin syndrome)

This rare condition is a dominantly-inherited form of thalamic dementia, characterized by subacutely progressive memory loss, psychotic behaviour, frontal release signs, hallucinations, and myoclonus over a period of up to 2 years.

Corticobasal degeneration

This rare, slowly progressive degenerative disease of unknown cause affects adults who present with features of parkinsonism and dementia with added pyramidal signs, limb apraxia, alien limb phenomena, dysphagia, chorea, focal reflex myoclonus, postural-action tremor, limb dystonias, rigidity, and cortical sensory loss. The response to levadopa is slight. Neuronal achromasia (swelling of the cell body and resistance to stains), gliosis, and neuronal loss in frontoparietal regions and in the substantia nigra are notable features (Rinne *et al.*, 1994; Rebeiz *et al.*, 1968).

Mesolimbocortical dementia

Mesolimbocortical dementia is another rare, degenerative disorder characterized by neuronal loss and gliosis affecting structures of the limbic system, substantia nigra, caudate nucleus, and inferior olive, and giving rise to features of a subcortical dementia (Verity *et al.*, 1990). Clinically, the late onset of slowly progressive personality changes, 'frontal release signs', and intellectual deterioration, usually without parkinsonism, are major features. Altered consciousness is described.

Subacute diencephalic angioencephalopathy

This syndrome of rapidly progressive impairment of intellect and memory, emotional symptoms, and myoclonus is associated with bilateral destructive lesions of the thalamus due to proliferative inflammatory lesions of the small blood vessels. The cause is unknown.

Heidenhain disease

Heidenhain disease is an insidious, progressive spongy degeneration of the adult cortex with neuronal loss and gliosis, causing severe dementia, cortical blindness, rigidity, athetosis, ataxia, dysarthria, cerebellar signs, and myoclonus leading to death within months of the onset of the illness. The condition strongly resembles Creutzfeldt–Jakob disease but manifests a slower course and shows more pyramidal and extrapyramidal features. Pathologically, there is marked occipital lobe involvement and the frontal lobes are relatively spared (Heidenhain, 1929).

Gerstmann–Straussler–Scheinker syndrome

This condition is a transmissible encephalopathy of humans caused by an unusual pathogen (prion) and presenting with spinocerebellar ataxia, pyramidal signs, and dementia with plaque-like deposits containing the kuru-type amyloid protein and also resembling those of Alzheimer's disease (Kuzuhara *et al.*, 1983). This condition, described first by Gerstmann in 1936, may be a (dominantly-inherited) variant of Creutzfeldt–Jakob disease in which inheritance is of a gene conferring susceptibility to an environmental agent.

Amyotrophic lateral sclerosis–Parkinson–dementia syndrome

The association of these three entities occurs sporadically or as a familial disease, most commonly on Guam but also in Europeans, in whom it may be inherited as a recessive trait (Schmitt *et al.*, 1984).

Multisystem degenerations

This term refers to all of the adult-onset degenerative conditions of unknown cause which show selective involvement of various combinations of defined nuclei and long tracts within the central nervous system. Such structures have included the retina, optic, thalamic and pyramidal pathways, cerebellar cortex and deep nuclei, inferior olives, vestibular nuclei, posterior columns, spinocerebellar and spinothalamic tracts, and anterior horn cells.

Clinically, any combination of extrapyramidal, pyramidal, cerebellar, and autonomic features may occur; gaze palsies and other disturbances of eye movements are described, as is the phenotype of amyotrophic lateral sclerosis. The response to levodopa is transient and incomplete.

This is a clinically and biochemically heterogeneous group of syndromes with adult onset, characterized clinically by any combination of ophthalmoplegia, parkinsonism, cerebellar and pyramidal signs, athetosis, anterior horn cell involvement, and sensory and autonomic neuropathy. Muscle biopsy may reveal ragged red fibres, suggesting the presence of a mitochondrial encephalopathy.

The olivopontocerebellar atrophies, idiopathic orthostatic hypotension, the Shy–Drager syndrome, and striatonigral degeneration are all subsumed under this general heading. The phenotypes include:

Striato-nigral degeneration type (predominant parkinsonism): sporadic, adult-onset parkinsonism, non- or poorly-responsive to levodopa without dementia, down-gaze progressive supranuclear palsy, with severe symptomatic autonomic failure, with or without cerebellar or pyramidal signs.

Olivo-ponto-cerebellar atrophy type (predominantly cerebellar): sporadic, adult-onset cerebellar and/or pyramidal symdrome with severe symptomatic autonomic failure and/or parkinsonism.

Genetic disorders which may present with dementia in late life

These are potentially many, most of which usually present in early life. Some have recognizable 'adult forms' whilst in others the typical juvenile syndrome may occasionally present in later life. The following list includes conditions representative of this group.

Adrenoleukodystrophy

This X-linked disorder presents in adult life with upper and lower motor neurone signs and sometimes cortical signs, including hemianopias and seizures. In some cases, dementia is a notable feature. Female carriers may also show some signs. Diagnosis requires determination of Very Long Chain fatty acid levels.

Alexander disease

This is a dysmyelinative disease which presents rarely in adult life with features resembling multiple sclerosis; or with mental retardation and later ataxia, dementia, and dysarthria. Diagnosis is achieved by brain biopsy.

Fabry disease

The clinical features of this uncommon genetic disorder include painful peripheral neuropathy, angiokeratoma, trunk papules, corneal opacities, cataracts, cardiac disorders, stroke, renal failure, and, rarely, dementia. Diagnosis relies on showing α-galactosidase deficiency.

GM₁ gangliosidosis type III (chronic form)

This condition is recessively inherited and presents in infancy, childhood, or adult life with chorea, tics, dystonia, dementia, and spasticity without viscero-megaly or skeletal signs (Nakano, 1985). Hexosaminidase levels are low.

GM₂ Gangliosidosis—adult (chronic) type

This condition represents a heterogeneous collection of phenotypes reflecting partial deficiency of hexosaminidase A and inherited recessively. They in-clude a spinocerebellar form, another resembling motor neurone disease, and a third with manifestations of each of these conditions, dystonia, dementia, seizures, sensory neuropathy, internuclear ophthalmoplegia, or psychiatric disorders. Diagnosis requires finding low hexosaminidase levels.

Glucosylceramide lipidosis

The Type 1 (**adult**) form is characterized by hypersplenism, jaundice, thrombo-cytopenia, anaemia, arthropathy, and retinal and skin pigmentation. Dementia, seizures, myoclonus, rigidity, ataxia, and sensory neuropathy have been re-ported occasionally, but this type is not ordinarily associated with neurologic dysfunction. Deficient β-glucocererosidase levels in the blood is diagnostic.

Krabbe (globoid cell) leukodystrophy

Krabbe disease is a recessively-inherited, lysosomal diffuse dysmyelinating disease with a fatal course. The **late infantile type** is characterized by optic atrophy, dysarthria, dementia, hypotonia, cerebellar signs, spasticity, myo-clonus, and motor neuropathy. An **adult** presentation with dementia is also recognized. The diagnosis is made by finding globoid cells in demyelinated brain and nerve biopsy specimens, and demonstration of deficiency of galactosylceramidase and the deposition of galactocerebroside.

Kufs' disease (adult amaurotic familial idiocy)

Kuf disease is the dominantly-inherited adult form of **neuronal ceroid lipofuscinosis** in which there is deposition in neurons and other cells of an abnormal lipoprotein with characteristic ultrastructural patterns. Clinically, the disease presents with photosensitive progressive myoclonic epilepsy or with progressive mental deterioration, seizures, and facial dyskinesias but without pigmentary retinal degeneration. Biopsy is required for diagnosis.

Metachromatic leukodystrophy

This disorder is a group of recessively-inherited, lysosomal storage diseases characterized by deficiency of arylsulfatase A. The **adult** form is rare; clinical features include insidious dementia, psychoses, optic atrophy, ataxia, pyramidal and extrapyramidal signs, and neuropathy with onset after the age of 16 years allows diagnosis.

Mucolipidosis (sialidoses) type III

Also known as pseudo-Hurler polydystrophy, this is a recessively-inherited, sphingolipid and mucopolysaccharide lysosomal storage disease in which lipid-like and polysaccharide-like material is deposited in the tissues. Its clinical features include mild mental retardation, ataxia and deafness, with coarse facies, corneal clouding, visceromegaly, aortic or mitral valve disease, and dysostosis. Dementia was described in the 1930s in one family. Deficiency of β-galactosidase and neuraminidase allow the diagnosis.

Neuronal intranuclear (hyaline) inclusion disease

Neuronal intranuclear (hyaline) inclusion disease is a rare, slowly-progressive inherited neuronal storage disorder with onset in childhood, characterized pathologically by the presence of round, eosinophilic antifluorescent inclusion bodies in neuronal nuclei in both the central and peripheral nervous systems. In a **variant form**, the disorder presents in adult life with dementia and a choreic movement disorder.

Niemann–Pick disease type C, juvenile form

The term 'downgaze paralysis, ataxia, foam cell syndrome' was that originally applied to this condition, which has three phenotypical presentations. Type 3 is the delayed-onset form with a slow course, characterized by mild intellectual impairment, vertical gaze pareses, ataxia and variable dementia, seizures, and extrapyramidal defects. Sphingomyelinase deficiency is diagnostic.

Wilson disease

Generally liver disorder appears before the age of 10 years and neurological signs between the ages of 10 and 32 years. Low serum ceruloplasmin and copper and high tissue and urinary copper levels are diagnostic.

Miscellaneous neurological diseases

Cognitive deterioration is a feature of advanced **multiple sclerosis, muscular dystrophy**, **primary central nervous system lymphoma**, and some of the **genetic ataxias**, but is rare in the early stages of such disorders.

References

Key references recommended by the authors are marked with an *.

Adams, R.D., Fisher, C.M, Hakim, S., *et al.* (1965) Symptomatic occult hydrocephalus with 'normal' cerebrospinal fluid pressure; a treatable syndrome. *New England Journal of Medicine*, **273**, 117–126.

Albert, M.L, Feldman, R.G., Willis, A.L. (1974) The 'subcortical dementia' of progressive supranuclear palsy. *Journal of Neurology, Neurosurgery and Psychiatry,* **37**, 121–130.

Anderson, C., Dahl, C., Almkvist, *et al.* (1997) Bilateral temporal lobe volume reduction parallels cognitive impairment in progressive aphasia. *Archives of Neurology*, **55**, 1294–9.

Beal, M.F., Fisher, C.M. (1982) Neoplastic angioendotheliosis. *Journal of the Neurological Sciences,* **53**, 359–375.

Brown, R.G., Marsden, C.D. (1988) 'Subcortical dementia': The neuropsychological evidence. *Neuroscience*, **25**, 363–387.

Brun, A., Passant, U. (1996) Frontal lobe degeneration of non-Alzheimer type. *Acta Neurologica Scandinavica* Suppl. 168, 28–30.

Brun, A., Englund, B., Gustafson, L., *et al.* (1994a) Clinical and neuropathological criteria for frontotemporal dementia. *Journal of Neurology, Neurosurgery and Psychiatry,* **57**, 416–418.

Brun, A., Englund, B., Mann, D.M.A., Neary, D. *et al.* (1994b) Consensus on clinical and neuropathological criteria for fronto-temporal dementia. *Journal of Neurology, Neurosurgery and Psychiatry,* **57**, 416–8.

Coker, S.B. (1991) The diagnosis of childhood degenerative disorders presenting as dementia in adults. *Neurology*, **41**, 794–798.

Corsellis, J., Goldberg, G.J., Norton, A.R. (1968) 'Limbic encephalitis' and its association with carcinoma. *Brain,* **91,** 794–798.

Cumings, J.L. (1990) *Subcortical dementia.* New York: Oxford University Press.

Folstein, S.E., Leigh, R.J., Parhad, I.M., Folstein, M.F. (1986) The diagnosis of Huntingdon's disease. *Neurology, 36,* 1279–1283.

Gascon, G.G., Gilles, F.H. (1973) Limbic dementia. *Journal of Neurology, Neurosurgery and Psychiatry,* **36,** 421–430.

Graff-Radford, N.R., Godersky, J.C., Jones, M.P. (1989) Variables predicting surgical outcome in symptomatic hydrocephalus in the elderly. *Neurology,* **39,** 1601–1604.

Halperin, J.J., Landis, D.M.D., Kleinman, G.M. (1982) Whipple disease of the nervous system. *Neurology, 32,* 612–617.

Hauw, J., Daniel, S.E., Dickson, D., *et al.* (1994) Preliminary NINDS neuropathologic criteria for Steele-Richardson-Olszewski syndrome (progressive supranuclear palsy). *Neurology,* **44,** 2015–2019.

Heidenhain, A. (1929) Klinische und anatomische Untersuchungen uber eine eigenartige arganische Erkankung des Zentralnervensystems im Praesenium. *Zeitschrift Gesamte. Neurol. Psychiatr,* **118,** 49–114.

Jenkyn, L.R., Walsh, D.B., Culver, R.G. *et al.* (1977) Clinical signs in diffuse cerebral dysfunction. *Journal of Neurology, Neurosurgery and Psychiatry,* **40,** 956–966.

Kaplan, H.I., Sadock, V.J. (1991) Geriatric psychiatry. In: *Synopsis of Psychiatry.* Anonymous. Baltimore: Williams and Wilkins.

Knight, R.S.G., Anslow, P., Theaker, J.M. (1987)Neoplastic angioendotheliosis: a case of subacute dementia with unusual cerebral CT appearances and a review of the literature. *Journal of Neurology, Neurosurgery and Psychiatry,* **50,** 1022–1028.

Kuzuhara, S., Kanakawa, I., Sasaki, H., *et al.* (1983) Gerstmann-Straussler-Scheinker's disease. *Annals of Neurology,* **14,** 216–225.

Lishman, W.A. (1988) *Organic Psychiatry.* Anonymous. Oxford: Blackwell Scientific Publications.

Masters, C.L., Harris, J.O., Gajdusek, D.C. *et al.* (1979) Creutzfeldt-Jakob Disease: patterns of worldwide occurrence and the significance of familial and sporadic clustering. *Annals of Neurology,* **5,** 177–188.

Mendez, M.F., Selwood, A., Mastri, A.R., *et al.* (1993) Pick's disease versus Alzheimer's disease: A comparison of clinical characteristics. *Neurology,* **43,** 289–292.

Mesulam, M.M. (1982) Slowly progressive aphasia without generalized dementia. *Annals of Neurology,* **11,** 592–598.

Moss, M., Albert, M., Butters, N., *et al.* (1986) Differential patterns of memory loss in patients with Alzheimer's disease, Huntingdon's disease and alcoholic Korsakoff's syndrome. *Archives of Neurology,* **43,** 239–246.

Nakano, T., Ikeda, S., Condo, K. *et al.*, (1985) Adult GM gangliosidosis. *Archives of Neurology*, **35**, 875–880.

Nott, P.N., Fleminger, J.J. (1975) Presenile dementia: the difficulties of early diagnosis. *Acta Neurologica Scandinavica,* **51**, 210–227.

Pick, A. (1892) Ueber die Beziehungen der senilen Hirnatrophie zur Aphasie. *Prag. Med. Wschr.,* **17**, 165–167.

Price, R.W., Brew, B.J. (1988) The AIDS-dementia complex. *Journal of Infectious Diseases,* **158**, 1079–1083.

Rebeiz, J.J., Kolodny, E.H., Richardson, E.P.J. (1968) Corticodentatonigral degeneration with neuronal achromasia. *Archives of Neurology,* **18,** 20–33.

Rinne, J.O., Lee, M.S., Thompson, P.D., *et al.* (1994) Corticobasal degeneration: A clinical study of 36 cases. *Brain*, **117**, 1153–1196.

Rossor, M. (1990) Miscellaneous causes of dementia. In: *Neurology in Clinical Practice* (eds WG Bradley, RB Daroff, GM Fenichel, CD Marsden). Boston: Butterworth-Heinemann.

Schmitt, H.P., Emwer, W., Heimes, C. (1984) Familial occurrence of amyotrophic lateral schlerosis, parkinsonism, and dementia. *Annals of Neurology,* **16**, 642–648.

Shulman, R. (1967) Psychiatric aspects of pernicious anaemia: A prospective controlled investigation. *British Medical Journal,* **1**, 266–270.

Snowden, J.S., Neary, D., Mann, D.M.A., *et al.* (1992) Progressive language disorder due to lobar atrophy. *Annals of Neurology,* **31**, 174–183.

Tyrell, P.J., Warrington, E.K., Frackowiak, S.J., *et al.* (1990) Heterogeneity in progressive aphasia due to focal cortical atrophy. *Brain*, **113**, 1321–1336.

Verity, M.A., Roitberg, B., Kepes, J.J. (1990) Mesolimbocortical dementia: clinical-pathological studies on two cases. *Journal of Neurology, Neurosurgery and Psychiatry,* **53**, 492–495.

Wexler, N. (1998) Huntingdon's disease. *Current Opinion in Neurology and Neurosurgery*, **1**, 319–323.

3 Management

16 Carer support

J. Gilliard and P. V. Rabins

Introduction

It is estimated that dementia affects approximately one in ten of the population over the age of 65, one in five of those over the age of 80, and a smaller proportion of younger people (Alzheimer's Disease Society, 1995). This means that there are about 640 000 people with dementia in the United Kingdom and approximately 3 900 000 in the United States. Most of these are cared for by a family member, so that when we consider the numbers of people who are affected by dementia we should probably at least double the above figures.

The impact of dementia on family members cannot be overlooked because the majority of people with dementia remain in their own homes for most of the course of the condition, and are cared for by family members. Care in the community means care by the community—those family members or friends who are referred to as 'informal carers', but who may not perceive themselves as a carer. They may be supported by professional service providers, whose own needs are often overlooked in the focus on the 'stress' and 'burden' of family care.

Caring for someone with dementia is very isolating (Mace and Rabins, 1985). It becomes harder to go out and socialize, and people stop visiting because of their own fears, ignorance, or prejudice. Caring for a person with dementia can cause many feelings which we are not proud to own. The importance of an impartial, non-judgmental listener should be recognized. In a small survey of carers from the Bristol Memory Disorders Clinic (Gilliard, 1991 unpublished), 85 per cent said they had other members of their family to whom they could turn in case of difficulty, but 82 per cent also said they felt isolated in their caring role. We should not underestimate the loneliness, concerns, and stress of those who care for a person with dementia.

The caring career

The stress and burden experienced by carers of people with dementia varies from day to day, according to the pattern of the patient's dementia. It is more

Table 16.1 A medical model of the progression of dementia (Jacques, 1988)

Healthy	
Questionable dementia	the person is beginning to behave oddly and relatives are wondering if something may be wrong
Mild dementia	there is definitely a problem, but the person with dementia is still able to maintain independence
Moderate dementia	help is required with the tasks of daily living; the person may wander, become aggressive and cause other difficulties; this is often the hardest stage for carers
Severe dementia	the person becomes gradually more frail until they are chair- or bed-bound

Table 16.2 A nine-stage 'social model' informed by listening to the experiences of people who have dementia (Keady *et al.*, 1995)

Slipping	The person with dementia often notices that
Suspecting	he/she is having difficulties, but keeps this
Covering up	concern private
Revealing	Sharing concerns with another
Confirming	Sharing concerns with a professional and reaching a diagnosis
Maximizing	Making the most of the abilities which remain
Disorganization	
Decline	
Death	

closely allied to behavioural disturbance than degree of dementia (Gilleard *et al.*, 1982), and may be dependent on the premorbid relationship between the caregiver and the cared-for person. There are peaks of distress during the caring career, for example on confirmation of the diagnosis or on having to let the person with dementia go into residential care.

The early stages—'slipping, suspecting, covering up'

Dementia is an unusual condition in that it is often first identified and reported by family members rather than the patient. There is evidence that some people with dementia are aware of their difficulties very early on, and often in private activities, so that they think they can conceal their problems from those who surround them (Keady *et al.*, 1995). Inevitably, as the condition progresses, family members become concerned and initiate the seeking of help. At this very early stage, there may be unawareness or denial on the part of the patient that there is a problem and an attempt to conceal the losses.

Keady *et al.* call the first three stages of early dementia 'slipping, suspecting, covering up'. For the family, there is uncertainty about whether the patient is becoming more cantankerous as they age, changing from the familiar spouse or parent into a stranger. Without the knowledge that a diagnosis can confirm, it is possible that there is simply a personality change associated with ageing. Relatives, who will not yet perceive themselves as 'carers', worry that they have done something to cause these problems. Gradually, as the situation deteriorates to the stage where help is requested, the concern shifts from fear of having to live with a stranger to fear of what is causing the problem. Many relatives consult a memory disorders team to have their worst fears confirmed. In these early stages there is often no one to turn to for support because there is no identified problem, just concern.

This prediagnosis stage may also cause difficulties for relatives who can only access services when there is a confirmed diagnosis of dementia. In many localities, the diagnosis opens the gates to service provision. Any delay in reaching a diagnosis, caused for example by the difficulties in making an accurate assessment, may result in continued lack of support for families and friends. This period may last for a year or more, with resultant increased stresses for carers in terms of their coping, and their physical and mental well being. (A medical model of the progression of dementia (Jacques, 1988) is shown in Table 16.1 and a 'social model' (Keady *et al.*, 1995) is shown in Table 16.2.)

Reaching a diagnosis

Finally, the situation reaches a stage at which the relative decides that help must be sought. This may be precipitated by a crisis, for example getting lost while shopping or driving dangerously. The relative seeks help from the general practitioner who may refer on to a memory disorders team. Confirmation of the diagnosis may be a relief, providing an explanation for the personality and behavioural changes and allowing carers to make sense of what is happening. They no longer need to blame themselves. Nevertheless, hearing the diagnosis may be a time of great stress for carers, a time when they can no longer deny that there is something seriously wrong with their relative, when their last vestiges of hope are removed, and when they have to face the future of living with someone with dementia and shifting into the caring role. It is also a time of uncertainty. Many people have heard of dementia, but many still do not understand exactly what it means. Confirmation of the diagnosis is a time for sharing information and carers often find themselves on a fast learning curve.

Having heard the diagnosis themselves, carers are then often faced with the dilemma of sharing this news with the patient. Many people would not want their relative to be told, although they would want to be told if they were themselves the patient (Maguire *et al.*, 1996). The role of the professional at this time is to support the carer, who is often very protective of their relative. The carer may need encouragement to allow disclosure of the information. Even when the diagnosis is imparted by the team, carers will be in the front line in helping the patient to come to terms with its implications, and will often be the mainstay for on-going support, having to explain or repeat the information.

At this stage, most relatives still regard themselves as the patient's spouse or child, or whatever the relationship is. They need to be introduced to the concept of becoming a caregiver. Confirmation of the diagnosis will open the gates to service provision for the patient. Acknowledgement of their role as carer allows access to services for the relative. There will be some relatives who may choose that they do not wish to care, or to continue to care. Society, and governments, assume that families will provide the care and there is tacit condemnation of those who do not wish to take on the role. Occasional carers may go as far as announcing their intention to divorce their partner, rather than provide care. Other carers will relinquish the care to an institutional setting at an early stage. Everyone has a caring threshold, and it is important to recognize that the ability and willingness to care is individual. Younger carers may find it especially difficult when they are trying to balance a career and their caring duties.

Sharing the caring

Most carers regard it as their duty to care and take on this new role with commitment. This makes it hard for them to accept help when they first need it. Perhaps this accounts, in part, for why community help is not sought. The Canadian Study of Health and Aging, for example, found that formal help was rarely used (Canadian Study of Health and Aging, 1994). If caring is seen as a duty and an act of love, it becomes difficult to allow another to take over the caring. Many carers feel that no one can care for their relative as well as they, the carer, can. Any outside help is seen as second best. However, carers should be encouraged to accept help when they feel they need it. Inevitably, all carers of a person with dementia will need some support as the condition progresses. To accept help sooner may obviate a crisis. Our role is to understand how difficult it is to let go, but to encourage the sharing of caring in order to optimize the carer's capabilities so that they can continue to care for as long as they wish.

Allowing someone into one's home in order to share the care is often the first, and very difficult, step. The next stage is usually to permit the person with dementia to go to a day centre, and then move towards longer respite care of a week or two. Most people with dementia are eventually admitted to some form of residential or nursing home care, and this is often the hardest step of all for carers. It may feel as if they are relinquishing their responsibilities completely and failing the person to whom they have devoted much time, energy, and love. Carers frequently require 'permission' to take this step. It can be helpful if a professional from the memory disorders team can explain that it is in the best interests of both parties if the person with dementia is allowed to enter institutional care. Carers are often at their lowest ebb at this point—overwhelmed by the stress of caring and the distress of having to let go—but studies show that admission to residential care is the one factor that can make a permanent and significant difference to carers' perceptions of burden (Levin *et al.*, 1990) and emotional state (Rabins *et al.*, 1990). Many carers report that their relationship with the person with dementia improves when they are admitted to residential care. With the stresses of daily care removed, they can rebuild their relationship at an emotional level. It can be helpful to reframe the decision to allow admission to residential care in this way, so that carers are able to focus on the positive benefits from taking this step.

Bereavement

Finally, there will be a peak of distress when the person with dementia dies. Caring for a person with dementia is more than a full-time job (Mace and Rabins, 1985) and, no matter how difficult it has been, their death leaves a void in the carer's life. Studies suggest that carers will manage their bereavement better if the caring relationship was good. Caring for a person with dementia has been described as a 'living bereavement' (Taylor, 1987), and for some carers the death of the person with dementia marks the beginning of the end of the grief process. For others it is simply a beginning, a time to rebuild their lives without the person for whom they have been caring. Many continue to work with organizations such as the Alzheimer's Disease Society or Alzheimer's Association, using the experience and expertise they have gained from caring to enable others who are still travelling along the caring road.

Support for carers

The need for information

We must listen to carers in order to understand what support they need to help them through their caring (Keady and Nolan, 1995). It seems that, in the early stages at least, they have an insatiable appetite for information. Carers need information to be provided:

♦ clearly;
♦ in language which they can understand—that is without the use of jargon;
♦ repeatedly.

Although they will almost certainly have heard of Alzheimer's disease, caregivers want and need to know the diagnosis and what this really means. They want to hear the prognosis, and they want to know what to expect from this condition called dementia (Gilliard, 1996a). The theory of learned help-lessness suggests that when we are faced with a new situation we often feel helpless; this leads to low morale and poor performance; and this becomes a vicious circle (Seligman *et al.*, 1968; Lubinski, 1991). In the case of carers, hearing the diagnosis from a memory team for the first time, they too feel unsure about how they can cope with the enormity of their new situation. Armed with a library of information, they are better able to cope with what the future holds in store for them. Because the consequences of the diagnosis are pervasive, they may not hear everything that is said to them the first time. The information needs to be given to them repeatedly, and perhaps in writing so they can refer back to it. They also need information about the services and benefits to which they are entitled. Giving carers this information can help to soften the blow because we are telling them that there is help available. It may be helpful to encourage them even from this earliest stage to prepare themselves to accept this help when they need it. Information should be given in the most accessible and acceptable forms. There should be a willingness to talk and listen to new carers, and to answer their questions. This can be followed up with written information, or audio- and video-taped information.

Carers need information about:

♦ the diagnosis;

♦ the prognosis;

♦ the practical implications for the person with dementia and the family;

♦ the health and social services which may be able to help;

♦ financial entitlements;

♦ legal affairs.

Listening support and counselling

Many carers feel isolated, even when they have a relative to whom they can turn. It helps to talk to an impartial and non-judgmental person. Some carers accept counselling to help them come to terms with their new situation and the losses involved in it. But many only require someone who can listen. Volunteers who have been trained and who are supervised and supported are able to provide the sort of befriending which many carers report that they find helpful. Recent research has shown this to be an effective way of supporting carers (Gilliard 1996b). The volunteers require a basic training course with information about dementia and the issues about which carers are concerned, together with teaching on basic listening skills. They are then able to visit and befriend carers, provided that they have supervision on a regular basis and know that they can ring someone for emergency support if necessary.

Some carers will also benefit from qualified counselling. These may be carers who have additional problems within their own family, or they may be carers whose relationship with the cared-for person was difficult before the diagnosis. In our experience, a time-limited series of counselling sessions early in the course of the dementia is often effective at helping carers take on this new role and come to terms with the changed relationship with the cared-for person. A recent study has shown that such a programme can delay early term care placement by one-third over 3 years (Mittelman *et al.*, 1996).

Self-help and support groups

Many carers find it helpful to talk to others who are in the same position, or who have had personal experience of caring for a person with dementia. Self-help support groups are now fairly widespread and accepted as a means of enabling carers (Toseland and Rossiter, 1989). The group may be facilitated by a professional or a volunteer, or it may be run exclusively by and for carers. Some groups have a speaker to provide a focus for meetings; some have a social programme giving carers an opportunity to enjoy some respite; other groups meet to allow carers to talk to each other with no particular focus; and some are a mixture of the above. It must be recognized that there will always be some carers who do not wish to go to a support group. They feel that they would rather use an opportunity for respite to escape completely from their caring duties and pursue other interests.

Written information

Written information which carers can dip into again and again when they feel the need and when time allows, is often welcome. There is, however, little evaluation of written information. Fortinsky and Hathaway asked about services which caregivers reported as 'extremely important' at the time of diagnosis (Fortinsky and Hathaway, 1990). More than 72 per cent (and easily the largest group) wanted written material about Alzheimer's disease. A study by Toner in 1987 evaluated a programme in which a group of carers was given written information about caring for a person with dementia (Toner, 1987). They were compared with a control group who received assessment visits only. The carers who read the booklet reported a reduction in stress levels and said that their attitude towards the person they cared for had changed as a result of reading the booklet. But, as Chris Gilleard points out, knowledge and understanding are not necessarily synonymous, and advice without counsel may not be the best way to proceed (Gilleard, 1990). Written information should complement other efforts to meet carers' needs, and not be seen as a replacement for services. Any written information given to carers needs to respond to them at a personal level, taking account for example of their first language and any impairments which they may have. There is a paucity of information available on audio- or videocassette, or in large print, or in the languages of ethnic minorities (Gilliard, 1996a). Some work has been carried out in America to consider the use which can be made of information technology, and this seems to be helpful for some carers (Brennan *et al.*, 1992, 1995; Smyth and Harris, 1993).

Carers with special needs

It should also be remembered that carers are not a homogeneous group. Most people with dementia are older, and many are cared for by their spouse, so there is an assumption that carers are also older people. This may be true in the majority of cases, but others are also affected by having a relative with dementia, and some of these may be young people. It would help them to have information presented to them in a way which they find acceptable—for example in cartoon form for very young children—but there is little available for them (Evans, undated; Gilliard, 1995; Fearnley, 1996). Similarly, carers of a person with a less usual form of dementia, like Creutzfeldt–Jakob disease or AIDS related dementia, may find it helpful to have information which speaks directly to them in addition to more general information about dementia and caring.

Information about services and benefits

Carers also need, and indeed deserve, to receive information about their entitlements, both in terms of service provision and benefits which they can claim. This will vary according to locality, but the sort of services which carers require information about will include domiciliary care, sitting services, day care, respite care, and residential facilities. Carers need to build a 'library of knowledge' about service provision so that they can dip into this library and access information and services when they are required. In our experience carers often find it difficult to allow themselves to accept help and even harder to ask for it. They need to be encouraged and supported through the difficult stage of seeking assistance for the first time.

Carers also need to develop a knowledge of the benefits which exist to support them. This may be financial help which the person they care for is entitled to claim, as well as the benefits which are paid to them as carers. Again they may be reluctant to claim this help, often saying that they feel others are more deserving than they are. They need gentle support to see them through this, ranging from information giving to practical help in form filling. Carers also need information about their legal rights and in particular how to manage the affairs of the person with dementia. There is a growing trend towards discussion of the diagnosis with the person with dementia (Erde *et al.*, 1988; Drichamer and Lachs, 1992; Gilliard and Gwilliam, 1996; Maguire *et al.*, 1996) (see Chapters 18 and 19), and it is therefore often appropriate to talk to carers about living wills or advanced directives.

Training for carers

There is evidence that carers do well if they are offered some form of education or training (Brodaty and Gresham, 1989; Magni *et al.*, 1995). This refers back to the theory of learned helplessness. As well as giving carers support by means of personal contact, they can be assisted through attending training programmes. The most successful format for this seems to be a course spread over a number of weeks, for a couple of hours each week. This is sometimes combined with a group for the person with dementia at the same time (Brodaty and Gresham, 1989). This allows the cared-for person to feel that they are also involved with something positive to help them, and allows for the carer to attend their training without the worry of leaving their relative alone. Training courses usually contain elements of basic instruction in what dementia is; how to manage challenging behaviours; how to manage with physical difficulties, such as lifting; information about services and benefits; and information about legal rights. By allowing some informal time, for example a refreshment break, the training sessions also become a form of early support network for new carers.

A sample training programme for carers consists of:

Session 1—What is dementia?

Session 2—Managing challenging behaviour

Session 3—Activities for the person with dementia

Session 4—Looking after oneself—e.g. stress management, relaxation

Session 5—Legal affairs and state benefits

Session 6—Services available to offer support

Recognizing oneself as a carer

We have already noted that, at the early stage when they present to a memory disorders team, most relatives will not have identified themselves as the patient's carer. So how do they make the transition in this perception of self? Keady and Nolan have identified a gap in longitudinal research studies which might answer this question, and have suggested their own temporal model (Keady and Nolan 1994; Nolan *et al.*, 1996a). This work builds on that of

Wilson who suggested an eight-stage model of caring (Wilson, 1989a, 1989b). In this model, 'taking it on', the stage at which a carer might be said to recognize their role as a caregiver, is the sixth stage. It is preceded by noticing (a gradual awareness), discounting or normalizing, suspecting, searching for explanations, and recounting—a retrospective reappraisal of behaviour and events. One can postulate, therefore, that carers have often been responsible for the care of another for some time before they perceive themselves as a 'carer' as well as spouse/child/sibling etc.

It may be worth considering this model in greater detail because it is confirmed by similar work by Willoughby and Keating, who identify five key stages in caring (Willoughby and Keating, 1991). This model starts with a gradual recognition of unusual or bizarre behaviour, which may be denied at first, before there is a gradual acknowledgement. Secondly, carers seek out as much information as they can in an attempt to gain control of their situation. Then there is the stage of seeking more formal support systems and outside help. And finally there is the act of letting go, of allowing someone else to provide the care so that the carer can move on.

Models which provide staging systems should, however, be regarded with caution. Individual carers will have their own reactions and commonly combine stages, going back and forth as mood and circumstances vary. Nevertheless, there is a subtle change in role when one becomes a carer, when the nature of the relationship changes, and many carers find this transition difficult, and in some case unacceptable.

From the point of view of staff working in memory disorders teams, it is clear that we should recognize that relatives attending with the patient may not perceive themselves as caregivers, and may need to be introduced to this concept. This is important because such self-perception may open the doors to service provision when it is needed. Some countries, for example, have legislation which requires an independent assessment for a caregiver in their own right.

Who are the carers?

Gender

There is evidence to suggest that carers are most likely to be female, that men are likely to spend less time caring than women, and that they are less involved in personal care (Parker and Lawton 1990a, 1990b), and that men and women cope differently with caring (Fisher, 1994). Men may be more reluctant to ask for help, but are more likely to succeed in obtaining help when they ask for it (Fitting *et al.*, 1986). The hypothesis for this is that men are perceived to be less able to care and therefore in greater need of support than women. Women are socialized to care and many spend a great part of their lives caring for another—their partner, their children, and other dependants. Men who have worked all their lives and who may have limited experience of caring, often cope with this new role by putting it into an occupational frame (Fisher, 1994). They take it on as a 'job of work' which legitimizes their calls for support (Twigg and Atkin, 1994). By this means they are more able to separate themselves emotionally from the caring than women and allow themselves time off and holidays. However, Fisher also argues that the gender of the cared-for person may also affect the demand for support—that women often prefer that personal care is provided by another woman (Fisher, 1994). Others have pointed out that men may undertake caring as a 'labour of love' or 'a sense of duty' as well as the worker model (Harris, 1993).

Age

Gender is an important influence in caring, but is only one factor in understanding the dynamics of care. Age is also an important determinant, and we should be aware that not all carers of people with dementia will be older people themselves. Approximately two-thirds of carers are spouses, and most of the remaining one-third are adult 'child carers' (although some will be other relatives, friends, or neighbours). The youngest carer we have seen was the 15-year-old son of a single parent who had early-onset dementia. The needs of young carers are often overlooked. They may be in full-time education and find it difficult to get to school or make the space for studying at home. They may be about to embark on further education or training and reluctant to leave home because they feel they are abandoning their caring responsibilities. They may want to work but find it difficult to leave the cared-for person. Young people often find it hard to share their fears and concerns, or even the truth behind their relative's condition, with their friends because there is pressure on young people to conform with their peers. They may find it difficult to get out and enjoy themselves doing the sorts of things that young people enjoy (Gilliard 1996c,1997). In addition, as we have already noted, there is little information which is aimed specifically at helping young people understand dementia.

Many middle-aged female carers find themselves facing a recently labelled phenomenon—the 'care trap' or the 'sandwich generation' (Brody, 1981). Many women are choosing to develop careers and delay having a family until they are older. Their children are then just reaching independence when the oldest generation is demanding support because of frailty associated with ageing. Women are caught in a trap—just as they become independent from caring for a family they are caught in caring for older relatives. They are torn between their duty to the generation above and the generation below, and the demands of their partner and their career. In some cases it may not be their own parent for whom they feel obliged to care—it may be a parent-in-law.

Professionals must be careful that they are non-judgmental of those who have to face difficult and painful decisions about the future of their caring responsibilities.

Towards a balanced view

The language and attitudes of many professionals who work with carers suggests a negative stereotype. We talk, for example, of the 'burden' of care. We place great emphasis on the stress of carers. We reflect on their difficulties. We label carers, and although we have argued that this may be necessary in order to access service provision, we should be cautious that this does not result in carers being seen as homogeneous. Indeed, we have indicated the differences between carers in age and gender. Work is still to be done which considers the needs of carers of different race and sexuality. Behind each caring situation is an individual relationship, and at least two individual people. Perhaps this is why carers do not recognize themselves as 'caregivers' until well into their caring career—they do not wish to lose their individuality.

Recent findings suggest that the benefits or satisfactions of caring are actually more important determinants of ability to care than perceived difficulties (Nolan *et al.*, 1996b; Cohen *et al.*, 1994). By using two complementary indices (the Carers' Assessment of Difficulties Index and the Carers' Assessment of Satisfactions Index) Nolan has shown that a high difficulties score can be balanced out by a high satisfactions score. The scenario which should give cause for concern is where a carer experiences a high number of difficulties in caring and expresses little satisfaction. This carer may well be struggling and their concerns should be addressed with urgency. Similarly, a positive balance of mood was found in more than 50 per cent of carers in a small study in the United States.

Conclusion

All those who work with people with dementia, whether in a memory disorders team or elsewhere, should be alert to the fact that dementia affects more than just the patient. The impact of the diagnosis has been described as 'ripples in a pond', radiating out from the person with dementia, through the main or primary carer to those who might be described as secondary carers (those who support the primary carer) and then on outwards to all those who know the person (Tibbs, 1995). It might be considered that dementia affects everyone who knows the person who has it. We must take their needs and feelings into account in our work, as well as those of the person with dementia. Dementia is indeed a family affair.

References

Key references recommended by the authors are marked with an *.

Alzheimer's Disease Society (1995). *Right from the start: primary health care and dementia.* ADS, London.

Brennan, P., Moore, S. and Smyth, K. (1992). Alzheimer's disease caregivers' uses of a computer network. *Western Journal of Nursing Research,* **14**, 662–73.

Brennan, P. Moore, S. and Smyth, K. (1995). The effects of a special computer network on caregivers of persons with Alzheimer's disease. *Nursing Research,* **44**, 166–72.

*Brodaty, H. and Gresham, M. (1989). Effect of a training programme to reduce stress in carers of patients with dementia. *British Medical Journal,* **299**, 1375–9.

Brody, E.M. (1981). 'Women in the middle' and family help to older people. *Gerontologist,* **21**, 471–80.

Canadian Study of Health and Aging (1994). Patterns of caring for people with dementia in Canada. *Canadian Journal on Aging,* **13**, 470–87.

Cohen,C.A., Gold, D.P., Shulman, K.I. and Zucchero, C.A. (1994). Positive aspects in caregiving: An overlooked variable in research. *Canadian Journal on Aging,* **13**, 378–91.

Drichamer, M. and Lachs, M. (1992). Should patients with Alzheimer's disease be told their diagnosis? *New England Journal of Medicine,* **326**, 947–51.

Erde, E., Nadal, E. and Scholl, T. (1988). On truth telling and the diagnosis of Alzheimer's disease. *Journal of Family Practice,* **26**, 401–6.

Evans, E. (undated). *It's me, Grandma! It's me!* Alzheimer's Disease Society, Bridport, UK. ISBN 0–9518329–0–5.

Fearnley, K. (1996). *Understanding dementia: a guide for young carers.* Health Education Board for Scotland. ISBN 1–873452–96–1.

Fisher, M. (1994). Man-made care: community care and older male carers. *British Journal of Social Work,* **24**, 659–80.

Fitting, M., Rabins, P., Lucas, M. and Eastham, J. (1986). Caregivers for dementia patients: a comparison of husbands and wives. *Gerontologist,* **26**, 248–52.

Fortinsky, R. and Hathaway, T. (1990). Information and service needs among active and former family caregivers of persons with Alzheimer's disease. *Gerontologist,* **330**, 604–9.

Gilleard, C. (1990). Self-help information for carers: does it help? *Geriatric Medicine,* February, 13–14.

Gilleard, C., Boyd, W., and Watt, G. (1982). Problems in caring for the elderly mentally infirm at home. *Archives of Gerontology and Geriatrics,* **1**, 151–8.

Gilliard, J. (1995). *The long and winding road: a young person's guide to dementia.* Wrightson BioMedical Publishing Ltd., Petersfield, Hants.

Gilliard, J. (1996a). *Caregiver literature.* Presentation at European Conference on Alzheimer's disease and related disorders, Limerick, Eire.

Gilliard, J. (1996b*). Counselling and alternative support for caregivers of people with dementia.* Presentation at Alzheimer's Disease International conference, Jerusalem.

Gilliard, J. (1996c). Ripples of stress across the generations. *Journal of Dementia Care,* **4**, 16–18.

Gilliard, J. (1997). Between a rock and a hard place: the impact of dementia on young carers. In *State of the art in dementia care* (ed. Marshall, M.). Centre for Policy on Ageing, London.

Gilliard, J. and Gwilliam, C. (1996). Sharing the diagnosis: a survey of memory disorders clinics, their policies on informing people with dementia and their families, and the support they offer. *International Journal of Geriatric Psychiatry,* **11**, 1001–3.

Harris, P. (1993). The misunderstood caregiver? A qualitative study of the male caregiver of Alzheimer's disease victims. *Gerontologist,* **33**, 551–6.

Jacques, A. (1988). *Understanding dementia.* Churchill Livingstone, Edinburgh.

Keady, J. and Nolan, M. (1994). Younger-onset dementia: developing a longitudinal model as the basis for a research agenda and as a guide to interventions with sufferers and carers. *Journal of Advanced Nursing,* **19**, 659–69.

Keady, J. and Nolan, M. (1995). A stitch in time. Facilitating pro-active interventions with dementia caregivers: the role of community practitioners. *Journal of Psychiatric and Mental Health Nursing,* **2**, 33–40.

Keady, J., Nolan, M., and Gilliard, J. (1995). Listen to the voices of experience. *Journal of Dementia Care,* **3**, 15–17.

*Levin, E., Sinclair, I., and Gorbach, P. (1990). *Families, services and confusion in old age.* Avebury, Aldershot.

Lubinski, R. (1991). *Dementia and communication.* Decker, London.

*Mace, N. and Rabins, P. (1985). *The 36-hour day.* Age Concern, London.

Magni, E., Zanetti, O., Bianchetti, A., Binetti, G. and Trabucchi, M. (1995). Evaluation of an Italian educational programme for dementia caregivers: results of a small-scale pilot study. *International Journal of Geriatric Psychiatry,* **10**, 569–73.

Maguire, C., Kirby, M., Coen, R., Coakley, R., Lawlor, B. and O'Neill, D. (1996). Family members' attitudes toward telling the patient with Alzheimer's disease their diagnosis. *British Medical Journal,* **313**, 529–30

Mittelman, M.S., Ferris, S.H., Shulman, E., Steinberg, G. and Lvein, B. (1996). A family intervention to delay nursing home placement of patients with

Alzheimer's disease. *Journal of the American Medical Association*, **276**, 1725–81.

Nolan, M., Grant, G. and Keady, J. (1996a). *Understanding family care.* Open University Press, Buckingham.

Nolan, M., Keady, J. and Grant, G. (1996b). Assessing carers' needs: responding to the challenge of the new legislation. Presentation at British Society of Gerontology annual conference, Liverpool, September 1996.

Parker, G. and Lawton, D. (1990a). *Further analysis of the 1985 General Household Survey data on informal care. Report 1: a typology of caring.* Social Policy Research Unit, Working Paper DHSS 716, 12.90, University of York.

Parker, G. and Lawton, D. (1990b). *Further analysis of the 1985 General Household Survey data on informal care. Report 2: the consequences of caring.* Social Policy Research Unit, Working Paper DHSS 716, 12.90, University of York.

Rabins, P., Fitting, M., Estham, J. and Zabora, J. (1990). Emotional adaptation over time in caregivers for the chronically ill elderly. *Age and Ageing,* **19**, 185–90.

Seligman, M., Maier, S. and Geer, J. (1968). Alleviation of learned helplessness in the dog. *Journal of Abnormal Psychology,* **73**, 256–62.

Smyth, K. and Harris, P. (1993). Using telecomputing to provide information and support to caregivers of persons with dementia. *Gerontologist,* **33**, 123–7.

*Taylor, B. (1987). The confused elderly: a living bereavement . .. Alzheimer's disease. *Nursing Times,* **83**, 27–30.

Tibbs, M.A. (1995). Getting it right together. *Journal of Dementia Care,* **3**, 20–2.

Toner, H. (1987). Effectiveness of a written guide for carers of dementia sufferers. *British Journal of Social and Clinical Psychiatry,* **5**, 24–6.

Toseland, R. and Rossiter, C. (1989). Group interventions to support family caregivers: a review and analysis. *Gerontologist,* **29**, 438–48.

*Twigg, J. and Atkin, K. (1994). *Carers perceived: policy and practice in informal care.* Open University Press, Buckingham.

Willoughby, J. and Keating, N. (1991). Being in control: the process of caring for a relative with Alzheimer's disease. *Qualitative Health Research,* **1**, 27–50.

Wilson, H.S. (1989a). Family caregivers: the experience of Alzheimer's disease. *Applied Nursing Research,* **2**, 40–5.

Wilson, H.S. (1989b). Family caregiving for a relative with Alzheimer's dementia: coping with negative choices. *Nursing Research,* **38**, 94–8.

17 Therapeutic intervention in dementia

Françoise Forette and Kenneth Rockwood

We are on the threshold of a new era in the treatment of dementia, in that pharmacological therapy is becoming available for palliation of cognitive symptoms. Until now, only the depressive symptoms, often seen in the early stages of dementia, and behaviour problems, more characteristically seen in the later stages, have been amenable to pharmacological treatment. This chapter will review standard methods of treatment of such problems and will also outline the current possibilities for the treatment of cognitive symptoms. In addition, it will discuss prescription of such medications in the setting of a multidisciplinary memory disability team.

Treatment of depressive symptoms in patients with cognitive impairment

For some time there has been controversy over the interpretation of coincidental symptoms of depression and of cognitive impairment. It seems clear that some patients who have depression will manifest cognitive symptoms. Others with cognitive impairment will become depressed in association or in consequence. In other words, some patients with depression will have dementia and some patients with dementia will have depression. A controversy has arisen, however, over whether treatment of depression can result in amelioration of dementia and whether, if it does, dementia follows (Wragg and Jeste 1989).

For a long time it was common practice to give patients with dementia who had symptoms of depression 'the benefit of the doubt' by prescribing an antidepressant (Jenike 1989). Sometimes this resulted in worsening of cognition, due to the anticholinergic side-effects of many of the older antidepressant medications. When no other potentially ameliorative cognitive therapy was available, such an approach might have been reasonable, but with the emergence of treatment of cognitive symptoms, current thinking favours the use of cognitive agents and secondary tracking of changes in mood. Pending better studies, the precise approach will have to be individualized.

Depressive pseudodementia, as discussed in Chapter 5, clearly merits treatment. As the symptoms of depression in patients with dementia tend towards withdrawal and psychomotor retardation, a more activating antidepressant is most commonly appropriate. The selective serotonin reuptake inhibitors (SSRIs) are somewhat less likely than tricyclic antidepressant medications to cause anticholinergic side-effects. There is little published evidence to indicated whether SSRIs are better for depressive pseudodementia, despite theoretical advantages. None the less, SSRIs are increasingly being prescribed in dementia. If a tricyclic antidepressant medication is chosen, one with a low potential for anticholinergic side-effects, such as desipramine or nortryptiline, is probably the best choice.

Treatment of non-cognitive behavioural problems

Delusions and hallucinations

In Alzheimer's disease, delusions and hallucinations are common. While they tend more often to occur in the later stages of the illness, they can sometimes be seen in the earlier stages and indeed may be the reason the patient is first seen for assessment (Reisberg *et al.* 1987). Hallucinations occasionally arise as a consequence of acute medical illness (see below) but they are more commonly seen as part of the disease course. As discussed in Chapter 19, assessment of the patient and the environment forms the foundation on which treatment can be undertaken. After environmental and social manipulation has been attempted, neuroleptic medications have been the mainstay of treatment (Rockwood 1995).

In the choice of neuroleptics, the trade off is generally between potency and side-effects. Haloperidol is generally the most potent, followed by agents such as loxapin or trifluoperazine, and finally agents such as thioridazine. The frequency of side-effects occurs in the same order (*EPR, postural hypo - tension, sedation, and akathisia*). Although there are theoretical reasons to suspect that side-effect profiles differ at equipotent doses, the clinical significance of this is controversial (see below). As always, individualization is key, as there is not one neuroleptic which works best for all patients.

Whichever neuroleptic medication is to be used, several prescribing principles are best adhered to (see also Table 17.1):

1. It is important to treat to a specific end-point. The targeting of symptoms and some understanding of the likely treatment effect is important. Thus, for example, it is usually more important to make the delusions more manageable than to attempt a cure. In some circumstances, sedation may be a desirable side-effect. In others, it will be necessary to avoid sedation.

Table 17.1 Questions to ask when undertaking medical treatment of behavioural problems in dementia

1. Is a non-pharmacological treatment available?
2. Have medical precipitants been ruled out?
3. Have environmental precipitants be ruled out?
4. What is the goal of treatment?
5. Has the dose been adjusted downwards? (Start low go slow)
6. If agitation persists, has it been made *worse* by treatment? (Akathisia, neuroleptic sensitivity syndrome)
7. What is the plan for reassessment?

2. It is extremely important to use judicious doses and the maxim 'start low and go slow' should be accorded proper prominence.

3. Neuroleptic-induced akathisia (persistent motor restlessness caused by the neuroleptic) must be anticipated. A common and tragic prescribing error is the use of neuroleptic doses which are much too high and the mistaking of akathisia for agitation. As discussed below, in such circumstances the patients need less medication, not more.

4. Untreated hallucinations and delusions in dementia do not last forever. It is therefore likely that discontinuation of treatment can be attempted after 3 to 6 months for this indication.

5. The occurrence of a neuroleptic sensitivity syndrome has been described in patients with Lewy body disease, who are exquisitely sensitive to even small doses of neuroleptic medications (McKeith *et al.* 1992). Hallucinations occur early in the course of patients with Lewy body disease so that hallucinations with only mild cognitive impairment should suggest this possibility. Despite some initial anecdotal enthusiasm for risperidone (Allen *et al.* 1995), there is equal anecdotal need for caution (McKeith *et al.* 1995). In such cases, non-neuroleptic management may be successful.

Acute psychomotor agitation

The pharmacological management of acute episodes of psychomotor agitation in patients who have dementia deserves special comment. Such episodes can ultimately lead to referral for specialist advice or, more commonly, result in the primary care physician requesting advice on patients previously seen by the team. Abrupt worsening of cognitive function in patients with dementia suggests delirium, although this can sometimes be difficult to ascertain when the dementia is more advanced. In any event, abrupt worsening suggests a medical cause should be sought (Rockwood *et al.* 1991; Malone *et al.* 1993). In our experience, the medical cause can usually be detected by physical examination with routine laboratory screening tests, so that we would not endorse elaborate searches for medical precipitants if none are apparent after the initial investigations.

While investigations and initial treatment are being undertaken, a temporary treatment strategy should be put in place. A precise description of the problem and its precipitants (particularly changes in the environment) is very important and may allow for non-pharmacological treatment to be undertaken (see Chapter 18). Despite agitation in dementia being a very common problem, there is disappointingly little scientific evidence on which to make recommendations (Carlyle *et al.* 1993). In our experience, the combination of a low dose of neuroleptic (such as haloperidol in the dose of 0.5 to 1.5 mg two to three times a day, or an equivalent dose of loxapine, in either case combined with a short acting benzodiazepine, such as lorazepam in a dose of 0.5 to 1.0 mg, given simultaneously) can be given either orally or intramuscularly. To avoid pressure prematurely to increase the dose, one regimen has this order written for 3 days, reassessed daily. This regimen is usually successful and it is rare to need to add other medications or to go beyond these doses in elderly patients with dementia, although others commonly find that higher doses (e.g. haloperidol 2.5 to 5.0 mg intramuscularly) are needed (Michalon 1995). Some physicians will use other neuroleptics such as thioridazine. The natural history of acute medical problems on which treatment has been started is favourable, so that even without treatment, most psychomotor agitation seen in agitated delirium will settle within a few days (Rockwood 1993).

Chronic agitation and disinhibition

Chronic aggressive behaviour can occur in many of the dementias, in particular late-stage Alzheimer's disease (Reisberg *et al.* 1987; Teri *et al.* 1988; Lloyd *et al.* 1995). Again, the natural history of the disease means that such problems generally only last a few months, although exceptions are famously noted, and disinhibited behaviour commonly persists in frontotemporal dementia (Rockwood *et al.* 1991). There is a considerable degree of variation in what is counted as chronic aggressive behaviour, which can range from wandering (usually curable in the right environment) to faecal smearing or physical violence. An inventory of the more common causes is provided in Chapter 19 (Table 19.3). It is important to look for chronic precipitating conditions, such as those likely to cause pain. Untreated faecal impaction is the most common of the remediable causes in our experience, although any experienced consultant physician will be able to generate an inventory of conditions which were otherwise missed in patients with 'unexplained' agitation, ranging from pressure ulcers to fractures.

Once the decision to institute pharmacological treatment has been undertaken, a number of agents are available. For some time, neuroleptics were the main stay (see above) but increasingly a range of non-neuroleptic medications are available. Again, one notes with disappointment the paucity of scientific data comparing types of medications for the chronic treatment of behavioural problems in patients with dementia (Tune *et al.* 1991; Carlyle *et al.* 1993; Aurer *et al.* 1996). Haloperidol (or melleril), if given, can be prescribed to be taken by mouth in the same doses outlined above. As an alternative, loxapine, which in one controlled study was as efficacious as haloperidol but had fewer side-effects (Carlyle *et al.* 1993), can be started in a dose of 5 mg two times a day. The use of cholinergic agents may result in improvement in the behavioural symptoms of dementia but data on their efficacy, particularly in patients with the later stages of dementia (where the problems most commonly occur), are lacking.

Trazodone, a serotoninergic agent, has been used for many years to treat depression. However, its sedating side-effects sometimes limited its therapeutic usefulness. In the treatment of patients with dementia and agitation though, these same sedating effects can be helpful, and we have also found them particularly useful in frontotemporal dementia. Other anecdotal reports are summarized elsewhere (Raskind 1995). Common starting doses such as 50 mg given at bed time and up to 350 mg/day in divided doses is well tolerated. Another very common dose is 50 mg in the morning and 100 mg at night. Higher doses are more commonly needed in frontotemporal dementia.

Aurer and colleagues (1996) have presented data showing that fluoxetine (Prozac) is as effective as haloperidol and melleril, but has fewer side-effects in the treatment of agitated behaviour and dementia. Such data properly lead to questioning of the primacy of neuroleptics in the treatment of chronic agitation in dementia.

There are conflicting data on the use of benzodiazepines for the treatment of behavioural problems in dementia. While benzodiazepines can result in oversedation and, importantly, in worsening of cognitive function, their use is reasonable for severe agitation and for the disruption of the sleep/wake cycle (see above). A host of other medications including pindolol, carbamazepine, lithium, and buspirone have been said anecdotally to be useful in treatment in long-term management of patients with behavioural problems. These have been reviewed elsewhere (Raskind 1995).

Symptomatic treatment of cognitive symptoms

Cholinergic treatment

The development of cholinergic agents has been extremely important in the symptomatic treatment of Alzheimer's disease (see Table 17.2). As reviewed

Table 17.2 Possible treatments for cognitive symptoms in dementia

Cholinergic agents	Cholinesterase inhibitors
	Muscarinic agonists
Possible preventative therapies	Control of cardiovascular risk factors
	Non-steroidal anti-inflammatory drugs
	Oestrogen
Miscellaneous	Calcium channel blockers
	Nerve growth factor
	Antioxidants
	Cerebral activation
Future agents	Neural transplantation
	Cerebral anti-inflammatory agents
	Specific amyloid modifying drugs
	Ampakines

elsewhere, data point to the involvement of the cholinergic system in Alzheimer's disease and to depletion of acetylcholine (Forette 1996). Broadly, three strategies have been employed to increase the amount of acetylcholine available in the brain; acetylcholine precursors (such as lecithin); the inhibition of acetylcholinesterase, the chief enzyme responsible for the normal break down of acetylcholine (physostigmine, tacrine, and a host of newer agents) and; direct muscarinic agonists. At present, acetylcholinesterase inhibition is the most developed and effective approach.

Physostigmine is the classic acetylcholinesterase inhibitor, but its very short half-life has limited its usefulness. Tacrine (Cognex) is the furthest along in development, and indeed is already on the market in a number of countries. Donepizil (Aricept) has recently been licensed in several countries. Aricept has a long half-life and is highly protein bound, which may predispose it to drug interactions, although the initial experience with its safety has been positive. Tacrine is an inhibitor of acetylcholinesterase and was first used for this indication in the 1980s. While early reports were very encouraging (Summers *et al.* 1981; Kaye *et al.* 1982) in that they resulted in a modest, but statistically significant, improvement, it was the publication by Summers and colleagues (1986) of their impressive results which drew widespread public and scientific attention to the therapeutic potential of this strategy. Despite some initial controversy and failure to replicate results as clinically meaningful (Boller and Forette 1989; Gauthier *et al.* 1990; Eagger *et al.* 1991) later data have been more encouraging (Davies *et al.* 1992; Forette 1991; Forette *et al.* 1995; Farlow *et al.* 1992; Knapp *et al.* 1994). While many patients may have to withdraw due to side-effects (especially peripheral cholinergic problems such as gastrointestinal tract disturbance) and while some patients will not benefit, there is a proportion who can benefit from higher doses of the drug (120–160 mg/day). The elevation of transaminases, previously considered to be a serious potential adverse event, has proved manageable in most cases. The majority of patients being successfully rechallenged with tacrine after the enzymes have returned to normal. As yet, we have no routine way to determine which patients will be responders. There is some anecdotal evidence for patients with the Lewy body variant responding well to tacrine (Levy *et al.* 1994). In addition, some preliminary investigations have implicated non-Apo E4 phenotypes as more likely to respond (Poirier *et al.* 1996).

Donepezil was approved for use in the United States in November 1996, and subsequently in the United Kingdom and other countries. An early report on 161 patients demonstrated improved cognitive function after 12 weeks of treatment with 5 mg/day. This study also showed a relationship between the degree of acetylcholinestrate inhibition and changes in psychometric test scores (Rogers *et al.* 1996). Donepezil also has been evaluated under double-blind conditions for 24 weeks, in a trial which compared 162 patients on placebo with 154 on 5 mg/day and 157 on 10 mg/day (Rogers *et al.* 1998). Three-quarters of the patients (mean age 72–74) had mild Alzheimer's disease, judged to be otherwise uncomplicated by comorbid illness. On all standard measures, save a patient-rated quality of life measure, those on donepezil had significantly better scores than those on placebo. No persuasive dose-response treatment effect was demonstrated, although fewer patients in the 10 mg/day group completed the trial (68 per cent) than in the 5 mg/day (85 per cent) or placebo (80 per cent) groups. Side-effects were chiefly related to cholinergic mechanisms (e.g. diarrhoea, nausea) and were usually mild and transient. Donepezil is currently the main stay of treatment in many countries.

Metrifonate, an organophosphate which irreversibly inhibits acetylecholine is also being studied for the treatment of Alzheimer's disease. In a small series (50 patients) those treated with metrifonate showed a 2.6 point difference in Alzheimer's Disease Assessment Scale (ADAS-Cog) scores compared with placebo after 3months, with trends in other measures (Becker *et al.* 1996). Reports of large series are awaited with interest.

An alternate approach to enhancing cholinergic function is by the use of direct cholinergic agonists. Such a strategy, employing xanomeline, a selective muscarinic receptor agonist, has been reported in a double-blind, controlled trial. Compared with those receiving placebo, patients on xanomeline had improved ADAS-Cog scores, and the result was clinically detectable (Bodick *et al.* 1997). The most clear improvements were seen at highest doses, however, which also had limiting side-effects, including syncope. Of interest, treated patients had fewer behavioural disturbances, an observations which merits follow-up. Other specific muscarinic agonists remain in development, but none are yet approved (Cutler and Sramek 1995). There is also some interest in nicotinic cholinergic agonists, but again no data support their routine use (Sahakian *et al.* 1989). With respect to other cholinergic approaches, to date, the use of lecithin alone is not supported. It is likely that the next few years will see further development in this area.

Given that the biochemical defects in Alzheimer's disease involve neuro-transmitters other than acetylcholine, other neurotransmitter-based treatments have been employed. To date, pharmacological interventions aimed at the adrenergic systems (Coull 1994), somatostatin (Bissette and Myers 1992), and NMDA receptor function (Isquierdo 1991) have not been successful. Dossiers on several other compounds have been submitted for regulatory approval, but peer reviewed publications have not yet appeared.

Recently, Lovestone and colleagues in London proposed guidelines for the drug treatment of Alzheimer's disease (Lovestone *et al.* 1997). Briefly, these restricted use by physicians who are not dementia specialists to the precise indication to be derived from the dossiers submitted for regulatory approval. These included mild to moderately severe probable Alzheimer's disease (as supported by a Mini Mental State Examination score of between 10 and 24) of at least 6 months duration. It was suggested that response be evaluated early (at 2 weeks) for side-effects, later (at 3 months) for cognitive function, and then every 6 months. The drug would be stopped if deterioration continued at the pretreatment rate for 3 to 6 months, or if a drug-free period suggested that it was no longer helping. Clearly, these recommendations greatly rely on clinical judgement and it is likely that memory disorders teams can make an important contribution through careful clinical observations of patients on treatment.

Drugs with disease modifying potential

It should be noted at the outset that the distinction between symptomatic treatment and disease modifying treatment may be obsolete. It may be the case that altered pathophysiology in Alzheimer's disease is in fact dependent on the cholinergic system, so that manipulation of the cholinergic system may modify the disease course at the molecular level (Small 1991; Geula and Mesulam 1995). In this section, however, we will review attempts to modify the disease course not based on neurotransmitter replacement.

Control of cardiovascular risk factors

There are some data to support the careful control of cardiovascular risk factors in ameliorating the decline in cognitive function seen in patients with multi-infarct dementia (Meyer *et al.* 1995). On the other hand, despite a strong relationship between vascular dementia and hypertension (Forette and Boller 1991), the data about cognitive function in patients with hypertension are more equivocal (Prince *et al.* 1996; Applegate *et al.* 1994). Strict control is in any event unlikely to do no harm, despite concerns about the hazard of hypertensive medications on cognitive function in elderly people. Other medications, which have been reported to improve cognitive function in vascular dementia include buflomedil (Cucinotta *et al.* 1992), oxiracetam (Villardita *et al.* 1992), pentoxifylline (Black *et al.* 1992), nimodipine (Parnetti *et al.* 1993), and nicergoline (Herrmann *et al.* 1997).

Non-steroidal anti-inflammatory drugs

Long-term exposure to non-steroidal anti-inflammatory drugs (NSAIDs) has been amongst the most consistently reported protective factor in observational studies of the risks for Alzheimer's disease (Rozzini *et al.* 1996). Multiple theoretical mechanisms for protection have been proposed (McGeer *et al.* 1992). A limited number of clinical studies appear to support this association, although each has important methodological features which limit their generalizability (Bruce-Jones *et al.* 1994; Rich *et al.* 1995; Rogers *et al.* 1993). As is the case for oestrogen (below) a prudent protocol for use in memory clinics would include a detailed account of NSAID exposure. Routine use of NSAIDs cannot be recommended at this time.

Oestrogen

The favourable effect of oestrogen therapy on cognitive function has made this an exciting area of research (Fillit 1995). The beneficial effect of oestrogen on the memory of postmenopausal and aged women has been noted (Robinson *et al.* 1994; Henderson *et al.* 1994; Paganini-Hill and Henderson 1994; Schneider and Farlow 1995). Oestrogen has also been shown to have an important role in metabolism of the amyloid precursor protein, resulting in less of the toxic form of the β-amyloid protein (Jaffe *et al.* 1994) and may also be helpful in decreasing liberation of free radicals (Fillit 1995).

A recent report has helped further a growing interest in the potential use of oestrogen to protect against dementia, especially in elderly women (Tang *et al.* 1996). In the absence of controlled trials of oestrogen for prevention (an undertaking with special methodological challenges) (Kuller 1996), current inferences are made largely from observational studies. As reviewed elsewhere, the evidence of modest benefit is suggestive for its use in postmenopausal women (Birse 1996). In the setting of a memory clinic, oestrogen exposure should be quantified (age of menarche, age of menopause, use and duration of hormone replacement therapy). Current data do not support routine use of hormone replacement therapy for prevention of dementia.

Calcium channel blockers

Intraneuronal calcium overload is known to be important in neural death from a number of causes. Despite some initially promising data from salbeluzole and nimodipine (Tollefson 1990) this approach now seems less fruitful. There are currently no data to encourage the use of calcium channel blockers for this indication.

Nerve growth factor

Nerve growth factor has important interactions with cholinergic neurones and, given the importance of lost cholinergic projections in a patient with Alzheimer's disease, there has been some interest in nerve growth factor as a potential treatment. Nerve growth factor does not cross the blood–brain barrier (Olson 1993; Hefti and Schneider 1989) so that administration of nerve growth factor has only recently been tried experimentally in humans (Winkler and Thal 1994) and further investigation is required.

Neural transplantation

While there is some enthusiasm for this in the treatment of Parkinson's disease (Lindvall 1991), a number of factors have limited the use of this treatment, even on an experimental basis, in Alzheimer's disease (Dunnet 1991). One important consideration is the likelihood of an acute confusional state in association with surgery, which, in Alzheimer's disease, is an important risk. Given that some proportion of patients with dementia will have a permanent worsening after delirium, experimental treatment may involve a substantial risk, which could outweigh that of most therapy.

Antifree radical and other treatments

As the brain is particularly susceptible to oxidative stress, and as liberation of free radicals plays an important role in the development of the neurotoxic form of the amyloid protein (Iversen *et al.* 1995), antioxidant treatment is an important area of further development. In this regard, the use of idebenone appears to hold promise (Weyer *et al.* 1996). Angiotensin converting enzyme inhibitors have been used based on the observation of increased ACE activity in patients with Alzheimer's disease. Attempts to date have not yielded conclusive results (Moore and Gershon 1990). Other agents such as hydergine (Schneider and Farlow 1995) and *Gingko biloba* extract (Kleijnen and Knipschild 1992) have engaged lay use in some countries, but the data in support of their efficacy have not been persuasive, although some evidence is being sought.

Of note, vitamin E, in a dose of 2000 iu/day, has been found to be effective in double-blind conditions over 2 years in preventing disease progression (Sano *et al.*, 1997). While this study showed an increased incidence of falls in those on vitamin E compared to placebo, its low cost and generally safe profile is likely to make it a common adjunct to current treatments.

A standardized extract from the *Ginko biloba* tree was tested in the treatment of Alzheimer's disease in a randomized, controlled trial. After 12 months of treatment, the Alzheimer's Disease Assessment Scale-Cognitive scores of active treatment patients were significantly better than those of patients receiving placebo. This effect was small however (effect size less than 0.15) and was not clinically detectable (LeBars *et al.* 1997).

Prescribing and the memory disorders team

Prescribing in the setting of a memory disorders team will, of course, be dependent upon local practices. Briefly, the crucial decision is whether the team physician will operate as a consultant to primary care physicians, who will be expected to prescribe, or whether he or she will take on the responsibilities of prescribing. Each view has its proponents but whatever tack is taken the question of polypharmacy must be considered. While the determinants of polypharmacy are complex, multiple illness and multiple prescribers are common causes (Hogan *et al.* 1995). These considerations are important in dementia, as most patients are elderly and therefore prone to diseases accumulated during ageing. As physicians can sometimes prescribe in isolation, it is important that, whether as a consultant or a prescriber, the full spectrum of the patient's medications are taken into account when the new drugs are added. In as much as combination therapy (e.g. a cholinergic agent and an anti-inflammatory drug) may constitute the new therapeutic horizon in dementia, this consideration is likely to become increasingly important. Given the role of medication in disease presentation and exacerbation of dementia, precise tracking of all drugs (including those obtained without prescription) should be part of the standard of care of a memory team assessment.

As mentioned in Chapter 1, an important role for specialized memory disorders services in the near term will be to define our understanding of treatment expectations for the newer compounds. Given that no single drug is likely to cure Alzheimer's disease, it will be important to understand when treatment has been successful. It is likely that some symptoms will improve, but even in successful treatment, others will stay the same whilst others will become worse (Rockwood *et al.* 1996). Our understanding of the natural history of Alzheimer's disease is greatly shaped by our expectations of staging. As treatment may influence how stages develop, there will be a growing need for careful, systematic clinical observation of large numbers of treated patients. Memory clinics will be well positioned to capture such information, and ultimately to shape treatment expectations.

References

Key references recommended by the authors are marked with an *.

Allen, R.L., Walker, Z., D'Ath, P.J., and Katona, C.L.E. (1995). Risperidone for psychotic and behavioural symptoms in Lewy body dementia. *Lancet*, **346**, 185.

Applegate, W.B., Pressel, S., Wittes, J., Luhr, J., Shekelle, R.B., Camel, G.H. *et al.* (1994). Impact of the treatment of isolated systolic hypertension on behavioral variables. *Archives of Internal Medicine*, **154**, 2154–60.

Aurer, S.R., Monteiro, J., Turossian, C., Sinaiko, E., Boksyg, J., and Reisberg, B. (1996). The treatment of behavioural symptoms in dementia: Haloperidol, thiordazine and fluoxetine: A double-blind, placebo-controlled, eight month study. *Neurobiology of Aging*, **17**, 652.

Becker, R.E., Colliver, J.A., Markwell, S.J., Moriearty, P.L., Unni, L.K., and Vicari, S. (1996). Double-blind, placebo-controlled study of metrifonate, an acetylcholinesterase inbibitor, for Alzheimer's disease. *Alzheimer's Disease and Associated Disorders*, **10**, 124–31.

Birse, S. (1996). Is there a role for estrogen replacement therapy in the prevention and treatment of dementia? *Journal of the American Geriatrics Society*, **44**, 865–70.

Bissette, G. and Myers, B. (1992). Minireview. Somatostatin in Alzheimer's disease and depression. *Life Sciences*, **51**, 1389–410.

Black, R.S., Barclay, L.L., Nolan, K.A., Thaler, H.T., Hardiman, S.T., and Blass, J.P. (1992). Pentoxifylline in cerebrovascular dementia. *Journal of the American Geriatrics Society*, **40**, 237–44.

Bodick, N.C., Offen, W.W., Levey, A.L., Cutler, N.R., Gauthier, S., Satlin, A., *et al.* (1997). Effects of xanomeline, a selective muscarinic receptor agonist, on cognitive function and behavioural symptoms in Alhzeimer's disease. *Archives of Neurology*, **54**, 465–73.

Boller, F. and Forette, F. (1989). Alzheimer's diseases and THA: A review of the cholinergic theory and of preliminary results. *Biomedicine and Pharmacotherapy*, **43**, 487–91.

Bruce-Jones, P.N., Crome, P., and Kalra, L. (1994). Indomethacin and cognitive function in healthy elderly volunteers. *British Journal of Clinical Pharmacology*, **38**, 45–51.

Carlyle, W., Ancill, R.J., and Sheldon, L. (1993). Aggression in the demented patient: a double-blinded study of loxapine versus haloperidol. *International Clinical Psychopharmacology*, **8**, 103–8.

Coull, J.T. (1994). Pharmacological manipulations of the alpha2 noradrenergic system. Effect on cognition. *Drugs and Aging*, **5**, 116–26.

Cucinotta, D., Aveni-Casucci, M.A., Pedrazzi, F., Ponari, O., Capodaglio, M., Valdina, P, *et al*. (1992). Multicentre clinical placebo-controlled study with buflomedil in the treatment of mild dementia of vascular origin. *Journal of International Medical Research*, **20**, 136–49.

Cutler, N.A. and Sramek, J. (1995). Muscarinic M1-receptors agonists. Potential in the treatment of Alzheimer's disease. *CNS Drugs*, **3**, 467–79.

Davis, K.L., Thal, L.J., Gamzu, E.R., Davis, C.S., Woolson, R.F., and Gracon, S.I. (1992). A double blind, placebo-controlled multicentre study of tacrine for Alzheimer's disease. *The New England Journal of Medicine*, **327**, 1253–9.

Dunnet, S.B. (1991). Cholinergic grafts, memory and aging. *Trends in Neuroscience*, **14**, 371–6.

Eagger, S.A., Levy, R., and Sahakian, B. (1991). Tacrine in Alzheimer's disease. *Lancet*, **337**, 989–92.

Farlow, M., Gracon, S., Hersley, L.A., Lewis, K.W., Sadowsky, C. H., and Dolan-Ureno, J. (1992). A controlled trial of tacrine in Alzheimer's disease. *Journal of the American Medical Association*, **268**, 2523–9.

Fillit, H. (1995). Future therapeutic developments of estrogen use. *Journal of Clinical Pharmacology*, **35**, 25–8.

Forette, F. on behalf of the French Tacrine Collaborative Group (1991). The French THA multicentre trial: purpose, design and discussion of the methodology used. *European Neuropsychopharmacology*, **1**, 267–9.

Forette, F. (1996). Maladie d'Alzheimer. Un défi médical et social. *Bulletin de l'Académie Nationale de Médecine*, **7**, 1731–46.

Forette, F., and Boller, F. (1991). Hypertension and the risk of dementia in the elderly. *American Medical Journal*, **90** 3A, 14S–19S.

Forette, F., Hoover, T., Gracon, S. *et al*. (1995). A double blind placebo-controlled, enriched population study of tacrine in patients with Alzheimer's disease. *European Journal of Neurology*, **2**, 229–38.

Gauthier, S., Bouchard, R., Lamontagne, A., Bailey, P., Bergman, H., and Ratner, J. (1990). Tetrahydroaminoacridine-lecithin combination treatment in patients with intermediate-stage Alzheimer's disease. Results of a Canadian double blind, crossover, multicentre study. *The New England Journal of Medicine*, **322**, 1272–6.

Geula, C. and Mesulam, M.-M. (1995). Cholinesterases and the pathology of Alzheimer disease. *Alzheimer's Disease and Associated Disorders*, **9**, 23–8.

Hefti, R. and Schneider, L.S. (1989). Rationale for the planned clinical trials with nerve growth factor in Alzheimer's disease. *Psychiatric Developments*, **4**, 299–315.

Henderson, V.W., Paganini-Hill, A., Emanuel, C., Dunn, M.E., and Buckwalter, J.G. (1994). Estrogen replacement therapy in older women. Comparisons between Alzheimer's disease cases and nondemented control subjects. *Archives of Neurology*, **51**, 896–900.

Herrmann, W.M., Stephan, K., Gaede, K., and Apeceche, M. (1997). A multicenter randomized double-blind study on the efficacy and safety of nicergoline in patients with multi-infarct dementia. *Dementia*, **8**, 9–17.

Hogan, D.B., Ebly, E.M., and Tak, S.F. (1995). Regional variations in use of potentially inappropriate medications by Canadian seniors participating in the Canadian Study of Health and Aging. *Canadian Journal of Clinical Pharmacology*, **2**, 167–74.

Isquierdo, I. (1991). Role of NMDA receptors in memory. *Trends in Pharmacologic Sciences*, **12**, 128–9.

Iversen, L.L., Mortishire-Smith, R.J., Pollack, S.J., and Shearman, M.S. (1995). The toxicity in vitro of beta amyloid protein. *Biochemical Journal*, **311**, 1–16.

Jaffe, A.B., Toran-Allerand, D., and Greengard, P. (1994). Estrogen regulates metabolism of Alzheimer amyloid beta precursor protein. *Journal of Biological Chemistry*, **269**, 13065–8.

Jenike, M.A. (ed.) (1989). *Geriatric Psychiatry and Psychopharmacology. A Clinical Approach*. Year Book Medical Publishers, Chicago.

Kaye, W.H., Sitaram, N., Weingartner, H., Ebert, M.H., Smallberg, S., and Gillin, J.C. (1982). Modest facilitation of memory in dementia with combined lecithin and anticholinesterase treatment. *Biological Psychiatry*, **17**, 275–80.

Kleijnen, J. and Knipschild, P. (1992). Ginkgo biloba. *Lancet*, **340**, 1136–9.

Knapp, M.J., Knopman, D.S., Solomon, P.R., Pendlebury, W.W., Davis, C.S., and Gracon, S.I. (1994). A 30-week randomized controlled trial of high-dose tacrine in patients with Alzheimer's disease. *Journal of the American Medical Association*, **271**, 985–91.

Kuller, L.H. (1996). Hormone replacement therapy and its potential relationship to dementia. *Journal of the American Geriatrics Society*, **44**, 878–80.

LeBars, P.L., Katz, M.M., Bermin, N., Ititl, T.I., Freedman, A.M., Schatzberg, A.F. (1997). Placebo-controlled, double-blind, randomised trial of an extract of gingko biloba for dementia. *Journal of the American Medical Association*, **278**, 1327–32.

Levy, R., Eagger, S., Griffiths, M., Perry, E., Honavar, M., and Dean, A. (1994). Lewy bodies and response to tacrine in Alzheimer's disease. *Lancet*, **343**, 294.

Lindvall, O. (1991). Prospects in human transplants in human neuro-degenerative disease. *Trends in Neuroscience*, **14**, 376–84.

Lloyd, C., Hafner, R.J., and Holme, G. (1995). Behavioural disturbances in dementia. *Journal of Geriatric Psychiatry and Neurology*, **8**, 213–16.

Lovestone, S., Graham, W., and Howard, R. (1997). Guidelines on drug treatment for Alzheimer's Disease. *Lancet*, **350**, 232–3.

Malone, M.L., Thompson, L., and Goodwin, J.S. (1993). Aggressive behaviours among the institutionalized elderly. *Journal of the American Geriatrics Society*, **41**, 853–6.

McGeer, P.L., Harada, N., Kimura, H., McGeer, E.G., and Schulzer, M. (1992). Prevalence of dementia amongst elderly Japanese with leprosy: Apparent effect of chronic drug therapy. *Dementia*, **3**, 146–9.

McKeith, I., Fairbairn, A., Perry, R., Thompson, P., and Perry, E. (1992). Neuroleptic sensitivity in patients with senile dementia of Lewy body type. *British Medical Journal*, **305**, 673–8.

McKeith, I.G., Ballard, C.G., and Harrison, R.W.S. (1995). Neuroleptic sensitivity to risperidone in Lewy body dementia. *Lancet*, **346**, 699.

Meyer, J.S., Muramatsu, K., Mortel, K.F., Obara, K., and Shirai, T. (1995). Prospective CT confirms differences between vascular and Alzheimer's dementia. *Stroke*, **26**, 735–42.

Michalon, M. (1995). The acutely agitated patient. In *Therapeutic choices* (ed. J. Gray), pp. 2–8. Canadian Pharmaceutical Association, Ottawa.

Moore, R.C. and Gershon, S. (1990). The brain reninangiotensin system and behaviour. *Dementia*, **4**, 225–36.

Olson, L. (1993). Growth factors: therapeutic implications. In *Cerebral plasticity and cognitive stimulation* (eds F. Forette, Y. Christen, and F. Boller), pp. 32–44. Fondation Nationale de Gérontologie, Paris.

Paganini-Hill, A. and Henderson, V. (1994). Estrogen deficiency and risk of Alzheimer's disease. *American Journal of Epidemiology*, **140**, 256–61.

Parnetti, L., Senin, U., Carosi, M., and Baasch, H. (1993). Mental deterioration in old age: Results of two multicentre, clinical trials with nimodipine. *Clinical Therapeutics*, **15**, 394–406.

Poirier, J., Delisle, M., Qurion, M. *et al.* (1996). Apolipoprotein E4, cholinergic integrity, synaptic plasticity and Alzheimer's disease In *Apolipoprotein E and AD*, (ed. A.D. Roses, A. Weisgraber, and Y. Christen), pp. 20–8. Springer Verlag, New York.

Prince, M.J., Bird, A.S., Blizard, R.A., and Mann, A.H. (1996). Is the cognitive function of older patients affected by antihypertensive treatment? Results from 54 months of the Medical Research Council's treatment trial of hypertension in older adults. *British Medical Journal*, **312**, 801–5.

Raskind, M.A. (1995). Alzheimer's disease: Treatment of noncognitive behavioural abnormalities. In *Psychopharmacology: The fourth generation of progress* (eds F.E. Bloom and D.J. Kupfer), pp. 1427–35. Raven Press, New York.

Reisberg, B., Borenstein, J., Salob, S.P., Ferris, S.H., Franssen, E., and Georgotas, A. (1987). Behavioural symptoms in Alzheimer's disease: pharmacology and treatment. *Journal of Clinical Psychiatry*, **48**, 9–15.

Rich, J.P., Rasmusson, D.X., Folstein, M.F., Carson, K.A., Kawas, C., and Brandt, J. (1995). Nonsteroidal anti-inflammatory drugs in Alzheimer's disease. *Neurology*, **45**, 51–5.

Robinson, D., Friedman, L., Marcus, R., Tinklenberg, J., and Yesavage, J. (1994). Estrogen replacement therapy and memory in older women. *Journal of the American Geriatrics Society*, **42**, 919–22.

Rockwood, K. (1993). The occurrence and duration of symptoms in elderly patients with delirium. *Journal of Gerontology-Medical Sciences*, **48**, 162–6.

Rockwood, K. (1995). Dementia. In *Therapeutic choices* (ed. J. Gray), pp. 27–31. Canadian Pharmaceutical Association, Ottawa.

Rockwood, K., Stolee, P., and Brahim, A. (1991). Outcomes of admission to a psychogeriatric service. *Canadian Journal of Psychiatry*, **36**, 275–9.

Rockwood, K., Stolee, P., Howard, K., and Mallery, L. (1996). Use of goal attainment scaling to measure treatment effects in an anti-dementia trial. *Neuroepidemiology*, **15**, 330–8.

Rogers, J., Kirby, L.C., Hempelman, S.R., Berry, D.L., McGeer, P.L., and Kaszniak, A.W. (1993). Clinical trial of indomethacin in Alzheimer's disease. *Neurology*, **43**, 1609–11.

Rogers, S.L., Friedhoff, L.T. *et al.* (1996). The efficacy and safety of donepezil on patients with Alzheimers disease: Results of a US multicentre, randomized, double-blind, placebo-controlled trial. *Dementia*, **7**, 293–303.

Rogers, S.L., Farlow, M.R., Doody, R.S., Mohs, R., Friedhoff, L.T. *et al.* (1998). A 24-week, double-blind, placebo-controlled trial of donepezil in patients with Alzheimer's disease. *Neurology*, **50**, 136–45.

Rozzini, R., Ferrucci, L., Losonczy, K., Havlik, R.J., and Guralnik, J.M. (1996). Protective effect of chronic NSAID use on cognitive decline in older persons. *Journal of the American Geriatrics Society*, **44**, 1025–6.

Sahakian, B., Jones, G., Levy, R., Gray, J., and Warburton, D. (1989). The effects of nicotine on attention, information processing and short-term memory in patients with dementia of the Alzheimer type. *British Journal of Psychiatry*, **154**, 797–800.

Sano, M., Ernesto, C., Thomas, R.G., *et al.*, (1997). A controlled trial of selegiline, alpha-tocopherol or both as treatment for Alzheimer's disease. *New England Journal of Medicine*, **336**, 1216–22.

Schneider, L. and Farlow, M.R. (1995). Predicting response to cholinesterase inhibitors. Possible approaches. *CNS Drugs*, **4**, 114–24.

Small, D.H. (1991). A protease activity associated with acetylcholinesterase releases the membrane-bound form of the amyloid protein precursor of Alzheimer's disease. *Biochemistry*, **30**, 10795–9.

Summers, W.K., Viesselman, J.O., Marsh, G.M., and Candelora, K. (1981). Use of THA in treatment of Alzheimer-like dementia : pilot study in twelve patients. *Biological Psychiatry*, **16**, 145–53.

Summers, W.K., Majovski, L.V., Marsh, G.M., Tachiki, K., and Kling, A. (1986). Oral tetrahydroaminoacridine in long term treatment of senile dementia, Alzheimer type. *New England Journal of Medicine*, **315**, 1241–5.

Tang, M-X., Jacobs, D., and Stern, Y. (1996). Effect of oestrogen during menopause on risk and age at onset of Alzheimer's disease. *Lancet*, **348**, 429–32.

Teri, L., Larson, E.B., and Reifler, F.V. (1988). Behavioural disturbances in dementia of the Alzheimer's type. *Journal of the American Geriatrics Society*, **1**, 1–6.

Tollefson, G.D. (1990). Short term effect of the calcium blocker nimodipine in the management of primary degenerative dementia. *Biological Psychiatry*, **27**, 1133–42.

Tune, L.E., Steele, C., and Cooper, T. (1991). Neuroleptic drugs in the management of behavioral symptoms of Alzheimer's disease. *Psychiatric Clinics of North America*, **14**, 353–73.

Villardita, C., Grioli, S., Lomeo, C., Cattaneo, C., and Parini, J. (1992). Clinical studies with oxiracetam in patients with dementia of Alzheimer type and multi-infarct dementias of mild to moderate degree. *Neuropsychobiology*, **25**, 24–8.

Weyer, G., Erzigkeit, H., Hadler, D., and Kubicki, S. (1996). Efficacy and safety of idebenone in the long-term treatment of Alzheimer's disease: A double-blind, placebo controlled multicentre study. *Human Psycho - pharmacology*, **11**, 53–65.

Winkler, J. and Thal, L. (1994). Clinical potential of growth factors in neurological disorders. *CNS Drugs*, **6**, 465–78.

Wragg, R.E. and Jeste, D.V. (1989). Overview of depression and psychosis in Alzheimer's disease. *American Journal of Psychiatry*, **145**, 577–87.

18 Non-pharmacological approaches to treatment

Bob Woods and Mike Bird

What is treatment?

In the context of the dementias, a group of diseases with no known cure and none at present foreseeable, it is crucial to define the concept of 'treatment'. The conceptual basis adopted for this chapter is an assertion made by Woods and Britton in 1985:

> We need to break away from our pre-occupation with treatment in the sense of cure and recovery, and be aware of the different types of goals that are feasible, and the value of some of the more limited goals in improving the patient's quality of life (Woods and Britton, 1985, p. 217).

Unfortunately, 12 years on, the preoccupation with treatment in the sense of a grossly simplified medical model of which any self-respecting medical practitioner would be ashamed (Kitwood, 1990), remains apparent in non-pharmacological dementia care and research. It is reflected explicitly in the quest to produce generalized improvement in functioning, usually assessed by changes in cognitive performance, following prolonged training in various modalities such as cognitive stimulation (e.g. Breuil *et al.*, 1994), or Reality Orientation (e.g. Drummond, *et al.*, 1978).

Though plagued by methodological problems (Greene, 1984); failure to generalize to everyday difficulties (Breuil *et al.*, 1994; Holden and Woods, 1995); minimal improvements claimed as clinically significant (e.g. Beck *et al.*, 1988); or a plunge to baseline as soon as the 'treatment' is withdrawn (Hanley and Lusty, 1984); there are occasional encouraging signs and researchers will clearly continue mining this vein. However, more than 30 years after the first attempts via Reality Orientation, it remains to be demonstrated whether generalized improvement is a chimera, or whether the quest for it will eventually produce gains which translate to improved functioning in everyday life (Woods, 1994).

Another example of the over-simplified medical model is the ascendancy of the self-contained 'Therapy', such as Validation Therapy (Feil, 1993) or Three Phase Therapy (Giuliano, 1994). Many claims are made based only on anecdotal evidence, for example Validation Therapy is said to resolve unfinished life tasks (Feil, 1993).

We contend that those working with people with dementia, whether in a clinic or in the community, should certainly be familiar with the basic techniques forming the kernel of these therapies. For example it is undoubtedly useful to remember that people with dementia need to be listened to at all levels, as recommended in Validation Therapy. To expect, though, that what is essentially open empathic Rogerian listening, however well adapted to dementia sufferers, will deal with unresolved conflicts from the patient's past or delay the dementing process, is likely to lead to disappointment. In some cases correcting and orientating the client to some kind of reality may be essential; for example that he has not been kidnapped but is in a day-care centre and will return home later. The clinician should not be thus led to believe that regular Reality Orientation will lead to global improvements, or that it will be appropriate in other cases, or even in other situations with the same client. Similarly, the usefulness of other therapeutic practices is not necessarily questioned here. Rather, it is the notion of a panacea, of a generalized psychosocial pill, applicable to all or most case profiles, leading to generalized improvement, which is challenged.

In this chapter the emphasis will be on tailoring individualized techniques to the individual case. Persons with dementia do not form an homogeneous group. There is wide variation in cognitive deficits even within discrete diagnostic categories such as Alzheimer's disease (Hart and Semple, 1990; Martin, 1987). Patients are of widely differing ages, personality, and emotional response types, with an infinite variety of life experiences and widely differing ways of coping with difficulty, and live in widely differing circumstances. Further, most are dependent on others, so that the care network, which may consist of several players, inevitably forms part of the case profile. These factors mean that there is an almost infinite possible interaction of variables which produce the problems likely to lead to referral to a memory disorders team. No case profile is quite like any other. In this context, the blanket therapy or the one technique therapist is likely to have limited impact. We are not advocating therapeutic nihilism, the 'nothing can be done' syndrome. On the contrary, we believe that there is much which can be done which will prove invaluable to people with dementia and their caregivers, as long as interventions are carefully planned and are individualized, with realistic goals recognizing the complexity of the condition and its context.

The conceptual basis of this chapter, then, is that the purpose of treatment, medical and/or non-pharmacological, is to reduce distress and improve quality of life. The method is to work out, by careful assessment, what adjustments can realistically be made to the individual case profile which will achieve this purpose for the maximum number of stakeholders, including the carers. Thus, entirely dependent upon the needs and resources identified in any one case profile, the nature of the interventions required from the health professional will vary widely.

The remainder of this chapter describes in more detail some of the clinical, psychosocial interventions which have been used with this very difficult population. First it will outline the essentials of an individualized approach, emphasizing the importance of assessment, before addressing the role of the caregiver and the often-neglected aspects of the person's emotional response and attempts to cope with their memory difficulties. Examples of work showing that residual memory capacity can be utilized for clinical goals, including spatial orientation and some more difficult behaviour problems, will be presented, concluding with an outline of behavioural approaches.

Assessment

A wide range of questions need to be addressed to achieve the depth of understanding of the case profile required for a properly individualized approach. Areas covered should include:

♦ **cognitive function**—the emphasis of neuropsychological assessment in dementia has too often been in establishing a diagnosis, and delineating impairment, at the expense of identifying the person's strengths and residual areas of preserved function; it is the processes, modalities or materials showing lesser degrees of impairment that can be most useful in devising an intervention plan;

♦ the person's **style of coping** with what is happening, their emotional response and defence mechanisms;

♦ the person's **life story**—providing a context for the development of the current situation and insight/ understanding of the person's preferences and choices over a life time;

♦ the person's **social network**, including family caregivers and other supports; the resources available to the person; are family relationships good or is there conflict? Is the primary carer strong and coping well or frail and close to breakdown? Do the financial resources exist to fund additional inputs?

♦ **areas presenting difficulty or distress** to patient or caregivers.

Note that the assessment is not driven simply by presenting problems; only in this broader context can an individualized approach proceed. Having identified particular issues which may form target areas for intervention, the essential first step is to ensure that proper screening for possible medical causes for the difficulty has been undertaken, especially if it has emerged suddenly. Pain, infections, constipation, and adverse drug reactions are frequently implicated in behavioural problems, adding additional dysfunction to that arising from any dementia present. Assuming no such medical cause is identified, a number of further assessment questions follow.

Is the person's behaviour causing distress?

The purpose of any intervention is to reduce distress in the person with dementia and/or their caregivers, not necessarily to change the behaviour. If, however bizarre the behaviour may appear to be, it is neither distressing nor dangerous, it should not be considered a legitimate therapeutic target. Further, there is no need to treat phenomena such as benign delusions and hallucinations (Peisah and Brodaty, 1994).

What is the patient actually doing, when, and under what circumstances?

Labels such as 'agitation' are unhelpful. A precise description of the behaviour is essential; it may be necessary to observe the patient to obtain it. This defines and objectifies the target; say, to reduce the number of repetitive questions per hour to a more manageable level. It also provides information about aetiology and sometimes even suggests the intervention. For example detailed observation of a woman referred for screaming and violence at bath time suggested that her resistance was based not on 'stubbornness' (the referrer's diagnosis) but on panic. It also showed that her fear was aroused more by anticipatory anxiety than the bath itself, though hair washing was a major trauma. Shortening exposure time to bath time signals, using stroking and quiet talk to reduce physiological arousal prebath, and taking her to a salon for her hair wash produced the data shown in Fig. 18.1(a).

Why is the patient behaving in this way?

Without some ideas concerning aetiology, designing an effective intervention is much more difficult. 'Because he has dementia' is no explanation! We need to understand why this particular patient is behaving in this particular way, in these particular circumstances. Though absolute certainty is rare, reasonable hypotheses can be generated by gathering information from as many sources as possible, primarily the direct carers, the wider family, and from observation and/or direct questioning of the patient. In the example above, the panic hypothesis was supported by family members who remembered a traumatic swimming incident in the patient's youth, and a life-long fear of exposing her body for recreational bathing. Careful questioning of carers about the circumstances under which the behaviour does and does not occur (perhaps

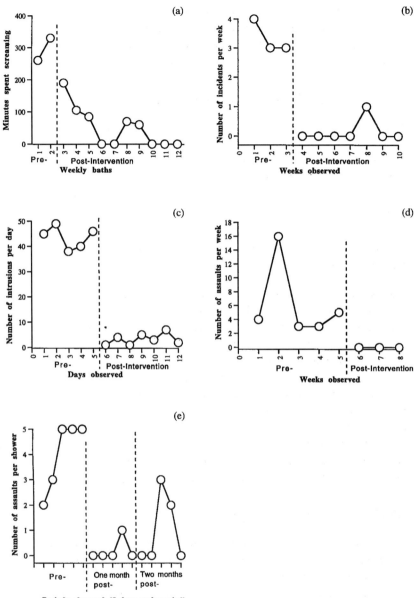

Fig. 18.1 Results of the use of cues to ameliorate clinical problems (Bird *et al.* 1995): (a) 'Mary' screaming and fighting during bathing; (b) 'Doris' accidentally overdosing on medication; (c) 'Una' intrusive behaviour and violence; (d) 'Paul' physical and verbal sexual assault; (e) 'Adrian' sexual assault during showering.

using monitoring sheets to record this) can also provide useful clues about aetiology and the intervention. These sources can be supplemented with behavioural experiments to determine whether certain stimuli produce the behaviour and others do not.

What can realistically be changed?

A complete cessation of the difficult behaviour is unusual; the more common goal is reduction to tolerable levels. An example of targeting what could be changed may be found in Bird *et al.* (1995), concerning a man with a chronic fear of soiling himself who demanded to go to the toilet, sometimes every few minutes. No attempt was made to change his fear of soiling; instead the intervention was focused on lengthening the intervals between his demands.

Working with caregivers

In our discussion we will not be covering methods of directly reducing care-giver stress, as this topic is covered in Chapter 16 (see also reviews by Brodaty, 1992; Knight *et al.*, 1993). In certain situations where the areas of difficulty are leading to distress only for the caregiver, with the person with dementia being quite untroubled, it may well be more appropriate to target the caregiver's distress rather than the patient's behaviour. In every case, the caregiver's perception of the problem and attributions regarding its development and maintenance are of great importance, and changes here may be sufficient to reduce strain.

Education

With some caregivers, simple education about dementia and brain–behaviour relationships will often be enough to achieve a reduction in their distress level by putting bizarre behaviour into context. Referral to support groups, de-scribed in Chapter 16, and organizations such as the Alzheimer's Association/ Alzheimer's Disease Society to gain this information can sometimes be the most valuable intervention. The professional worker's role is to encourage and enable the caregiver to attend, organizing the logistics of transport and relief care if needed. Such information, whether gained via formal education, literature and advice provided by the memory clinic worker, or mutual support groups, often also leads to the caregiver learning basic management principles such as the irrelevance of logic, the counter-productive nature of confrontation, the value of reassurance, and of 'going with the flow'. For example in a carer's group one man learned from other members not to argue and physically restrain his wife when, daily, she marched out of the house declaring that she was going home. He now asks if he may come with her, they do a few laps round the block holding hands and talking and, eventually, approach the house from an angle she recognizes and come 'home'. Another carer has reduced from an average of half an hour per day to 3 to 5 minutes the time it takes to remove his wife's dentures, a painful process for her because of a jaw injury. Instead of angrily arguing with her and trying physically to remove them, he now gently suggests it while cuddling and reassuring her and then removes his own dentures; she then follows suit.

Reframing

In some cases, asking 'Does it have to be seen as a problem?' may help the caregiver to reframe the situation—tackling more directly their distress regarding all the changes in the care recipient's behaviour and their own sense of loss, rather than struggling to change the person with dementia. For example a woman with dementia would only let her husband into their bedroom if he were wearing a particular hat; he chose to comply, rather than expending valuable energy in explaining over and over that he was indeed her husband, with or without the hat! Or a person with dementia whose motor coordination is declining chose to eat with a spoon, rather than with a knife and fork; his wife was upset at this evident decline in a previously well-mannered man, but decided that as he was eating effectively and with enjoyment it would be counter productive to insist on him using knife and fork.

Realistic targets

Not all 'problems' are readily accepted, of course; the key issue here is that if the plan includes efforts to change the person with dementia's behaviour, these should be carefully targeted on those areas where maximum benefit to the quality of life of the person with dementia and his/her supporters will accrue. The ability of caregivers to participate in an intervention plan may be reduced by their own strain and distress, or by pre-existing issues in the relationship, or by the habitual style of interaction. For example caregivers showing a high level of Expressed Emotion, characterized by a critical attitude to the person with dementia, would be predicted to have particular difficulty in adopting problem-solving approaches (Bledin *et al.*, 1990). In some circumstances an objectively successful intervention may not be perceived as useful by emotionally involved family caregivers. What is, say, a 10 per cent increase in communication, when so much in the relationship has been lost (Bourgeois, 1990).

If the plan does involve some attempt to change the patient's behaviour, as well as the carer's reaction to it, realistic expectations should be encouraged. Though rarely reported in the literature, failure directly to change the maladaptive behaviour of a patient with dementia—whether by pharmacological or psychosocial means—is only too common. Accordingly, it is important to give carers hope while being realistic about the possibilities of success—a delicate balancing act at times. Apart from pre-empting the dashing of unrealistic expectations, an honest and realistic approach can contribute directly to the therapeutic process, empowering carers who have come to see the situation as hopeless and that they are failures.

Collaboration

Working closely and sensitively with caregivers is vital. The plan will not be pursued if it is seen as an additional burden, or peripheral to the carer's concerns. In principle, memory-clinic-based interventions should succeed in engaging caregivers in interventions in a way that traditional services appear to have failed to do, as the earlier contact may come at a point where strain is less pervasive and problems less entrenched. However, each stage of the caregiving career (Aneshensel *et al.*, 1995) has its particular stresses, and around the time of diagnosis there are many adjustments to be made, much information to be absorbed, much to reflect on. Engaging others, less directly emotionally involved, in any intervention plan is recommended, rather than relying simply on a sole caregiver.

Collaboration is the key: family carers are, after all, the real experts on the patient and may already have developed by trial and error a number of successful management methods. The way forward is not to take management of the situation out of the carers' hands, but rather to assist them in refining and adding to their existing expertise. Engaging carers as cotherapist also helps them to start to objectify aspects of the problem, rather than viewing it as an overwhelming amorphous mass. By understanding the rationale for the intervention, they may apply it more flexibly and adaptively. Even if the intervention fails, the carer engaged from the outset will have gained more understanding about the person and their behaviour, which in itself may assist coping.

The response of the person with memory difficulties

Insight and coping

In understanding the response of the person with dementia, the interplay of cognitive changes, affective state and personality/coping style must be considered. Memory clinics have played a key role in the discovery of the person with dementia. Professionals have come into contact with many more people with mild dementia, more readily able to articulate their perspective. Several authors have recently drawn attention to the importance of the subjective experience of the person with dementia in understanding his/her response (e.g. Kitwood, 1997; Keady, 1996). Insight, the person's awareness of their condition, is being addressed (Mullen *et al.*, 1996) but raises complex issues. What is the person aware of? Alzheimer's, a memory problem, a loss of capacity in everyday life? To what extent does denial, as a defence mechanism, contribute to apparent lack of insight (see Bahro *et al.*, 1995)? Or is lack of insight another result of neuropathological damage—an example of anosognosia in fact?

Given that people with dementia are often not informed of the diagnosis (Rice and Warner, 1994), a lack of formal insight is perhaps to be expected. Opinions are divided as to what people with dementia should be told, or indeed whether they should be told at all (Gilliard and Gwilliam, 1996).

Caregivers are now nearly always told the diagnosis and are reported to want to protect the person with dementia, whilst acknowledging that if in the same position themselves they would want to be told (Maguire *et al.*, 1996). The debate is reminiscent of the situation with cancer 20 years ago; to tell or not to tell? In the future will we likewise look back and wonder what all the concern was about, that of course people with dementia will be informed of their diagnosis? Part of the difficulty clinically at present is what to tell: diagnosing the specific dementia is not yet straightforward; the prognosis in the individual case remains uncertain, for example in terms of speed of progression and areas of function likely to be impaired. Tackling sensitively the specific practical implications of the diagnosis, for example in terms of ability to drive and competence to make financial decisions, may help the broader discussion of an uncertain future.

The variation in response style of people with dementia is beginning to be documented. Kitwood *et al.* (1995) report a cluster analysis of the current personality profiles of 112 people with dementia, with six clusters emerging, reflecting quite different responses to their situation, ranging from the 'happy socialite' to the person 'fighting the system', stubborn and fiercely wanting independence, through the vulnerable and anxiety prone. Bahro *et al.* (1995) report clinical observation of a series of seven patients in the period after diagnosis. Coping strategies including denial, externalization, somatization, and self-blame were identified in various combinations in individual cases. These clusters and case descriptions raise questions as to the optimal style of coping with a dementia; self-blame is clearly likely to lead to greater distress; minimizing the importance of what has been lost—a more subtle form of denial—seems to be adaptive for some. Different styles may be effective at different stages or in different situations; denial may be adaptive, but the effort required can become unbearable. Showing sorrow and grief for what has been lost may appear the natural response, but we have as yet little understanding of whether a point of acceptance, of resolution, may be reached, or at least a lessening of grief-related distress to balance the pain of experiencing grief. The continuing losses of function, and the loss of ability to articulate experiences clearly, add to the complexity of this process.

Depression and anxiety

It is well-established that substantial numbers of people with dementia in addition have symptoms of depression and/or anxiety. For example Ballard *et al.* (1996) reported that, in a memory clinic sample, 30 per cent of patients diagnosed as having dementia had one or more anxiety symptoms, with 38 per cent reporting tension. Three sub-groups were identified: those whose anxiety arose in the context of depression; those who also suffered hallucinations or delusions; and finally a group who showed some insight into their problems, who were anxious they would be embarrassed in particular situations because of their cognitive lapses. Depression coexisting with dementia has perhaps received less attention over the years than its due, probably because of an over emphasis on distinguishing the two conditions, rather than recognising depression as a common concomitant of dementia. Reifler and Larson (1990) report a prevalence of between a quarter and a third of dementia patients with a coexisting depression in their outpatient studies. They describe the mood disorder as a major source of 'excess disability' in dementia, reducing function below the level which the neuropathological impairment would necessitate. In an attempt to reduce the level of disability, depressed patients were randomly allocated to receive either antidepressant medication or a placebo; both groups showed reduced depression, with the placebo group's improvement attributed to increased support and attention during the treatment trial.

Psychological therapies

There is increasing interest in offering psychological therapies for anxiety, depression, and adjustment to loss to people with dementia. An early report (Yesavage *et al.*, 1982) described the successful application of a relaxation therapy; Thompson *et al.* (1990) describe the applicability of Cognitive Behaviour Therapy to depression in dementia, and accounts of psycho-dynamic therapies are also appearing (e.g. Hausman, 1992; Sinason, 1992). Hausman recommends beginning the therapeutic relationship as early as possible in the course of the dementia, and ideally continuing until the person dies, so that the therapist does not become another of the person's losses. A clear sense emerges of the progression of the dementia forming a back-drop to what can be achieved, and the goals of such work require careful consider-ation. However, there is no doubt that this growth of interest is a welcome antidote to the all too common assumption that all such approaches must be inappropriate for anyone with the diagnosis of dementia. It is always the individual case profile that indicates suitability—not the diagnostic category. Groups for people with memory difficulties, offering opportunities for peer support as well as development of problem-solving, coping strategies have also been described, particularly for early-stage patients (Yale, 1995; Allen, 1996; Birnie, 1997).

An example of the application of a structured counselling approach is provided by the case of a mildly dementing man who vehemently refused, over 2 years, to go into respite care when his wife of necessity took brief breaks. He was frequently found wandering the streets or ringing the police while she was away. Encouragement to discuss his fears over three supportive counselling sessions in his home made it possible to reduce the main issues to a digestible formula, namely: though he hated the thought of going into respite, the alternative was full-time residential care because his wife would be worn out. Expressed in three short sentences printed in large type, these issues were posted in two prominent places in the house and the clinician also phoned him twice a day to remind him to look at them. Having grasped and remembered the core issue by these means, and with plentiful support and reminders of the short length of his 'sentence', it has now proved relatively easy to persuade him to accept respite regularly.

Attempting to understand the basis of the person's fears and concerns is always worthwhile, and may suggest useful approaches to care. Not uncommonly, fears relate to basic concerns of rejection, of being alone, of insecurity, or of losing control. Good listening skills, such as those learned in counselling—or in psychotherapy—training are invaluable, assisting the helper to 'tune in' to the affective component of the communication, to the meaning behind the actual words spoken (Stokes and Goudie, 1990). This is the aspect of 'Validation Therapy' that we would commend, as a way of opening up good communication. Similarly, individualized reminiscence work can be utilized in the assessment process, to inform and guide the individual plan, helping all concerned to keep the whole person firmly in mind (Gibson, 1994). In a life-span developmental context, the person's attachment style, with its roots in early childhood, may emerge in dementia in late life, for example in the familiar phenomenon of 'parent fixation', where the person frequently searches for and talks about a lost parent (Miesen, 1992).

In seeking to reduce distress through 'treatment' the impact of the environment should not be forgotten. Both the physical and social surroundings may serve to increase agitation, for example through noise, discomfort, and interactions perceived as hostile or threatening. The patient described above who resisted in the bath is a good example. Shortening the exposure time to arousing bathroom stimuli and washing her hair in a different environment were important ingredients of the intervention. The sensory environment (touch and quiet talk) was also manipulated, and there is now more than anecdotal evidence that changes to the sensory environment, for example music or pleasant sounds (Gerdner and Swanson, 1993; Burgio *et al.*, 1996), can calm patients who are behaving maladaptively. However, it is our experience that it is most often necessary to adjust the social environment, frequently the understandable but counter-productive responses by carers. The family carer described above who learned to prompt his wife to take her dentures out, or the carer who learned to accompany his wife when she marched out both managed to change their spouse's behaviour. Approaches espoused in communication techniques like Validation Therapy may best be seen not as cure-alls, but as efforts to change the social environment and make it more humane and thus less likely to cause behavioural counter-reactions.

Cognitive strategies

Reducing cognitive load

As suggested above, any cognitive strategies to be included in the plan should be drawn from a detailed assessment of strengths and weaknesses in cognitive function. Some suggestions are beginning to emerge from the research literature as to how the cognitive profile might be the basis for useful intervention. The emphasis has been largely on memory and learning; the major more general cognitive strategy adopts the simple principle of reducing the cognitive load as far as possible. This has implications for interacting with people with dementia individually and in groups (Woods, 1996). Distractions must be reduced to avoid divided attention and short, simple sentences used. The spoken word may be supplemented with relevant pictures and objects to provide a context for what is said (Bourgeois, 1990,1992).

Applying this simple principle to memory suggests the use of external memory aids, to reduce the load on memory, and cues and prompts have enjoyed widespread clinical use, for example in Reality Orientation programmes (Holden and Woods, 1995). Environmental cues and prompts need to be obvious or salient if they are to enhance quality of life. For example even moderately impaired patients are likely to find a picture of a toilet on a door more effective than, say, a symbolic figure; a whiteboard with important information is likely to be more effective than a diary, especially when placed where the patient often comes face to face with it. Unfortunately, these basic principles are often overlooked, as if any cue must be a good thing. One frequently comes across scrawled reminders to patients which they never look at and, often, are unable to read anyway!

Illustrating the good use of a cue which was sufficiently obvious in itself, McEvoy and Patterson (1986) 'cured' a patient with a history of hiding her dirty linen by having an open laundry basket prominently placed where she undressed. An example of a salient cue can be seen in work with an Alzheimer's patient who frequently took multiple doses of anxiolytic medication from her week's supply by mistake. Hiding or removing the medication box was not an option, because she was anxious about her medication and would spend all day agitatedly looking for it. Reminder notes in prominent locations that outreach workers would be in to supervise her medication were also unsuccessful. The case was only solved (see Fig. 18.1(b)) by fixing a large notice actually on the dispenser:

Doris! Wait for the girls to come before you take your pills.

That is, the cue/prompt was in the exact place where she was sure to see it when there was a risk of overdosing.

Training and cues

Cues used sensibly can sometimes then be effective in themselves, without further training. Frequently, however, they are ineffective, especially when less obvious. For example painting toilet doors in nursing homes a particular colour is a practice probably more therapeutic for architects than dementia sufferers. It requires the learning of a rather obscure association: 'red door = toilet'. Hanley (1981) and Gilleard *et al.* (1981) demonstrated in classic ward orientation studies that even signposts are not very effective for dementia patients in the absence of systematic training in what they relate to. That is, the patient must usually be assisted to learn the association between the cue (e.g. red door) and the information whose retrieval the cue is meant to prompt (e.g. this is the toilet). Without such learning, a red door is just a red door. Though the cue is meant as a retrieval aid, learning the association is actually an acquisition problem, a critical point rarely mentioned in texts extolling the use of cues.

This reflects a general principle emerging from the literature on memory retraining in dementia: substantial assistance must be provided at the two most commonly impaired stages of the learning process—acquisition (or input) and retrieval (or output). That is, if the person is systematically assisted to acquire or learn a piece of information, there is an increased chance that he/she will be able to remember it if (and only if) retrieval assistance is also provided when that information is required (Bird and Luszcz, 1991, 1993; Bäckman, 1992). Camp and associates (e.g. Camp and McKitrick, 1992) and Bird and Kinsella (1996), and Bird *et al.* (1995) have demonstrated how this may be accomplished. They have also shown that cues may assist patients in recalling and performing desired behaviour, as well as information (such as the location of the toilet) which will affect behaviour. The technique used to teach the association between the cue and the information or action the cue is meant to prompt is spaced retrieval combined with fading cues. It is based on the robust finding that the act of recalling a piece of information (i.e. retrieval) helps to consolidate it in memory (Bjork and Bjork, 1992). This holds true for people with mild to moderate dementia, though they require many more retrieval trials than normal individuals. Essentially the patient is told the association between the cue and the information it is intended to prompt, and then is immediately tested. For example:

'This beeper sound means it's time to go to the toilet. . ... What is this beeper reminding you to do?'

The intervals between test trials are then slowly increased at the patient's learning rate (spaced retrieval) and, where failure occurs, the patient is given extra hints and cues as necessary (fading cues) until they do retrieve the information.

Bird *et al.* (1995) reported the use of this technique in detail in five cases to ameliorate clinical problems including, as well as orientation, more serious difficulties such as intrusive aggressive behaviour and obsessive toileting. In each case the patient was taught the association between a cue and a desired behaviour. For example the intrusive patient was an ex-missionary who went into other patient's bedrooms many times a day to 'help' them and, when they resisted, became aggressive. She was taught the association between a large red STOP sign and the action 'Stop and walk away'. The STOP sign was then placed at eye height on door frames in all the rooms she frequented and intrusions and violence ceased (see Fig. 18.1(c)). The model used for this and similar interventions undertaken by the authors appears in Table 18.1.

Other recent cases include a community-resident woman with chronic faecal incontinence who was trained to associate a beeper with going to the toilet and two separate cases of gross sexual disinhibition. The men concerned were taught, using spaced retrieval and fading cues, to respond to the cue: What's the ward rule? with: 'Don't touch women' They both eventually internalized this association and the behaviour ceased; one is reported in Alexopoulos (1994); the data for the other is in Fig. 18.1(d).

There are important caveats. Firstly, the technique requires sensitive clinical skills to apply. Patients must not feel harassed or irritated during training trials, which are best casually introduced into general conversation, for example: 'By the way, what does that beeper sound mean?'. Secondly, it is

Table 18.1 Model of cued recall of behaviour

Acquisition	Patient taught, using spaced retrieval and fading cues, the association between a cue, and the information the cue is meant to prompt (e.g. cat picture on door = my room; beeper = it's time to visit toilet)
Retrieval	Patient encounters cue (e.g. cat picture) in the environment or cue (e.g. beeper) is activated and information is recalled
Maintenance	Because of the retrieval effect, each naturalistic encounter with the cue where successful recall occurs is a fresh learning trial, maintaining the association

important to understand the underlying principle; rote application will surely fail. Thirdly, only single associations can be taught at a time, and only a few to any one patient. This is not generalized memory improvement; it is focused use of a technique to ameliorate particular identified problems. Finally this is not a panacea. It is simply a technique like all others which sensibly and sensitively adapted to the case profile will be appropriate to some situations, and completely inappropriate in others.

Behavioural approaches

Operant conditioning

Stimulus control methods are frequently used, in that the responsiveness of behaviour to the environment—physical and social—is a central feature of many plans. However, the other technique most often associated with traditional behaviour modification—operant conditioning—is also often advocated in texts on psychosocial interventions (e.g. McGovern and Koss, 1994; Rapp *et al.*, 1992). Despite this, there are almost no cases reported in the literature on the use of differential reinforcement to ameliorate behavioural problems in dementia. The memory clinic worker who wants to develop expertise on non-pharmacological methods should be familiar with the idea of changing behaviour by systematically adjusting the consequences, and is directed to appropriate texts (e.g. Kazdin, 1984). Used selectively, by clinicians who understand the principles (not always the case), it can be of benefit.

As an example, in another case of sexual disinhibition, a stroke victim who verbally and sexually assaulted a female nurse in the shower eventually learned that he would obtain company during the day if he desisted. The nurse was trained to say: 'No, none of that!' very sharply each time he looked like offending, but then immediately promise him a visit later if he abstained. Any time he abstained for longer than a minute she praised him and promised that she would come and talk to him later because he was 'behaving like a gentleman'. This illustrates the necessity for selective and focused use of operant conditioning. The intervention was only possible because the patient's memory was not too badly impaired, and because the best hypothesis for the aetiology of his behaviour was loneliness and low social stimulation. That is, the reinforcer also addressed the posited cause.

It should be noted (see Fig. 18.1(e)) that although more effective than neuroleptic medication in controlling this problem, the behaviour was not eliminated completely by operant conditioning. This is the kind of outcome memory disorders team workers can most realistically expect when attempting to change patient behaviour, whether by pharmacological or behavioural means. A reduction in behaviour to more manageable proportions is a more realistic target than cessation of that behaviour. Success, when it occurs, is far more commonly partial rather than total.

Problem prevention

A further behavioural approach involves preventing the problem behaviour, by interrupting the habitual sequence of actions leading to it. A common example is locks which require memory and/or problem solving skills to operate to prevent certain forms of wandering. Hussian and Brown (1987) found that a grid pattern painted on the floor was perceived by some wandering patients as a solid barrier. A curtain across a door or door handle, or disguising a door as a window have been equally effective in our experience. This is an area where the ingenuity of the clinician can be used to good effect, to find ways of avoiding problems without precipitating a counter-productive response of agitation and frustration. As an example, a man who obsessively showered, fully clothed, was 'cured' by removing the tap heads. Even though they remained in the bathroom, he was unable to make the connection and screw them on again, or to find another showering source. In another example, a woman who was telephoned scores of times daily by her mother put an answer-phone on the original line, and obtained a new number for all other calls. The answer-phone message told the mother the three times each day the daughter would call back, which she faithfully did. The repetitive telephoning soon stopped, probably because it was not reinforced by direct contact with the daughter each time it occurred (i.e. operant conditioning).

Summary

In summary, when undertaking non-pharmacological treatment of distressing symptoms in dementia some helpful principles emerge:

(1) the problem should be clearly defined;

(2) treatment should be individualized, based on a thorough assessment;

(3) treatment should address factors in the environment alleviating or exacerbating the problem;

(4) simple learning and behavioural principles, sensitively employed, may be helpful in alleviating the difficulties;

(5) collaboration with carers is essential;

(6) seeking to understand the perspective of the person with dementia is perhaps the most important aspect of planning an intervention.

However, we have made it clear that research into optimal ways of working with people with dementia and their families non-pharmacologically is under-developed, a major indictment of the clinical research community given that the problem has been recognized since Alzheimer's time. In reality we need to know a great deal more about the effectiveness of psychosocial methods (see Woods and Roth, 1996). It is not clear that they would be any less effective than pharmacological methods (Orrell and Woods, 1996), and used appropriately will certainly have fewer side-effects. Major tranquillisers have remarkably little efficacy with behavioural problems in dementia, out of all proportion to their widespread use. There is now a slowly growing clinical literature on psychosocial methods, as illustrated in this chapter. We would argue that it is often possible to provide significant assistance by psychosocial means, whether as alternatives or adjuncts to pharmacological methods, provided the clinician approaches each case in the systematic way described. This requires thorough assessment to define and understand the idiosyncratic, individual parameters of each case, and a range of clinical skills from the ability to impart basic information about dementia to carers, through knowledge of common drug side-effects in older people and ability to recognize cases where medical screening or medication is required, to a reasonably sophisticated understanding of techniques such as operant conditioning, environmental adjustments, and use of residual memory. All this must be achieved sensitively, ensuring that any intervention does not dehumanize or devalue the person with dementia or exploit the caregiver's good will.

Rather than expecting each individual clinician to be the repository of all wisdom, we have found it more useful to employ a team approach, with much cross-disciplinary discussion of difficult cases. This is an idea whose time appears to be approaching, and many recent authors have explicitly recommended an interdisciplinary approach to behaviour problems associated with dementia (e.g., Hinchliffe *et al.*, 1995; Teri *et al.*, 1992; Rapp *et al.*, 1992).

References

Key references recommended by the authors are marked with an *.

Alexopoulos, P. (1994). Management of sexually disinhibited behaviour by a demented patient. *Australian Journal on Ageing,* **13***,* 119.

Allen, C. (1996). The effectiveness of memory aid groups. *PSIGE Newsletter,* **56***,* 15–19.

Aneshensel, C. S., Pearlin, L. I., Mullan, J. T., Zarit, S. H., and Whitlatch, C. J. (1995). *Profiles in caregiving: the unexpected career.* San Diego: Academic Press.

Bäckman, L. (1992). Memory training and memory improvement in Alzheimer's disease: rules and exceptions. *Acta Neurologia Scandinavica,***139** (suppl.), 84–89.

*Bahro, M., Silber, E., and Sunderland, T. (1995). How do patients with Alzheimer's disease cope with their illness? A clinical experience report. *Journal of American Geriatrics Society,* **43**, 41–46.

Ballard, C., Boyle, A., Bowler, C., and Lindesay, J. (1996). Anxiety disorders in dementia sufferers. *International Journal of Geriatric Psychiatry,* **11**, 987–990.

Beck, C., Heacock, P., Mercer, S., Thatcher, R. N., and Sparkman, C. (1988). The impact of cognitive skills retraining on persons with Alzheimer's disease or mixed dementia.*Journal of Geriatric Psychiatry,* **21**, 73–88.

*Bird, M., Alexopoulos, P., and Adamowicz, **J.** (1995). Success and failure in five case studies: Use of cued recall to ameliorate behaviour problems in senile dementia. *International Journal of Geriatric Psychiatry,* **10**, 305–311.

Bird, M., and Kinsella, G. (1996). Long-term cued recall of tasks in senile dementia. *Psychology and Ageing,* **11**, 45–56.

Bird, M. J., and Luszcz, M. A. (1991). Encoding specificity, depth of processing, and cued recall in Alzheimer's disease. *Journal of Clinical and Experimental Neuropsychology,* **13**, 508–520.

Bird, M. J., and Luszcz, M. A. (1993). Enhancing memory performance in Alzheimer's disease: Acquisition assistance and cue effectiveness. *Journal of Clinical and Experimental Neuropsychology,* **15**, 921–932.

Birnie, J. (1997). A memory group for older adults. *PSIGE Newsletter,* **59**, 30–33.

Bjork, R. A., and Bjork, E. L. (1992). A new theory of disuse and an old theory of stimulus fluctuation. In A. F. Healy, S. M. Kosslyn, and R. M. Shiffrin (eds) *From learning processes to cognitive processes: Essays in honor of William K. Estes.* (pp. 35–67). New Jersey: Erlbaum.

Bledin, K., MacCarthy, B., Kuipers, L., and Woods, R. T. (1990). Daughters of people with dementia: expressed emotion, strain and coping. *British Journal of Psychiatry,* **157**, 221–227.

Bourgeois, M. S. (1990). Enhancing conversation skills in patients with Alzheimer's disease using a prosthetic memory aid. *Journal of Applied Behavior Analysis,* **23**, 29–42.

Bourgeois, M. S. (1992). *Conversing with memory impaired individuals using memory aids: a memory aid workbook.* Bicester: Winslow Press.

Breuil, V., Rotrou, J. D., Forette, F., Tortrat, D., Ganansia-Ganem, A., Frambourt, A., Moulin, F., and Boller, F. (1994). Cognitive stimulation of patients with dementia: preliminary results. *International Journal of Geriatric Psychiatry,* **9**, 211–217.

Brodaty, H. (1992). Carers: training informal carers. In T. Arie (ed.), *Recent advances in psychogeriatrics–2* (pp. 163–171). Edinburgh: Churchill Livingstone.

Burgio, L., Scilley, K., Hardin, J., Hsu, C., and Yancey, J. (1996). Environmental 'White Noise': An intervention for verbally agitated nursing home residents. *Journal of Gerontology: Psychological Sciences,* **51B**, P364–P373.

*Camp, C. J., and McKitrick, L. A. (1992). Memory interventions in Alzheimer's type dementia populations: Methodological and theoretical issues. In R. L. West and J. D. Sinnot (eds), *Everyday memory and aging: Current research and methodology* (pp. 155–172). New York: Springer.

Drummond, L., Kirchoff, L., and Scarbrough, D. R. (1978). A practical guide to reality orientation: A treatment approach for confusion and disorientation. *Gerontologist,* **18**, 568–573.

Feil, N. (1993). *The Validation breakthrough: simple techniques for communicating with people with 'Alzheimer's type dementia'.* Baltimore: Health Professions Press.

Gerdner, L., and Swanson, E. (1993). Effects of individualized music on confused and agitated elderly patients. *Archives of Psychiatric Nursing,* **7**, 284–291.

Gibson, F. (1994). What can reminiscence contribute to people with dementia? In J. Bornat (ed.), *Reminiscence reviewed: evaluations, achievements, perspectives* (pp. 46–60). Buckingham: Open University Press.

Gilleard, C., Mitchell, R. G., and Riordan, J. (1981). Ward orientation training with psychogeriatric patients. *Journal of Advanced Nursing,* **6**, 95–98.

Gilliard, J., and Gwilliam, C. (1996). Sharing the diagnosis: a survey of memory clinics, their policies on informing people with dementia and their families, and the support they offer. *International Journal of Geriatric Psychiatry,* **11**, 1001–1003.

Giuliano, B. (1994). *ThreePhase Therapy: A fresh approach to aged care in plain words.* Canberra: Australia: Patrick Allen.

Greene, J. G. (1984). The evaluation of Reality Orientation. In I. Hanley and J. Hodge (eds), *Psychological approaches to the care of the elderly* (pp. 192–212). London: Croom Helm.

Hanley, I. G. (1981). The use of signposts and active training to modify ward disorientation in elderly patients. *Journal of Behavioural Therapy and Experimental Psychiatry,* **12**, 241–247.

Hanley, I. G., and Lusty, K. (1984). Memory aids in reality orientation: a single-case study. *Behaviour Research and Therapy,* **22**, 709–712.

Hart, S., and Semple, J. M. (1990). *Neuropsychology and the dementias.* London: Taylor and Francis.

Hausman, C. (1992). Dynamic psychotherapy with elderly demented patients. In G. Jones and B. M. L. Miesen (eds), *Care-giving in dementia: research and applications* (pp. 181–198). London: Routledge.

Hinchliffe, A. C., Hyman, I. L., Blizard, B., and Livingston, G. (1995). Behavioural complications of dementia—can they be treated? *International Journal of Geriatric Psychiatry,* **10**, 839–847.

Holden, U. P., and Woods, R. T. (1995). *Positive approaches to dementia care.* (3rd edn). Edinburgh: Churchill Livingstone.

Hussian, R. A., and Brown, D. C. (1987). Use of two-dimensional grid patterns to limit hazardous ambulation in demented patients. *Journal of Gerontology,* **42,** 558–560.

Kazdin, A. (1984). Behavior modification in applied settings (3rd edn). Chicago: Dorsey Press.

Keady, J. (1996). The experience of dementia: a review of the literature and implications for nursing practice. *Journal of Clinical Nursing,* **5,** 275–288.

Kitwood, T. (1990). The dialectics of dementia: with particular reference to Alzheimer's disease. *Ageing and Society,* **10,** 177–196.

Kitwood, T. (1997). The experience of dementia. *Aging and Mental Health,* **1,** 13–22.

Kitwood, T., Buckland, S., and Petrie, T. (1995). *Brighter futures: a report on research into provision for persons with dementia in residential homes, nursing homes and sheltered housing.* Kidlington: Anchor Housing Association.

Knight, B. G., Lutzky, S. M., and Macofsky-Urban, F. (1993). A meta-analytic review of interventions for caregiver distress: recommendations for future research. *Gerontologist,* **33,** 240–248.

McEvoy, C.L., and Patterson, R.L. (1986). Behavioral treatment of deficit skills in dementia patients. *Gerontologist,* **26,** 475–478.

McGovern, R. J., and Koss, E. (1994). The use of behavior modification with Alzheimer patients: values and limitations. *Alzheimer Disease and Associated Disorders,* **8,** 82–91.

Maguire, C. P., Kirby, M., Coen, R., Coakley, D., Lawlor, B. A., and O'Neill, D. (1996). Family members' attitudes toward telling the patient with Alzheimer's disease their diagnosis. *British Medical Journal,* **313,** 529–530.

Martin, A. (1987). Representation of semantic and spatial knowledge in Alzheimer's patients: Implications for models of preserved learning in amnesia. *Journal of Clinical and Experimental Neuropsychology,* **9,** 191–224.

Miesen, B. M. L. (1992). Attachment theory and dementia. In G. Jones and B. M. L. Miesen (eds), *Care-giving in dementia* (pp. 38–56). London: Routledge.

Mullen, R., Howard, R., David, A., and Levy, R. (1996). Insight in Alzheimer's disease. *International Journal of Geriatric Psychiatry,* **11,** 645–651.

Orrell, M., and Woods, R. T. (1996). Tacrine and psychological therapies in dementia—no contest? *International Journal of Geriatric Psychiatry,* **11,** 189–192.

Peisah, C., and Brodaty, H. (1994). Practical guidelines for the treatment of behavioural complications of dementia. *Medical Journal of Australia,* **161,** 558–564.

Rapp, M. S., Flint, A. J., Herrmann, N., and Proulx, G.B. (1992). Behavioural disturbances in the demented elderly: phenomenology, pharmacotherapy and behavioural management. *Canadian Journal of Psychiatry*, **37**, 651–657.

Reifler, B. V., and Larson, E. (1990). Excess disability in dementia of the Alzheimer's type. In E. Light and B. D. Lebowitz (eds), *Alzheimer's disease treatment and family stress* (pp. 363–382). New York: Hemisphere.

Rice, K., and Warner, N. (1994). Breaking the bad news: what do psychiatrists tell patients with dementia about their illness? *International Journal of Geriatric Psychiatry*, **9**, 467–471.

Sinason, V. (1992). The man who was losing his brain. In V. Sinason (ed.), *Mental handicap and the human condition: new approaches from the Tavistock* (pp. 87–110). London: Free Association Books.

Stokes, G., and Goudie, F. (1990). Counselling confused elderly people. In G. Stokes and F. Goudie (eds), *Working with dementia* (pp. 181–190). Bicester: Winslow Press.

Teri, L., Truax, L., Logston, R., Uomoto, J., Zarit, S., and Vitaliano, P. (1992). Assessment of behavioral problems in dementia: the Revised Memory and Behaviour Problems Checklist. *Psychology and Aging*, **7**, 622–631.

Thompson, L. W., Wagner, B., Zeiss, A., and Gallagher, D. (1990). Cognitive/behavioural therapy with early stage Alzheimer's patients: an exploratory view of the utility of this approach. In E. Light and B. D. Lebowitz (eds), *Alzheimer's disease: treatment and family stress* (pp. 383–397). New York: Hemisphere.

Woods, R. T. (1994). Management of memory impairment in older people with dementia. *International Review of Psychiatry*, **6**, 153–161.

*Woods, R. T. (1996). Cognitive approaches to the management of dementia. In R. G. Morris (ed.), *The cognitive neuropsychology of Alzheimer-type dementia* (pp. 310–326). Oxford: Oxford University Press.

Woods, R. T., and Britton, P. G. (1985). *Clinical psychology with the elderly*. London: Croom Helm / Chapman Hall.

Woods, R. T., and Roth, A. (1996). Effectiveness of psychological interventions with older people. In A. Roth and P. Fonagy (eds), *What works for whom? A critical review of psychotherapy research* (pp. 321–340). New York: Guilford Press.

Yale, R. (1995). *Developing Support groups for individuals with early stage Alzheimer's disease: Planning, implementation and evaluation*. Baltimore: Health Profession Press.

Yesavage, J. A., Rose, T. L., and Spiegel, D. (1982). Relaxation training and memory improvement in elderly normals: correlation of anxiety ratings and recall improvement. *Experimental Aging Research*, **8**, 195–198.

19 Management of common problems

D. O'Neill and D. Carr

Introduction

In this chapter we will discuss class-specific management (i.e. for dementia of any cause), assuming that dementia-specific treatment (i.e. cholinesterase inhibitors for Alzheimer's disease, or blood pressure control and smoking cessation for vascular dementia) will be initiated. The evidence-based literature in dementia is heavily biased towards i) the aetiopathology of the dementias, ii) their accurate diagnosis, and iii) pharmacological interventions, particularly those aimed at the cholinergic system. While these are issues of great importance, there is a relative lack of formal evaluation of the assessment and management of problems by dementia services as well as the efficacy and appropriateness of commonly used strategies for intervention. There are also differences between memory disorders teams as to the emphasis and structure of management strategies for those patients and caregivers who consult them. It is important that existing strategies should be evaluated and where shown to be effective should be incorporated into routine service provision. A lack of controlled studies should not prevent the use of common-sense strategies but should spur on research programmes on their efficacy, a need recognized by the European Union (O'Neill, in press) and the National Institute on Aging in the United States.

These initiatives may help to dispel some of the nihilism associated with the management and treatment of patients with dementia. This is in stark contrast to other progressive diseases where traditional medical management potential is limited, such as cryptogenic fibrosing alveolitis or cancers with no potential for medical or surgical intervention. For such patients a wide range of supports are available and it is important that a similar approach is adopted for patients with dementia. As patients and their families are assessed by memory disorders teams, not only for advice and assessment on diagnosis but perhaps more often for concerns about management, it is critical that management strategies should be given a more prominent emphasis. Such services have an important educational role for other health-care providers, and it is important that they place as much priority on intellectual rigour in management issues as they would on assessment policies.

Needs of patients and caregivers

Surveys of distress among patients and caregivers cite different inventories of problems: the difficulties of making an accurate assessment of prevalence of symptoms has been described in one review which provides estimates of problem behaviours in dementia (Collenda, 1995) (Table 19.1). It is important that an approach is taken which includes the needs of both the patient and the caregiver.

Table 19.1 Mean prevalence of problem behaviours in dementia, from eight studies (Collenda, 1995)

Problem behaviour	%
Physical aggression/agitation	42
Verbal aggression/threats	54
Restlessness	38
Wandering	30
Sleep disturbances	38
Apathy/withdrawal	27

Principles of management

Six broad principles can be discerned:

♦ **Management should be based on problems rather than abnormalities** (Winograd and Jarvik, 1986). This is not a semantic nicety: cognitive abnormalities form the basis of most diagnostic strategies but non-cognitive problems, particularly behavioural, cause the most troublesome problems for caregivers. This highlights the different emphasis of diagnostic and management strategies.

♦ **Increasing attention to the subjective experience of the patient is required** (Bahro *et al.*, 1995a; Kitwood, 1997): this is a relatively new area of research and has, to a certain extent, been overshadowed by the very important development of emphasis on the needs of the caregivers.

♦ **An individualized package of care is required in each case.** The impact of dementia will vary enormously between individuals and families (Brody, 1990). This means that assessment of problems and their management will have to be caried out in a phenomenonological fashion.

♦ **Some interventions can cause more harm than good**: the use of 'as-required' (PRN) sedation with neuroleptics is associated with an increased incidence falls (Aisen, 1992), and physical restraints are associated with injury and death.

♦ **Memory disorders teams need to integrate their intervention with existing primary care services**. Management strategies which are initiated need to be shared with the primary care services, a process which is a two-way educational experience. Defining the responsibilities for service provision is an important component of the contact between the patient, caregivers, and the memory clinic.

♦ **It may take a number of visits to formulate the most successful manage-ment strategies** for a disease with a such a wide range of manifestations and problems, just as it may take several visits to provide an accurate diagnosis of a dementia.

♦ **An interdisciplinary format is essential:** ideally this should take advantage of the skills of the interdisciplinary team, all of whom may have something to offer, and none of whom can work effectively without a knowledge of the other's expertise (Cunningham *et al*., 1996). Physicians, nurses, social workers, occupational therapists (Corcoran and Gitlin, 1992), and psycho-logists are among the professionals who can contribute to management of common problems. In view of the strong interplay between physical and psychological aspects of dementia, it is important that the memory dis-orders team should have strong links between physicians and psychiatrists, and a social worker/ counsellor position is invaluable. Interdisciplinary case conferences and continuing professional development are important in fostering good team work.

Assessment strategies

A thorough problem-based assessment of the patient and family is the foundation of management. The first step is to detect and catalogue problems. Just as the detection of cognitive impairment improves with the routine use of brief cognitive screening schedules, there is increasing support for using inventories of common problems in dementia. One of the earliest and most widely quoted is that of Winograd and Jarvik (1986) (Table 19.2).

While this should be seen as a first attempt, and open to future revision, it offers a useful check list of common problems. It has not been shown that use of a check list improves the therapeutic yield of a clinical encounter but it does not seem unreasonable to use an aide memoire like this, particularly bearing in mind a strong tradition of nihilism within the health-care professions when faced with chronic neurodegenerative disease. More specific inventories include the BEHAVE-AD (Reisberg *et al.* 1987), the Cohen-Mansefield Agitation Inventory for behavioural and psychiatric symptomatology (Cohen-

Table 19.2 Checklist for patients with dementia (Winograd and Jarvik, 1986)

I. Medical and psychiatric condition	**III. Social supports**
A. Medications	A. Living arrangements
B. Coexistent medical illnesses	1. housing
C. Nutrition	2. financial resources
D. Anorexia	
E. Sleep disturbance	B. Human resources
F. Neurological changes	1. available family
G. Incontinence	2. available friends
H. Sexual problems, disinhibition	3. counselling
I. Depression	4. in-home services
J. Agitated, restless, irritable behaviour	
K. Inappropriate affect	**IV. Caregiver needs**
L. Suspicious, paranoid thoughts	A. Social supports
M. Hostility, verbal and physical threats	1. respite services
N. Dental conditions	2. support group
O. Foot problems	3. financial aid
	4. available friends and family
II. Care needs of patient	
A. Activity and functional status	B. Psychological issues
1. what is patient's daily schedule?	1. evidence of depression
2. does patient wander? get lost?	2. evidence of other psychopathology
3. activities of daily living	3. abuse by patient
4. instrumental activities of daily living	4. abuse of patient
5. does patient drive? problems?	
6. does patient use or abuse drugs or alcohol?	C. Medical issues
	1. symptoms of physical illness?
7. who supervises medications?	2. use of drugs/ alcohol?
8. who handles finances?	3. sleep disturbance
	4. health habits?
B. Social skills	
1. what are the patients social activities?	D. Legal issues
2. with whom does the patient have relationships?	1. property
	2. durable power of attorney
3. how does the patient react to visitors?	3. arrangements for decisions
4. how does the patient react to change in environment (e.g. panics in a restaurant)	regarding medical treatment, durable power of attorney for health, living will

Mansfield 1986), and the Consortium to Establish a Registry for Alzheimer's Disease Behaviour Rating Scale Revised Memory and Behaviour Problems checklist (RMBPC) (Teri *et al.*, 1992). It is worth noting that there are also incidences of positive features such as the Pleasant Event Schedule (Teri and Logsden, 1991). This is a reminder that we need to ask relatives about what things they believe to be important in promoting quality of life for the patient with dementia. This positive approach can be effectively harnessed for dementia care, for example by participation in musical activities (Pollack and Namazi, 1992).

A positive response on a check list should trigger a response from the team. There will need to be a detailed interview with the caregiver and the patient to identify the problems and to determine:

♦ What is the relationship between the caregiver and patient and how does this influence the occurrence and treatment of behavioural problems?

♦ What are the realistic goals for non-drug intervention?

♦ What are the resources of the patient and caregiver?

♦ What can be expected based on the cognitive level of the patient and the degree of stress on the caregiver?

♦ If agitated, whose problem is the agitation? Is it disruptive or not?

A thorough physical examination should be undertaken to rule out any underlying medical condition, drug, or medication side-effects which may be causing behavioural or cognitive problems. The examination may include a full blood count with differential, electrolyte levels, hepatic or renal profile, urinalysis, and/or chest radiograph.

Sharing the diagnosis

Informing the patient

Informing caregivers has been recognized as integral to success in management for many years; a less well-recognized core issue is how to help the patient deal with the illness. Until recently it was recognized that patients suffer from distress in the early stages of the disease but it was rare to consider sharing the diagnosis with the patient. The involvement of the patient in the assessment and management programme has largely tended to be achieved by working around the patient. Most older people state a preference to be told the diagnosis should they develop the disease (Holroyd *et al.*, 1996; Maguire *et al.*, 1996). However, the majority of relatives of patients with Alzheimer's disease would not want the patient to be told the diagnosis, but would themselves wish to know if they develop the condition (Maguire *et al.*, 1996). This inconsistency may reflect a generational difference in the perception of the disease, a paternalistic desire by family members to protect patients from the harsh reality of their condition, or a reluctance of relatives to deal with the patient's knowledge and possible grief.

Most of those who opposed disclosure of the diagnosis to the patient felt that it could precipitate symptoms of anxiety and depression. However, Bahro *et al.* have shown that when the diagnosis is given, both patients and family members often use denial as a defence mechanism to deal with it (Bahro *et al.*, 1995a). Many patients are aware of their progressive cognitive deficits, regardless of whether or not a diagnosis of Alzheimer's disease has been given. Insight may be an important determinant of reaction to disclosure, with lack of insight providing a degree of psychological protection. Retention of insight varies from patient to patient. Some studies have found it to be unrelated to degree of cognitive deterioration, though related to 'frontal' dysfunction (Michon *et al.*, 1994); others have shown that, at least in moderate or severe dementia, insight declines with increasing severity (McDaniel *et al.*, 1995). In insightful patients, the risk of depressive reactions or even suicide must be seriously considered after disclosure of any major illness. This seems no different in Alzheimer's disease. Two cases of suicide in patients told their diagnosis have recently been described (Rohde *et al.*, 1995). In one study, 10 family members said that they would consider committing suicide if they were diagnosed as having Alzheimer's disease (Maguire *et al.*, 1996).

In 1961, 90 per cent of physicians expressed a preference for not telling cancer patients their diagnosis. By 1977 a complete reversal of opinion had occurred with 97 per cent of physicians favouring disclosure of the diagnosis (Novack *et al.*, 1979). The reasons for not telling cancer patients their diagnosis in 1961 were similar to those quoted for not telling patients with Alzheimer's disease their diagnosis today. The change in policy among doctors coincided with advances in the management and treatment of cancer. Similar advances are being made with Alzheimer's disease today, so clinicians must decide whether to respect the wishes of family members not to tell patients their diagnosis, or to respect individual autonomy, inform patients, and involve them in the management of their condition.

We would agree with a recent review which advocated disclosure of diagnosis but which also emphasized that clinicians must evaluate each situation individually (Drickamer, 1992). Family members as well as patients respond in a variety of ways to the psychological threats presented by the diagnosis of Alzheimer's disease, and the issue of disclosure needs to be dealt with on a patient by patient basis. It is likely that the disclosure by recent prominent figures in public life that they suffer from Alzheimer's disease will help to reduce the difficulties that health-care providers and caregivers have with disclosure of the diagnosis. Positive developments in this regard include self-help groups for the patients and their families with early stage disease run by the Alzheimer's Association in the United States.

Informing the caregiver

Informing the family of the diagnosis and possible management strategies has been an implicit part of clinical practice. Reinforcement has been given by an Australian study which showed positive benefits from a 4-day residential educational programme for caregivers (Brodaty and Gresham, 1989). This intensity of training is not realistic for most services and the challenge is to develop the most time and cost effective way to inform, train, and support caregivers. Among the options are: information, individual counselling, caregiver support groups, family meetings, and training courses. Information may be way of brochures, books, videos, or over the internet (references below). Family meetings have the potential to be a valuable two-way process, with clinicians learning more about the patient and his milieu and families learning more about the condition. Short courses have been proposed and preliminary results are encouraging, although there can be practical problems in terms of the caregiver getting time to get to the course. Caregiver support groups are helpful for some caregivers, but the lack of a formal core structure and variations in leader training make it difficult to generalize about their utility or overall acceptability.

Behavioural and psychiatric disturbances

Types of disturbances

Behavioural or psychiatric symptoms are common in patients with all dementias and in Alzheimer's disease (Table 19.1). These may include depression, hallucinations, delusions, agitation, screaming, wandering, sleep disturbances, suspiciousness, violent episodes, and sexually inappropriate behaviour among others. The phenomenology of some of the symptoms are further complicated in that they do not exactly follow the criteria or typology of psychiatric symptoms as defined in psychotic illness; for example the relatively common phenomena of not recognizing oneself in the mirror (mirror sign) or mistaking members of one's own family may well reflect cognitive changes rather than a pure delusional state. Behavioural symptoms are a significant source of caregiver or family stress and this relates not only to the behaviour of the patient but also to the relationship with the caregiver and caregiver characteristics.

Assessment

Careful assessment is the key to determining the cause of any behavioural disorder such as agitation, to deciding which behaviours to target for change, and to designing specific integrated management approaches. Agitation is one of the most common reasons for admission to a nursing home for people with dementia and may be defined as a syndrome of pathological arousal, usually repetitive, compulsive motor activity of verbalization which occurs either as acute, discrete episode or as a subacute chronic state (Spar and La Rue 1990). There clearly may be a good deal of licence in the interpretation of this definition. Agitation tends to be the result of multiple factors and it is important for the memory clinic team to work systematically through various possible contributing elements. These include physical illnesses or conditions which affect psychological state. It is important to treat comorbidity, minimize medications which may cause delirium or agitation and treat coexistent depression. It is also important to interview the family with regard to social and environmental conditions which may trigger the behaviour.

A useful concept is the ABC model of behaviour management to guide caregivers in coping with agitated patients with dementia. 'A' is the antecedent or triggering event that precedes the problem behaviour; 'B' is the behaviour itself; 'C' is the consequence of the behaviour which reinforces and maintains the behaviour. An example is that of a loud, irritated caregiver trying desperately to feed a soon-to-be-agitated older demented woman in a room filled with people, resonant with loud noises, and the table with the patient's food is cluttered with other objects. By modifying the environment, both physically (removing clutter and engaging in feeding at a less crowded time) and interpersonally (caregiver softening her voice and attitude), the patient evidenced less agitated behaviour and was able to eat more calmly. Thus, the antecedent (caregiver's tone and stressful environment) was identified, and the problem behaviour (agitation and potential violence) was consequently mitigated (Teri, 1997).

Agitation-manifested behaviours need to be catalogued; those behaviours causing the most problem should be targeted for change. Table 19.3 charts possible causes of behaviour disturbances and broad management strategies.

Table 19.3 Management guidelines

Possible cause	Management guidelines
Physical illnesses or conditions	
Pain/distress	Physical exam and medical interventions
Delirium	Medical evaluation, check drug history, treat underlying problems, behavioural intervention
Sensory Impairments	Hearing aids, glasses, constant illumination, quiet surroundings
Psychological state	
Depression	Antidepressants, pleasurable tasks, behaviour modification
Psychosis	Neuroleptics, carbamazepine
Anxiety	Behaviour modification methods, pharmacology if necessary
Cognitive impairment/functional decline	
	Behaviour modifications, environmental modification, walking exercise, pleasurable tasks, regular routine

Depression

Depression is a frequent occurrence in dementia and may exacerbate cognitive and non-cognitive dysfunction. For example agitated behaviour has been linked with depressed affect in nursing home patients with dementia

(Teri and Wagner, 1992). There should be a high index of suspicion of de-pression in patients with agitation, particularly in the presence of anxiety. In older people in general, there is evidence that depression is detected but under-treated: it is likely that this is also true for depression in dementia. Aids in detection are the Geriatric Depression Scale which has been shown to be useful in mild to moderate dementia (O'Riordan *et al.*, 1990) and the Cornell scale (although the rating of this would seem to limit its use to those with psychiatric training) (Alexopoulos *et al.* 1988). The detection of depression in severe dementia can be more difficult and one potential solution is a 'gestalt' rating of depression in severe dementia (Greenwald and Kramer, 1991). Certain medical conditions as well as a family or personal history of de-pression may be helpful pointers. In mild to moderate dementia, there is little evidence to suggest that depression is commonly atypical: in more severe dementia, it may present as behavioural disturbance or disruption of behavioural patterns. We recommend a high index of suspicion as well as a low threshold for a psychogeriatric consultation for such cases.

Treatment should take into account social and psychological factors which may be precipitating or exacerbating a depression, for example carer stress and negative caregiver–patient interaction. Certain common medications such as β-blockers can have a depressive effect, and a medication review is critical. Pharmacological opportunities for depression in dementia may be enhanced by the selective serotonin re-uptake inhibitors (SSRIs) as the anticholinergic activity of tricyclic antidepressants (TCA) is associated with cognitive and behavioural deterioration. The only controlled trial of TCAs in depression associated with Alzheimer's disease showed no difference between TCAs and placebo (Reifler *et al.*, 1991). However, both groups improved, and it is reason-able to interpret this as supportive of psychotherapy in depression associated with dementia. Other possible modalities include reversible inhibitors of monoamine oxidase A (RIMA) and electroconvulsive therapy: the latter seems to be effective in Alzheimer's disease (Nelson and Rosenberg, 1991).

Non-pharmacological management

After comorbidities such as depression have been eliminated and/or treated, there are several avenues of treatment for behavioural problems. In the first instance non-pharmacological management should be tried. The efficacy of medications for behavioural disturbance is uncertain, even for medications as widely used (or over-used) as neuroleptics (Schneider *et al.* 1990); many of these medications also have troublesome side-effects which occur more frequently in dementia. Pharmacological approaches should be viewed as supportive to behavioural and environmental approaches. This is a common-sense position, supported by small studies and clinical experience rather than by placebo-controlled studies.

One useful scheme for behavioural management (Chandler, 1987) is to divide interventions into four main categories. These are work with the family, environmental control, maintenance of routine, and environmental safety. Ideally, caregivers should be educated about how to look for triggers of behavioural disturbance, aided in interpreting non-verbal clues, and instructed in monitoring the efficacy of the treatment plan. Communication is particularly important between the caregiver and the patient and body language may constitute an important part of this. Many of the lay manuals on dementia care have chapters dedicated to these techniques (Mace and Rabins 1992, Wilcock, 1990); putting these concepts into clinical practice in a concise training package must be a goal for future research. Non-pharmacological strategies are considered in more detail in the preceding chapter.

Pharmacological management

Early data indicates that therapy with cholinomimetic agents may improve difficult behaviours, and many drug companies are pursuing these studies to determine efficacy (Gorman *et al.* 1993). Other pharmacological therapies addressed at control of behavioural problems can be divided into four groups: neuroleptic agents; benzodiazepines; agents enhancing serotoninergic system; and a miscellaneous group including β-blockers and anticonvulsants. There are two main issues to prescribing these drugs: i) appropriate prescribing philosophy and practice and ii) appropriate choice of agent and dose. Overuse and overdosage of medications is common in dementia, and can contribute to a worsening of cognitive impairment. The philosophy of prescribing psychoactive agents is careful assessment of need, as rational a choice of medication as possible, and to 'start low, go slow, review as you go'. This dictum emphasizes low starting doses, gradual titration of dose against symptoms, and review with the goal of reducing the dosage and, ideally, eventual withdrawal of the agent. This in itself implies a sensitization of health-care staff and caregivers in the detection and monitoring of both behavioural symptomatology and troublesome side-effects. It also requires good communication between the memory disorders team and the family physician and community health-care workers to avoid inappropriate therapy. Some form of supervision is almost always necessary for compliance with psychoactive medication.

The choice of agent depends on the underlying neuropathology, symptomatology, comorbidity, and tolerance of side-effects. Neuroleptics are among the most commonly prescribed agents, and a useful guide to positive indications for neuroleptic therapy are outlined in the OBRA 87 criteria—a United States law designed to prevent abuse of neuroleptics in nursing homes (Table 19.4 is an abbreviated summary of the guidelines). More specific recommendations are covered in Chapter 17.

Benzodiazepines have a useful role when the phenomenology is marked by

Table 19.4 OBRA 87 Interpretive guidelines for the use of antipsychotic drugs in nursing homes

Specific conditions for which antipsychotic drugs are appropriate
Organic mental syndrome (including dementia and delirium) with associated psychotic and or agitated behaviours:

which have been quantitatively and objectively documented;

which are not caused by preventable reasons;

which cause a danger to the agitated individual or others;

which cause the agitated individual to cry, scream, yell, or pace and thereby create functional impairment;

which cause the agitated individual distress or impairment.

Symptoms or indications for which antipsychotic drugs are inappropriate

Wandering	Indifference to surroundings
Poor self care	Fidgeting
Restlessness	Nervousness
Impaired memory	Depression
Anxiety	Unco-operativeness
Insomnia	Agitation (that is not a danger)
Unsociability	

PRN antipsychotic use should be restricted to appropriate conditions and limited to five doses in 7 days.

anxiety, agitation, or insomnia (Leibovici and Tariot, 1988), assuming that other comorbidities which cause these symptoms are treated. They may also be helpful in patients where neuroleptics are virtually contra-indicated; those with severe parkinsonism, Lewy body dementia, or a history of previous malignant neuroleptic syndrome. Their effectiveness is limited by tolerance, worsening of cognitive impairment and anterograde amnesia, dependency, sedation, and an increased tendency to fall with chronic administration. In most countries they are licensed for relatively short periods, usually up to 6 weeks at a time, although this is often ignored.

Agents affecting serotonin (5-HT) may have a beneficial effect on behaviour disturbance, possibly through their antidepressant properties (Nyth and Gottfries 1990). Selective serotonin reuptake inhibitors citalopram, or mixed agents such as trazodone (serotonin agonist, antagonist, and uptake inhibitor) are the main agents studied and preliminary reports are encouraging (Lebert *et al.*, 1994). Trazodone can cause sedation or postural hypotension, and may be helpful in patients without frank psychotic symptoms.

Medication compliance

The difficulties of treating a behaviourally disturbed older patient who lives alone is a classic example of the difficulties experienced with compliance in dementia. Non-compliance or inappropriate use of medication may occur for several reasons in patients with dementing illnesses, including; complex medication regimens or polypharmacy, loss of memory with no compensatory dispensing system, inadequate finances and expensive medication, lack of insight into the need for medication, or inability to allow oversight. Taking medications reliably is a major factor in the health of a patient for a variety of reasons. Of medications available specifically to treat Alzheimer's disease, Tacrine (Cognex) requires administration four times a day, which is often difficult to administrate in a memory impaired patient in the outpatient setting. Donepezil (Aricept) can be given once a day and is likely to assist with compliance. Treatment of psychosis, depression, dementia, and other medical conditions often require daily administration of medications. Iatrogenic illness and drug toxicities are not an uncommon cause for hospitalization in elderly people (Bero *et al.*, 1991). Strategies to assist with medication compliance include; pillboxes, reducing the number of medications, prescribing affordable drugs, supervision, and phone calls or other reminders to take pills.

Caregiver stress

Caregiver stress may be defined as events or circumstances that are attributable to the patient's dementing illness which have a direct or indirect adverse effect on the psychological or physical well being of the caretaker. Since dementing illnesses can affect the physical, psychological, functional, and social domains of the patient and family, it is not surprising that this stress may be the initiating event for having the patient assessed or moved to another level of care. A growing body of literature has focused on areas surrounding the efficacy of interventions and treatments in improving health of the caregiver and/or postponing nursing home placement. The role of the memory disorders team to detect or anticipate caregiver stress, and where possible to initiate strategies to alleviate it, and to give support is discussed in further detail in Chapter 16.

Precipitants of stress

Caregiver stress may be brought on by the psychological aspects of the disease, which may include; frustration over lost memories, aggravating repetition, catastrophic reactions, or the loss of recognition of a spouse or close family member. Agitation and psychosis can be especially troubling. Delusions may increase suspicions towards family and friends and hallucinations may provoke anxiety for both patient and caregiver. Insomnia may lead to sleep deprivation for both parties. Verbal or physical abuse directed toward the caregiver may result in arguments and actual physical abuse to either patient or caregiver. Lack of insight into the disease process may lead to confrontation while attributing difficult behaviours to personality traits or stubbornness. A further potential source of caregiver burden is the fear of genetic implications of the disease. Many children of the affected patient are interested in knowing their risk of developing the disease.

Even in the early stages of a dementing illness, the caretaker may have to take on many responsibilities such as medication supervision, finances, shopping, cooking, and cleaning. This may be especially difficult if the spouse or caregiver were previously not familiar with these activities or at least had assistance from the patient. As the disease progresses, urinary or faecal incontinence, difficulty with ambulation or transfers, and assistance with dressing, bathing, or feeding may also add to caregiver burden. In order to diminish stress and provide additional care in the home or nursing home setting, financial savings are typically depleted or exhausted.

Manifestations of caregiver stress

Caregiver stress can manifest itself in many forms. Emotional reactions that can occur intermittently or consistently may include; anger, loneliness, frustration, embarrassment, or grief from observing the loss of intellect in a loved one. Guilt may arise when allowing others to assist in managing the care. Anxiety and/or depression often accompany caregiving of the demented patient (Fleming *et al.* 1995) and can present in a variety of ways. Caregivers may have new difficulties with other family relationships or while performing duties in other roles or occupations. Separation, divorce, or disagreements amongst family members may occur in those settings that were 'dysfunctional' prior to the onset of the illness. Impairments in physical health may occur from actual worsening of already existent medical conditions or precipitate previously unrecognized subclinical disease. Fatigue is another common physical manifestation that may occur from both psychological and physical caregiving.

It is imperative to determine how the disease is affecting caregivers. Memory disorders teams may be in an unique position to provide this type of assessment. Physicians will benefit from the assistance of social workers, nurse specialists, or geriatric care managers to assess the degree of caregiver burden in these areas. Brief clinical tools are available that quantify caregiver stress and may be helpful to clinicians (Zarit *et al.* 1985, Robinson 1983). These may not only be useful for assessing the presence of stress, but repeat measurements can determine whether interventions have been effective.

Interventions for caregiver stress

Interventions to alleviate caregiver stress have been grouped into four themes: information, emotional needs and self-care, improvement of interpersonal relationships, and communications and development of support systems. This process is started through assessment by clinicians who make the time, and develop the expertise, to listen and provide education about the disease process. This is in itself a form of psychotherapy; this may be the best 'medicine' for early-stage caregiver stress. The caregiver needs to be instructed that patients may make statements or perform actions that are due to the disease and not a desire of the patient to be 'difficult'. An accurate diagnosis and discussion of the prognosis may help with disease acceptance and planning for future needs. Non-pharmacological and pharmacological treatment of the patient may also be useful in alleviating caregiver stress, as outlined above. Caregivers and family members should be encouraged to learn about this disease, since there are excellent books available (Mace and Rabins, 1992; Wilcock, 1990).

Fears about genetic susceptibility should be cautiously explored as described above and, where necessary, appropriate genetic counselling provided. A liaison with a clinical genetics service is very important, and not only for those dementias classically recognized as genetic, such as Huntington's disease. With advances in our understanding of genetic contribution to Alzheimer's disease, guidelines are being developed for advising patients about genetic issues in Alzheimer's disease (Lennox *et al.*, 1994). Currently, genetic testing for late-onset/ sporadic Alzheimer's disease is still experimental. Apo E testing is not recommended for clinical use at this time (Continuum, 1996). For most sporadic or late-onset disease, the immediate family members should be reassured that though their risk is increased (probably 3–4 times the normal rate), it is still unlikely they would contract the illness (Breitner, 1991).

The emotions the caregiver has been expressing should be identified and discussed in an understanding manner. If the caregiver has anxiety and/or depression, psychotherapy and pharmacological intervention may be useful. Referral to their primary care physician or psychiatrist will be necessary under some circumstances. However, relief efforts that utilize family and community resources should be encouraged so as to alleviate or reduce caregiver stress.

Local government services, community groups, or organizations may provide useful support services, and a medical social worker is best qualified to match patient's and caregiver's need to local resources. These may include the Alzheimer's disease associations, support groups for the patient and/or caregivers, day care programmes, chore workers (United States)/home helps (United Kingdom), nurses aids, visiting nurses, assisted living centres, respite care, and long-term care facilities. National or local Alzheimer's disease associations are often to the fore with service initiatives such as education, referral sources for diagnosis and treatment of dementing disorders, phone lines or help centres to answer questions, and support groups. In some countries they run day-care centres and respite services, often with transportation and sliding scales for payment depending on the financial resources of the family. Many care organizations can provide chore workers/ home helps for oversight of medication, assistance with cooking and cleaning, and also the basic activities of daily living. Respite care (unfortunately, unavailable in some European countries) is a system of admitting the patient to a skilled nursing facility for short periods to give the caregiver respite from the task of caring. Although there may be some difficulty with patient consent and also disruption of behaviour by the changes of environment, early data suggest that this is a cost-effective intervention (Koloski and Montgomery, 1995).

Eventually, as more support is required to continue at home, the cost and/or stress of providing care will make home care a less viable option. Long-term care facilities can usually provide less expensive care and are often the final choice of placement for many patients.

Abuse and neglect

A dysfunctional and unsupported relationship between patient and caregiver can result in abuse and neglect, terms that may apply to the caregiver and/or patient. Much of the knowledge base for abuse and neglect in dementia stems from the considerable body of literature on elder abuse (O'Neill *et al.*, 1990). Abuse is a complex issue and more commonly occurs when both patient and caregiver are compromised, for example a patient with dementia and a caregiver suffering from alcohol dependency. There may be a background of violence within a family and it is probably best to avoid terminology such as 'victim', which is not only judgmental but suggests a passive role in what may be a two-way process.

Abuse may be physical, involving kicking, biting, scratching, hitting, or sexual assault. It may be psychological, involving emotions of hate and anger and can manifest as screaming, shouting, insults, cursing, etc. Financial abuse may also be relatively common. Neglect is probably a more common phenomenon, and may be defined as a deficiency in basic care (the provision of adequate hygiene, adequate food, or social isolation) from the caregiver or caregivers. It should be mentioned that many demented patients will resist assistance in these areas, making caregiving extremely difficult.

Detection of abuse requires a sensitivity to the possibility of its existence, and a positive attitude to help both patient and caregiver. Many caregivers do not have the skills or resources to deal with these situations. Some couples have had long-standing marital strife and may be unable or unwilling to address and correct these problems. Clinicians who evaluate demented patients should inquire about these issues and look for signs of neglect or abuse on physical examination. A supportive and understanding interdisciplinary approach in addressing these highly charged emotional issues can be the first step in assisting a family. Working with the patient and caregiver, we should aim to relieve stress and empower both parties to make their own decisions.

Aids in this process are optimization of dementia management, including a programme for managing behavioural problems, and maximization of support structures for the caregiver. This may involve counselling, maximizing support from other family members, or utilizing community resources such as day care, respite care, home service, or chore workers/ home helps. If these measures do not work, institutionalization may be required in the event of a risk to either party; this is usually a very unhappy experience for all parties.

Reporting of elder abuse is mandatory in all states in the United States; in the absence of clearly helpful intervention by the state in many cases, it is likely that significant under-reporting occurs. On a more positive note, many state departments and other jurisdictions have phone hotlines and agencies that can be contacted to deal with suspected or actual cases of abuse or neglect of elderly patients.

Communication

In the early stages of Alzheimer's disease, language problems are often not a major problem. Subtle word finding difficulties are often noted by the collateral source, but usually do not interfere with function. The 'lost' word will often return or the patient can provide enough description to continue the train of thought or conversation. As the disease progresses, the patient with DAT has more difficulty in 'talking around' forgotten words, and eventually will develop expressive language disorders and paraphasic errors (Morris, 1995). Caregivers will often have to finish the sentence or provide the appropriate word or words. Bilingual patients will often revert back to their first learned language. Problems with comprehension will occur in the latter phases of the disease. Eventually, the patient will develop a global aphasia. Only nonsensical or inappropriate phrases may remain or they can become mute.

Atypical or rare degenerative dementing illnesses such as Pick's disease, primary progressive aphasia, cortical-basal ganglionic degeneration, or Creutzfeld–Jakob disease may present with language impairment in the early stages of these diseases (Kertesz et al. 1994). These dementing illnesses will often initially manifest as word finding problems but eventually progress and patients exhibit impairments in both expression and comprehension of language. Ischaemic vascular dementias, specifically large strokes or multi-infarct dementia, may also affect language depending on the anatomic site of injury.

Management of communication disorders

Management of communication disorders is often difficult and can be frustrating; liaison with a speech therapist (pathologist) can be helpful.

Table 19.5 Communication strategies in patients with dementia

Identify or correct visual or hearing deficits
Communicate one thought or idea at a time
Use of written notes in addition to verbal information
Speak slowly
Communicate in an environment free of distracting noise
Have the patient use gestures if they are unable to find the right word
Provide reassurance
Assist in completing the sentence
Change the subject and revisit it later
Consider speech therapy evaluation

Attempts should be made to identify or correct any hearing deficits, but patients may not manage, or may resist, hearing aids. Phrases should be short, concise, and simple. Communicating only one thought or idea at a time to individuals with memory problems can be helpful. Written notes, explanations, or reminders can be useful adjuncts to oral information that may not be retained or understood. Speaking slowly in an environment free of distracting noises should enhance communication. Asking the patient to describe what they mean or point to the object may diffuse a tense situation. Providing reassurance during times of frustration can be helpful, in addition to assisting the patient with the rest of the phrase if it can be determined by the context of the sentence. Demonstrating what behaviour you would like done can also be a useful strategy. Distraction and changing the subject may be helpful when the patient has become very frustrated over the inability to communicate or the caregiver is upset about repetitive questions. Those with vascular dementia may have other communication disorders such as dysarthria which may also benefit from a speech pathology referral. These strategies are summarized in Table 19.5 (see also Chapter 9).

Activities and instrumental activities of daily living

Functional assessment is one of the cornerstones in providing adequate evaluation of dementing illnesses. A more detailed account of the theoretical and practical aspects of functional assessment is found in Chapter 10. It is not only a fundamental component of the diagnosis of dementia but also forms the basis for quantifying dementia severity in many dementia scales (Hughes *et al.* 1982).

There are many excellent books and articles which describe or review various functional assessments (Kane and Kane, 1981). From a caregiver standpoint, it is usually functional impairment that triggers a visit to the physician.

Impairments in a patient's ability to perform important functions will depend on the previous ability to perform the skill, the ability or willingness of the caregiver to allow a portion of the task (or a subpar performance) to occur, and the extent of the cognitive impairment. Functional measures can be obtained by subjective report from a caregiver, family member, or close friend or by direct observation of abilities. The latter usually requires special training or equipment but may be a more reliable measure of a patient's capabilities.

A home assessment by an occupational therapist should be considered in addressing areas of support that are needed in maintaining the patient with dementia in the home setting. There are times when the demented patient will refuse entry of an unfamiliar person such as a homemaker into their house. We recommend that the caregiver is present during the first few visits from these individuals in order to establish a routine and a rapport with the worker.

Impairments in instrumental activities

Instrumental activities of daily living may include; shopping, cooking, cleaning, finances, medications, driving, and hobbies. One of the early findings in dementia is impairment in the ability to handle money. Balancing the cheque book, remembering to write and document cheques, comparing cheques book balances to bank statements, making change or leaving a tip, and preparing tax returns are often affected by impaired memory, executive function, and problem solving abilities. Patients with dementia may be the target for insurance scams and may make repeat donations to charity organizations. Families should be questioned about these specific issues and, where applicable, a durable power of attorney for finances should be encouraged. Most jurisdictions recognize a clinical judgement of financial competency by a senior clinician, and it may be helpful to families to point out that in mild dementia, valid financial decisions may be made by the patient. Options available may be some form of enduring power of attorney or guardianship; where this is not available, assigning financial resources and residence in joint names may be the most positive solution. This manoeuvre will avoid the more complex task of assigning court protection to the incompetent patient, a procedure which is usually more lengthy and often more costly.

Cooking is a complex task and many individuals with dementing illnesses will no longer be able to perform at their previous baseline. Initially, this may become evident during times of increased stress, that is holidays. As the disease progresses, only simple meals can be prepared. Many patients will no longer be able to operate the oven or microwave, or learn how to use new appliances. Many individuals may be able to prepare certain aspects of the meals, and caregivers should be encouraged to allow some participation. Special supervision should be provided around gas burners, since many elderly people who suffer from burn injuries or are victims of smoke inhalation suffer from a dementing illness (Hogue, 1982). Shutting off access to the stove by removing the knobs or having the gas company shut off or provide a turn-off valve for the gas may be necessary.

Direct observation of food in the refrigerator and pantry items may reveal duplicate or missing items and spoiled or unused food. Inspection of bathrooms may reveal untidy or unkempt conditions. At this point, many patients will benefit from family or chore workers/ home helps that can provide shopping needs, house cleaning, or cooking services. Meals on wheels are popular and may provide a valuable source of nutrition. Driving issues will be discussed in the section below on hazards.

Impairments in basic activities

Basic activities of daily living may include; bathing, dressing, walking, toileting, transferring, and eating. These functional tasks are usually affected later in the course of the dementing illness and often result in additional caregiver stress, additional costs for supportive care, or nursing home placement. However, neglect of personal hygiene and reminders to wear appropriate clothes or change clothes can occur relatively early in the disease. In the middle stages of the disease more assistance will be necessary with bathing and dressing. Apraxia may make it difficult to shave, dress, or walk. Gait problems from apraxia and parkinsonism may affect mobility, and dementia is a major risk factor for falls and hip fractures (Birge *et al*. 1994). An occupational therapy home evaluation can be beneficial to safety-proof the home and suggest assistive devices (i.e. grab bars in the bathroom) that will assist safety and transfers. Physical therapy may not be successful in advanced cases due to the lack of training ability and cognitive faculties needed to learn to use assisted devices appropriately.

In the latter stages of DAT, eating may become difficult. Helpful strategies may include; a supportive environment, adding flavouring to meals, avoiding plates with confusing patterns, using only one utensil, tolerating messy behaviour, using finger foods, adding verbal reminders to keep eating, cooking favourite foods, assuring appropriate food temperatures, and focusing on one portion at a time (Table 19.6). Nutritional supplements may provide additional calories. Weight loss may contribute to ill fitting dentures that may need adjustment. Dysphagia can occur and may be alleviated by a soft diet, thickened liquids, and special attention to positioning. Speech therapy may be helpful in difficult cases.

When incontinence occurs early in the disease, other causes for dementia (predominantly vascular but occasionally normal pressure hydrocephalus) should be considered, along with other mechanisms (i.e. overflow from prostatic enlargement). Incontinence in dementia is often due to detrusor hyperactivity (but not to the same degree as previously assumed) (Skelly and

Table 19.6 Feeding strategies for caregivers of patients with dementia

Eat in a non-distracting environment
Add flavouring and spices to meals
Avoid plates with confusing patterns
Use only one utensil or allow eating with hands
Use finger foods
Prepare favourite meals
Add verbal reminders to keep eating
Serve the food at appropriate temperatures
Focus on one portion at a time
Consider nutritional supplements
Use small portions and thickened liquids if dysphagia is present
Consider speech therapy (pathology) referral for dysphagia

Flint, 1995) and can be an especially aggravating condition. If a patient also develops mobility impairment, functional incontinence can compound the problem. Ruling out reversible or transient causes for incontinence is appropriate. A trial of low-dose anticholingeric agents can often be initiated if post void residuals are normal, but may also worsen their cognitive state. Referral for urodynamic studies are rarely necessary. In the absence of a specialist continence advisor, a toileting regimen, attention to aggravating medications, and continence aids can often make incontinence manageable. Indwelling catheters should only be used in the presence of pressure sores or in males with retention where effective medical or surgical intervention is not possible.

Hazards

As cognitive and functional impairment increase, the risk for certain hazardous events can occur. Psychosis can result in combativeness and injury to the caregiver, or conversely result in an injurious response to the patient. Mobility problems may result in falls and fractures. Delusions or suspicions may result in accidental injury if firearms or knives are within reach. Motor vehicle crashes with injuries may result from slow processing time, impairment of memory, visuospatial skills, or disorientation and concerns about driving ability may prompt the initial referral for assessment.

Driving

It is important that the policy of a memory clinic or community team should take into account the complexities of dealing with this topic. At a population level, drivers with dementia may contribute little, if anything, to traffic accidents; this counter-intuitive finding is probably due to the limitation of driving by patients, family, and physicians (Trobe *et al.*, 1996). Not only is there evidence that the crash rate among drivers with dementia during the first 2 years of dementia is similar to age-matched controls, but up to 30 per cent of drivers with early dementia may pass an appropriate driving test (Dobbs, personal communication). Another aspect of driving is its importance to older people—rated third after health and finances (O'Neill, 1996a). Giving up driving is not akin to giving up smoking; it has more resemblance to giving up food, and the lack of satisfactory alternative transport (paratransport) is a major bar to persuading those who should not drive to stop.

The task is to detect the presence of continued driving, to evaluate mobility needs of the patient and caregiver, and to assess driving ability. There is no simple, quick assessment (Lundberg *et al.*, 1997); this is still a clinical assessment, aided by an interdisciplinary assessment (especially neuropsychology and occupational therapy), taking into account comorbidities and medications, and may require an appropriate on-road driving assessment (Carr, 1991, O'Neill, 1996b). If the patient is considered fit to drive, this should be reviewed at regular intervals, and the patient and family should be advised i) that the patient should always be accompanied when driving (Bédard 1996), ii) to inform the driving licensing authority and insurance company depending on local legislation.

In the event of the driver being unfit to drive, this should be worked out with the patient and family. A case report by Bahro *et al.* (1995b) described a successful psychotherapeutic and behavioural intervention which helped a patient to make the transition from driving to not driving. The key principles included sharing the diagnosis with the patient, treating the patient as a collaborator in the process, and exploring other activities and mobility options with the patient. This approach needs to be generalized, and holds promise for the future. Some patients may prove resistant to all persuasion and subterfuge may be required, such as immobilizing the car. Responsibility for withdrawal of a driving licence varies between jurisdictions; in some countries in Europe, only a court order can withdraw a driving licence.

The legal position regarding disclosure of a diagnosis of dementia to driver licensing authorities varies from one jurisdiction to another. It is mandatory for physicians to report drivers with dementia in California and several provinces in Canada, whereas in the United Kingdom, the physician is bound to inform the patient of the patient's duty to inform the driving licensing authority. There may be a clear conflict between patient confidentiality and concern about risk to third parties; in most countries, it is considered reasonable to breach confidentiality if a) there is clear evidence of dangerous driving, b) the patient refuses to curtail driving despite discussion with the patient and family. In all cases, it is prudent to advise all patients and their carers about driving and mobility, and to document carefully the advice given.

Additional hazards

Smoking can be problematic; ideally, smoking should only occur with supervision, and the patient with memory loss should not have independent access to matches and cigarettes. Burn injuries or smoke inhalation can occur with inappropriate use of the stove. Patients with dementing illnesses may not be able to respond appropriately to fire alarms or smoke detectors. Wandering can result in exposure to intolerable weather conditions or unsafe crime areas.

Intervention for hazards is often a compromise between the changes that a patient will tolerate in his/her environment and the caregiver's perception of hazard. Providing supervision or use of 'safe return' identification bracelets may be beneficial. Inability to manage thermostats can result in too warm or cold temperatures at home. Hot water heaters should be set to low temperatures and the home environment should be uncluttered. Gas supplies can usually be fitted with an isolator switch so that caregivers can use the gas cooker but not the patient. Inappropriate medication administration may lead to untreated medical conditions or drug toxicity. Poisonings can occur if glasses or jars are mistaken for digestible fluids, or if poisonous plants are consumed. Power tools and heavy machinery require complex skills and should be monitored and access removed once skills have diminished.

Ethical problems

Dementia presents a range of ethical problems to health-care providers. The recent academic emphasis on competency to consent for medical treatment and on end-of-life issues, particularly tube feeding, do-not-resuscitate orders, and advance directives, reflects a common clinical concern. Unfortunately this has diverted attention from other ethical issues, two of which we present.

The ethics of adequate care and the role of advocacy

The greatest ethical and moral dilemma surrounding dementia is the lack of universal access to high quality assessment and management, and it is very likely that far more suffering is caused to patients with dementia and their caregivers by undertreatment than by overtreatment. It is particularly worrying that a recent textbook of ethics in neurology should support discrimination against access to high-technology life support on the basis of age (ageism) and dementia (perhaps we could call this dementiaism) rather than on functional or physical status (Bernat, 1994). Access to appropriate neuroradiology may be circumscribed due to these influences, and some health-care provider organizations in the United Kingdom may refuse to provide funding for cholinesterase inhibitor therapy. Those who care for patients with dementia should understand the potency of ageism and dementiaism in health and social services, and assume a role of advocacy to ensure adequate assessment and care facilities for their patients.

Ethical aspects of the patient–clinician relationship in dementia

One of the most subtle and less well-recognized effects of dementia is the tendency for the cognitive decline to alter the patient–physician relationship (Cassel and Jameton, 1981). In contrast to other illnesses, the patient may not initiate the consultation, and may be a reluctant participant in the assessment/management process. While the cognitive traffic is disproportionately, but not entirely, skewed in the favour of the physician, the emotional and human elements are preserved. In the past, patients with dementia and their care-givers complained of insensitive assessment whereby the physician did not interview the patient alone and talked to the caregiver as if the patient was not in the room. It is a challenge to our humanity and professional skills to ensure that the patient feels that they are at the centre of a relationship where their fears and problems will be professionally and confidentially handled. The emerging literature on the subjective experience of dementia should help us to respond to this need. At the very least, the patient should be interviewed on their own before any discussion with caregivers and, where feasible, permission should be sought for collateral history.

While many contributors to this book recognize the enormous impact of dementing illness on caregivers, this should not blind us to the potential conflict between the needs of the patient and caregiver. Interventions for behavioural disturbance need to balance limitations to the patient and re-duction of the caregiver's burden (Post, 1992). Similarly, respite care may cause upset and temporary worsening of cognitive state for the patient, but the long-term aim is to maximize the length of time for which the patient can stay in their own home before institutionalization.

Decision-making capacity

As decision-making capabilities decline with disease progression, early diag-nosis and attention to the issues gives an opportunity to capitalize on residual competency and to plan for the future. Assessment of capacity to consent for medical treatment is an issue which has attracted much attention (Cassel *et al.*, 1991). Apart from an understanding of the difficulties of assessing com-petency, a knowledge of the growing literature in this field is important as it will help in understanding the uncertainties and prejudices which may underpin our decisions and help us to respond positively to them.

Relatives consistently choose a lesser intensity of treatment than patients would themselves, nursing home residents state a majority preference for life-sustaining measures but discuss this with caregivers in only a minority of cases (O'Brien *et al.* 1995), health-care workers display negative treatment attitudes to older patients (ageism), economic hardship encourages a lesser intensity of medical therapy by proxy decision makers (Covinsky *et al.* 1996), and do-not-resuscitate orders tend to be made more common in groups who are discriminated against in other circumstances (Wenger *et al.*, 1996). These facts are not quoted to promote a charter of treatment of all diseases at a maximum intensity without regard to quality of life but rather to underline that families and health-care professionals are probably more likely to under treat than to over treat diseases in later life and dementia.

As in other areas of intervention in dementia, careful assessment is the key to success. The interdisciplinary team need to gauge the patient's communication ability, cognitive, and affective state; a psychosocial assessment of the patient and family should explore relationships, fears, and understanding of patient and family. Several competency instruments have been developed for capacity to consent for medical treatment (Janofsky *et al.*, 1992) or making advance directives (Molloy *et al.*, 1996), but these represent tentative steps in developing a knowledge base for the future. The decision of a senior specialist physician with appropriate interdisciplinary support, is the current standard measure of competency in virtually all jurisdictions. It is increasingly clear that it is best to view competency as decision specific; an excellent review on the subject is recommended (Glass and Silberfeld, 1996). Research on physicians' consistency in assessing competency is inconclusive. Although one study suggested that agreement was not good when assessing patients with mild Alzheimer's disease, this was on the basis of viewing videos of patients with a mean Folstein Mini-Mental State Examination of 24 (Marson *et al.*, 1997); it is debatable whether this is more widely applicable.

In the first instance the patient's own views must be canvassed as there may be sufficient insight to make a decision. Unless the patient is a ward of court or under guardianship, the primary responsibility lies with the patient and the physician, if the patient is adjudged incompetent. The views of the family should be canvassed along with appropriate psychosocial assessment; there is as yet little clear guidance for those without caregivers (Miller *et al.*, 1997). Any refusal by the patient should be treated with respect. The main clinical priority is to detect and treat any condition which may influence this refusal, particularly depression and pain. In the absence of these factors it would be rare for a clinician to over rule a refusal.

When a patient is no longer capable of participating in the decision-making process, clinicians need to confer with family to support the decision-making process, which usually hinges on issues of technical futility and quality of life issues. Technical futility may seem straightforward, but the impossible of today is the history of tomorrow (Marguerite Duras) and appropriate specialist referral is important. Quality of life is a difficult concept and in the event of dissonance between the family and the clinician, it may be wise to seek a second opinion; this is now the legal position in Ireland.

Advanced directives

Attitudes to advance directives vary between countries, races, and cultures and this may depend on many factors including the depth of the perceptions of over or under treatment at the end of life (Alemayehu *et al.*, 1991). In the United States, advanced directives on resuscitation are now required as part of federal regulations to be discussed at the time of admission to health-care facilities, including nursing homes. The difficulty of advance directives is illustrated by the commonest form of advance directive: 'Don't put me in a nursing home when I'm old'. Clearly it is very difficult for health providers and families to comply with this directive when living at home is no longer possible. Another difficulty is that advance directives are being promoted as a method of achieving health-care cost savings (Teno *et al.* 1997). This will set alarm bells ringing for those who look after older people with disabling illness.

Of more relevance to end-of-life issues is an understanding of the phenomenology of death in dementia and a more finely developed expertise in palliative and hospice care of dementia. This type of approach has been described (Volicer *et al.*, 1986), and will help to change a passive approach of non-intervention into a positive one of palliative care. Weight loss and swallowing disorders is one of the key areas and requires skilful handling. Once a full assessment has been carried out and other remediable factors treated such as depression or oral candidiasis, compensatory strategies such as semisolid feeding can be considered. It is the authors' experience that patients do not take kindly to modification of their fluid intake, and that free fluid intake and palliative care of the symptoms of aspiration may be more humane than modification and restriction of normal diet. Other alternatives such as feeding by percutaneous endoscopic gastrotomy can raise ethical dilemmas, as much by the relative ease and safety of performing the procedure. The current state of medical knowledge leaves unanswered the question of whether routine tube feeding of demented patients maximizes their interests (Ackerman, 1996); the benefits and disadvantages will have to be weighed in each individual case. For example the stroke-related dysphagia of a patient with early vascular dementia and reasonably preserved function is very different to the anorexia of advanced Alzheimer's disease, and percutaneous endoscopic gastrotomy feeding might be more clearly indicated in the former case.

Institutionalization and death

Helping to plan for the future is one of the major management goals of any dementia service. It is estimated that up to 50 per cent of nursing home patients have a dementing illnesses (Ouslander, 1989). Dementia may result in admission to long term care for a variety of reasons. Grief and sadness are typical responses among spouses, and disagreements between family members as to the need for placement are not uncommon. It is important that assessment should touch on the possible eventuality of institutionalization and appropriate liaison between family members and a social worker/counsellor initiated. Finances are a major issue and will need to be discussed extensively with the family and social services before admission. Guides are available to assist family members in choosing a long-term care setting (Alzheimer's Association, 1992). Although special dementia care units are often available, they should be closely scrutinized to determine how they will benefit the patient. Although patients may be upset with family members during and after placement, it is important to encourage regular visitations.

Many memory clinics have traditionally been involved at the time of death in liaising with families to encourage donation of brain tissue for post-mortem verification and research. Tissue donation is not only a scientific process; for many families there is comfort in the reassurance of definitive diagnosis. Consultation with the team in a formal manner may help to resolve grief if managed appropriately. Ideally, permission should occur after a few visits, when a relationship has been built up with the family, and should give plenty of time for reflection. The process of considering death and post-mortem issues may also help the family in preparing their consideration of end-stage issues which may be very stressful for family members.

The memory disorders team may not be directly involved in the patient's terminal care, but in conjunction with the primary care services may be able to steer the family towards resources such as hospice care. Even after a patient dies, it may be helpful to contact the family to discuss any lingering issues. Families need an opportunity to discuss their grief and concerns, and may need to ventilate regret or remorse regarding end of life decisions.

Recommended reading

Gauthier S (ed.) (1996). *Clinical diagnosis and management of Alzheimer's disease*. Martin Dunitz, London.

Lawlor BA (ed.) (1995). *Behavioral complications in Alzheimer's disease*. American Psychiatric Press, Washington DC.

Mace NL (ed.) (1990). *Dementia care. Patient, family and community*. John Hopkins University Press, Baltimore.

O'Neill D (ed.) (in press). *Practical management of dementia; an evidence-based approach*. Government Publications, Dublin.

Wilcock GK (1990). *Living with Alzheimer's disease and similar conditions.* Penguin, London.

Internet sites

http://www.alz.org/ — American Alzheimer's Association

http://www.alzheimer's.org.uk/ — United Kingdom Alzheimer's Disease Society

http://dsmallpc2.path.unimelb.edu.au/ad.html — Alzheimer Web Home Page

References

Key references recommended by the authors are marked with an *.

Ackerman TF (1996). The moral implications of medical uncertainty: tube feeding demented patients. *Journal of the American Geriatrics Society*, **44**, 1265–1267.

Aisen PS, DeLuca T, Lawlor PA (1992). Falls among geropsychiatry inpatients are associated with PRN Medication for agitation. *International Journal of Geriatric Psychiatry*, **7**, 709–712.

Alemayehu E, Molloy DW, Guyatt, GH, Singer, J, Penington, G, *et al.* (1991). Variability in physician's decisions on caring for chronically ill elderly patients: an international study. *Canadian Medical Association Journal*, **144**, 1133–1138.

Alexopoulos GS, Abrams RC, Young RC, *et al.* (1988). Cornell Scale for Depression in Dementia. *Biological Psychiatry*, **23**, 271–284.

Alzheimer's Association (1992). *Family guide for Alzheimer care in residential settings.* Alzheimer's Association, Chicago.

Bahro M, Silber E, Sunderland T (1995a). How do patients with Alzheimer's disease cope with their illness?—a clinical experience report. *Journal of the American Geriatrics Society*, **43**, 41–46.

Bahro M, Silber E, Sunderland T (1995b). Giving up driving in Alzheimer's disease—an integrative therapeutic approach. *International Journal of Geriatric Psychiatry*, **10**, 871–874.

Bédard M, Molloy DW, Lever JS (1996). Demented patients should not drive alone. *Journal of the American Geriatrics Society*, **44**, S9.

Bernat JL (1994). *Ethical Issues in Neurology*. Butterworth-Heinemann.

Bero LA, Lipton HL, Bird JA (1991). Characterization of geriatric drug-related hospital readmissions. *Medical Care*, **29**, 989–1003.

Birge SJ, Morrow-Howell N, and Proctor EK (1994). Hip fracture. *Clinics in Geriatric Medicine*, **10**, 589–609.

Breitner JC (1991). Clinical genetics and genetic counseling in Alzheimer disease. *Annals of Internal Medicine*, **115**, 601–606.

Brodaty H, and Gresham M (1989). The effect of a training programme to reduce stress in carers of patients with dementia. *British Medical Journal*, **299**, 1375–9.

Brody EM (1990). The family at risk. In *Alzheimer's disease treatment and family stress: directions for research* (eds E Light and B Lebowitz). Hemisphere, Washington.

Carr D (1991). A multidisciplinary approach in the evaluation of demented drivers referred to geriatric assessment centers. *Journal of the American Geriatrics Society*, **39**, 1132–1134.

Cassell CK, Jameton AL (1981). Dementia in the elderly: an analysis of medical responsibility. *Annals of Internal Medicine*, **94**, 802–807.

Cassell CK, Hays JR, Lynn J (1991). Alzheimer's: decisions in terminal care. *Patient Care*, **25**, 125–134.

Chandler JD (1987). Geriatric psychiatry. *Primary Care*, **14**, 761–772.

Cohen-Mansfield J (1986). Agitated behaviours in the elderly II: preliminary results in the cognitively deteriorated. *Journal of the American Geriatrics Society*, **34**, 722–727.

Collenda CC (1995). Agitation: a conceptual overview. In *Behavioural complications in Alzheimer's disease* (ed. BA Lawlor), pp. 3–17. APA Press, Washington DC.

Continuum. A Program of the American Academy of Neurology. *Dementia care*. Section IV: Genetic aspects of dementia: testing, education, and referral, pp. 115–144. Volume 2; July 1996.

Corcoran M, Gitlin LN (1992). Dementia management: an occupational therapy home-based intervention for caregivers. *American Journal of Occupational Therapy*, **46**, 801–807.

Covinsky KE, Landefeld CS, Teno J, Connors AF, Dawson N, Youngner S, *et al.* (1996). Is economic hardship on the families of the seriously ill associated with patient and surrogate care preferences? *Archives of Internal Medicine*, **156**, 1737–1741.

Cunningham C, Horgan F, Keane N, Connolly P, Mannion A, O'Neill D (1996). Detection of disability by different members of a multi-disciplinary team in a geriatric rehabilitation setting. *Clinical Rehabilitation*, **10**, 247–54.

Drickamer MA, Lachs MS (1992). Should patients with Alzheimer's disease be told their diagnosis? *New England Journal of Medicine*, **326**, 947–951.

Fleming KC, Evans JM, Weber DC, Chutka DS (1995). Practical functional assessment of elderly persons: a primary care approach. *Mayo Clinic Proceedings*, **70**, 900.

Glass KC, Silberfeld M (1996). Determination of competence. In *Clinical diagnosis and management of Alzheimer's disease* (ed. S Gauthier). Martin Dunitz, London.

Gorman G, Read S, Cummings JL (1993). Cholinergic therapy of behavioural disturbances in Alzheimer's disease. *Neuropsychiatry*, **6**, 229–234.

Greenwald BS, Kramer E (1991). Major depression in severe dementia. *Proceedings of 144th Annual meeting of the American Psychiatric Association*, New Orleans, p170.

Hogue CC (1982). Injury in late life: Part I. Epidemiology. *Journal of the American Geriatrics Society*, **30**, 187–88.

Holroyd S, Snustad DG, Chalfoux ZL (1996). Attitudes of older adults on being told the diagnosis of Alzheimer's disease. *Journal of the American Geriatrics Society*, **44**, 400–403.

Hughes CP, Berg L, Danziger WL, Coben LA, Martin RL (1982). A new clinician scale for the staging of dementia. *British Journal of Psychiatry*, **140**, 566–572.

Janofsky JS, McCarthy RJ, Folstein MF (1992). The Hopkins Competency Assessment Test: a brief method for evaluating patients' capacity to give informed consent. *Hospital and Community Psychiatry*, **43**, 132–136.

Kane RA, Kane RL (1981). *Assessing the elderly*. Lexington Books, Lexington MA.

Kertesz A, Hudson L, Mackenzie ERA, Munoz DG (1994). The pathology and nosology of primary progressive aphasia. *Neurology*, **44**, 2065–2072.

Kitwood T (1997). The experience of dementia. *Aging and Mental Health*, **1**, 13–22.

Kosloski K, Montgomery RJ (1995). The impact of respite use on nursing home placement. *Gerontologist*, **35**, 67–74.

Lebert F, Pasquier F, Petit H (1994). Behavioral effects of trazodone in Alzheimer's disease. *Journal of Clinical Psychiatry*, **55**, 536–538.

Leibovici A, Tariot PN (1988). Agitation associated with dementia: a systematic approach to treatment. *Psychopharmacology Bulletin*, **24**, 49–53.

Lennox A, Karlinsky H, Meschino W, Buchanan JA, Percy ME, Berg JM (1994). Molecular genetic predictive testing for Alzheimer's disease: deliberations and preliminary recommendations. *Alzheimer's Disease and Related Disorders*, **8**, 126–47.

Lundberg C, Johansson K, Ball K, Bjerre B, Blomqvist C, Braekus A, *et al.* (1997). Dementia and driving: An attempt at consensus. *Alzheimer's Disease and Associated Disorders*, **11**, 28–37.

Mace NL, Rabins PV (1992). *The 36-hour day*. The Johns Hopkins University Press, Baltimore.

Maguire C, Kirby M, Coen R, Lawlor B, Coakley D, O'Neill D (1996). Family members' attitudes toward telling the patient with Alzheimer's disease their diagnosis. *British Medical Journal*, **313**, 529–530.

Marson DC, McInturff B, Hawkins L, Bartolucci A, Harrell L (1997). *Journal of the American Geriatrics Society*, **45**, 453–457.

McDaniel KD, Edland SD, Heyman A. (1995) Relationship between level of insight and severity of dementia in Alzheimer disease. CERAD Clinical Investigators. Consortium to Establish a Registry for Alzheimer's Disease. *Alzheimer's Disease and Associated Disorders*, **9**, 101–104.

Michon A, Deweer B, Pillon B, Agid Y, Dubois B (1994). Relation of anosognosia to frontal lobe dysfunction in Alzheimer's disease. *Journal of Neurology, Neurosurgery and Psychiatry*, **57**, 805–809.

Miller TE, Coleman CH, Cugliari AM (1997). Treatment decisions for patients without surrogates: rethinking policies for a vulnerable population. *Journal of the American Geriatrics Society*, **45**, 369–374.

Molloy DW, Silberfeld M, Darzins P, Guyatt GH, Singer PA, Rush B, *et al*. (1996). Measuring capacity to complete an advance directive. *Journal of the American Geriatrics Society*, **44**, 660–664.

Morris JC (1995). Relationship of plaques and tangles to Alzheimer's disease phenotype. In *Pathobiology of Alzheimer's Disease* (eds AM Goate and F Ashall). Academic Press Limited, London, p. 198.

Nelson JP, Rosenberg DR (1991). ECT treatment of demented elderly patients with major depression: a retrospective study of efficacy and safety. *Convulsive Therapy*, **7**, 939–944.

Novack DH, Plumer R, Smith RL, Ochitill H, Morrow GR, Bennett JM (1979). Changes in physicians' attitudes toward telling the cancer patient. *Journal of the American Medical Association*, **241**, 897–900.

Nyth AL, Gottfries CG (1990). The clinical efficiency of citalopram in treatment of emotional disturbances in dementia disorders: a Nordic multicentre study. *British Journal of Psychiatry*, **157**, 894–901.

O'Brien LA, Grisso JA, Maislin G, *et al.* (1995). Nursing home residents' preferences for life-sustaining treatment. *Journal of the American Medical Association*, **274**, 1775–1779.

O'Neill D (1996a). The older driver. *Reviews in Clinical Gerontology*, **6**, 295–302.

O'Neill D (1996b). Dementia and driving: screening, assessment and advice. *Lancet*, **348**, 1114.

O'Neill D, McCormack P, Walsh JB, Coakley D (1990). Elder abuse. *Irish Journal of Medical Science*, **159**, 48–49.

O'Riordan T, Hayes J, O'Neill D, Shelley R, Walsh JB, Coakley D (1990). The effect of mild to moderate dementia on the Geriatric Depression Scale and on the General Health Questionnaire in the hospitalised elderly. *Age and Ageing*, **19**, 57–61.

Ouslander JG (1989). Medical care in the nursing home. *Journal of the American Medical Association*, **262**, 2582–2590.

Pollack NJ, Namazi KH (1992). Effect of music participation on the social behavior of Alzheimer's disease patients. *Journal of Music Therapy*, **29**, 54–67.

Post SG (1992). Behavior control and Alzheimer disease in perspective. *Alzheimer Disease and Related Disorders*, **6**, 73–76.

Reifler BV, Larson E, Teri L, *et al.* (1991). Double blind trial of imipramine in AD patients with and without depression. *American Journal of Psychiatry*, **139**, 623–626.

Reisberg B, Franssen E, Sclan SG, *et al.* (1987). BEHAVE-AD: A clinical rating scale for the assessment of pharmacologically remediable behavioural symptomatology in Alzheimer's disease. In *Alzheimer's Disease: Problems, Prospects and Perspectives* (ed H. Altman), pp. 1–16. Plenum, New York.

Robinson BC (1983). Validation of a Caregiver Strain Index. *Journal of Gerontology*, **38**, 344–348.

Rohde K, Peskind ER, Raskind MA (1995). Suicide in two patients with Alzheimer's disease. *Journal of the American Geriatrics Society*, **43**, 187–189.

Schneider LS, Pollock VE, Lyness SA (1990). A metaanalysis of controlled trials of neuroleptic treatment in dementia. *Journal of the American Geriatrics Society*, **38**, 533–563.

Skelly J, Flint AJ (1995). Urinary incontinence associated with dementia. *Journal of the American Geriatrics Society*, **43**, 286–294.

Spar JE, La Rue A (1990). Dementia and delirium. In *Concise Guide to Geriatric Psychiatry* (ed RE Hales), pp. 89–138. American Psychiatric Press, Washington DC.

Teno J, Lynn J, Connors AF, Wenger N, Phillips RS, Alzola C, *et al.* (1997). The illusion of end-of-life resource savings with advance directives. *Journal of the American Geriatrics Society*, **45**, 513–518

Teri L (1997). Address to the 150th Meeting of the American Psychiatric Association.

Teri L, Logsdon R (1991). Identifying pleasant activities for Alzheimer's disease patients: the Pleasant Event Schedule—AD. *Gerontologist*, **31**, 413–6.

Teri L, Wagner A (1992). Alzheimer disease and depression. *Journal of Consulting and Clinical Psychology*, **60**, 379–391.

Teri L, Truax P, Logsdon R, *et al.* (1992). Assessment of behavioral problems in dementia: the Revised Memory and Behaviour Problems Checklist. *Psychology of Aging*, **7**, 622–631.

Trobe JD, Waller PF, Cook-Flannagan CA, Teshima SM, Bieliauskas LA (1996). Crashes and violations among drivers with Alzheimer disease. *Archives of Neurology*, **53**, 411–416.

Volicer L, Rheaume Y, Brown J, Fabiszewski K, Brady R. (1986). Hospice approach to the treatment of patients with advanced dementia of the Alzheimer type. *Journal of the American Medical Association,* **256**, 2210–2213.

Wenger NS, Pearson ML, Desmond KA, *et al*. (1996). Epidemiology of do-not-resuscitate orders. *Archives of Internal Medicine,* **155**, 2056–2062.

Wilcock GK (1990). *Living with Alzheimer's disease and similar conditions.* Penguin, London.

Winograd CH, Jarvik LF (1986). Physician management of the demented patient. *Journal of the American Geriatrics Society*, **34**, 295–308.

Zarit SH, Orr NK, Zarit JM (1985). *The hidden victims of Alzheimer's disease: Families under stress.* New York University Press, New York.

20 The primary care physician's perspective

Jan Marcusson and John P. Sloan

Overview of the role of the primary care physician in dementia management

Epidemiological studies show that 5 to 15 per cent of persons over 70 years of age exhibit signs of dementia. Thus, the primary care or general practitioner often meets persons with possible dementia and is in an important position in the basic investigation and further management of the case (Fig. 20.1). The general practitioner, who often cares for the whole family, has unique opportunities to detect early cases of dementia through contact with the patient and his or her relatives. In many countries, the general practitioner also has the medical responsibility for special living facilities for elderly people where dementia often occurs. In recent years, specific treatments for Alzheimer's disease (tacrine and donepezil) have become available in North America and parts of Europe. As such treatments have been largely studied in patients with mild or moderate disease, it is important at the primary care level to detect possible Alzheimer patients early in the disease process.

Unfortunately, primary health-care professionals may not necessarily possess the skills to care for individuals with dementia. Studies from England, the Netherlands, and from Australia show that despite a high prevalence of dementia and depression in elderly people, too few of these conditions are diagnosed by the general practitioner (Glasser et al., 1994; Pond et al., 1994; Iliffe et al., 1994). Moreover, the interest general practitioners show in dementia investigation is highly variable (Pond et al., 1994; Lepeleire et al., 1994).

At what health-care level should dementia investigations be made?

It is difficult clearly to separate those parts of a dementia investigation to be carried out by general practitioners and those which perhaps best belong to

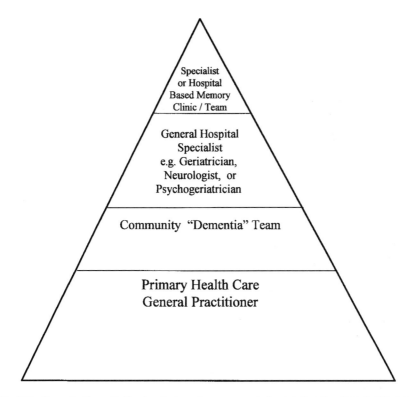

Fig. 20.1 Dementia: the reality. People with dementia are commonly dependent on the primary health care system for diagnosis, treatment, or rehabilitation. Relatively few patients are managed by hospital-based memory clinics. The remaining individuals are managed by specialists at general hospitals and by general practitioners. It is reasonable to believe that diagnostic competence varies among these three health-care levels. If diagnostic procedures at one level do not lead to a diagnosis (see Table 20.1), then the patient should be referred to a higher level for further investigations. △ represents the dementia population.

specialists. In most cases, the general practitioner is responsible for a basic investigation in order to detect conditions which may be confused with dementia such as depressive pseudodementia or delirium, or dementia secondary to treatable symptoms. Either specialists or general practitioners may then proceed with diagnosis of specific dementia causes. Irrespective of the health-care level at which the dementia investigation is made, the aims shown in Table 20.1 have to be met.

Which patients should be offered a complete dementia investigation?

All persons who exhibit signs or symptoms of dementia should undergo a medical evaluation. Even though it usually is not possible to offer curative treatment, many patients can, after a dementia investigation and following

Table 20.1 The aims of a clinical investigation of dementia

Verify the presence of dementia

Find treatable causes (e.g. cerebral tumour, depression, delirium, hypothyroidism)

Diagnose of the type of dementia (e.g. Alzheimer's disease or vascular dementia) and when available initiate pharmacological treatment

Clinically assess the nature and degree of cognitive impairment

Determine the nature and degree of functional disability

Describe functional abilities that are intact

Perform a medical examination and treat associated symptoms and diseases

Describe the social situation of the patient, including activities of daily living and relationships with family

Initiate an appropriate programme for rehabilitation and activities of daily living

Provide continuous competent medical care throughout progression of the disease

treatment and social interventions, have several years of an acceptable standard of life with only limited health-care needs. This results in both human and economic gains. The dementia investigation of course has to be individualized.

How can possible dementia be managed at the primary care level?

The management of persons with dementia at the primary care level most often involves both social and medical conditions. This means that intervention or management of the patient usually requires co-operation between community based or private care and medical care. Sometimes an apparently medical problem has its origin in a social condition. Therefore a broad approach to problem solving is best (Fig. 20.2).

The geriatric day hospital or outpatient clinic visit—investigations

Dementia investigation can advantageously be performed at a geriatric day hospital or other multidisciplinary clinic. In such circumstances, admission to hospital is only needed when unmanageable behavioural disturbance or somatic disease are present. See Chapters 4, 14 , and 15 for more detailed discussion of medical investigations.

In many services, the visit usually takes 1 to 2 hours, including full medical examination, but this varies according to local custom. As in all medical investigations, the management of each patient has to be individualized. In

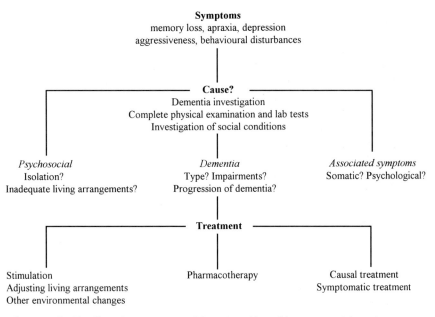

Symptoms
memory loss, apraxia, depression
aggressiveness, behavioural disturbances

Cause?
Dementia investigation
Complete physical examination and lab tests
Investigation of social conditions

Psychosocial
Isolation?
Inadequate living arrangements?

Dementia
Type? Impairments?
Progression of dementia?

Associated symptoms
Somatic? Psychological?

Treatment

Stimulation
Adjusting living arrangements
Other environmental changes

Pharmacotherapy

Causal treatment
Symptomatic treatment

Fig. 20.2 Algorithm illustrating management of the patient with possible symptoms of dementia. Dementia symptoms require a systematic approach to determining their underlying causes. In addition to a possible dementia, other conditions such as psychosocial difficulties or associated somatic conditions may contribute to the clinical picture.

addition, depending upon the practice in their own country and the facilities available in their area, primary care physicians will undertake different levels of assessment. Whatever level of assessment the general practitioner undertakes, he or she is ideally placed to detect early cases of dementia. When detecting cognitive symptoms, the general practitioner can always, after the primary investigation, refer the patient to a specialist for further evaluation.

History

The history must consider heredity and previous diseases that might have resulted in neurological or cardiovascular events. The exact history of the symptoms of the dementia condition, their time of onset, progression, and the actual disabilities must be carefully noted since they may contribute to the diagnostic evaluation. Especially important is the gathering of information which enables a differential diagnostic evaluation of symptoms. For example cerebrovascular events and stepwise progression of dementia symptoms increase the probability of vascular dementia, whereas an insidious onset and gradual progression of symptoms is more typical for Alzheimer's disease. Evaluation of mental and physical status is necessary. Undiagnosed medical conditions can exacerbate dementia (Table 20.2).

Table 20.2 Associated somatic conditions found in patients with known or suspected dementia who were admitted by general practitioners to the University Hospital of Linköping over a 2-month period (one patient can have several conditions), N = 49

Medical conditions	Number of patients
Lower urinary tract infection	17
Pneumonia	12
Depressive symptoms	8
Heart failure	7
Uncontrolled diabetes mellitus	5
Anaemia	4
Side-effects from drug treatment	4
Gastrointestinal bleeding	3
Constipation	3
Minor stroke/TIA	3

Neurological examination and mental status testing

Assessment of mental status and the neurological examination are of great importance since they provide the basis for differential diagnosis. The neurological examination is a prerequisite for an appropriate functional evaluation in which the patients impairments and abilities are described. Memory and other cognitive functions can be screened in several different ways. The most commonly used test is the Mini-Mental State Examination (Folstein *et al.*, 1975), but it is important to remember that simple screening instruments cannot be used as diagnostic instruments, though they complement diagnostic procedures.

Blood and urine tests

Basic laboratory analysis includes tests to detect diseases which may give rise to dementia (e.g. hypercalcaemia, hypothyroidism). These tests can also detect possible associated somatic diseases (e.g. infection, anaemia, malignancy) which may worsen a dementia. Low levels of vitamin B_{12} are a relatively common finding in elderly people, but the clinical relevance of this is not clearly established. Intracellular vitamin B_{12} deficiency can be detected as increased levels of methylmaleonate or homocysteine. Despite a lack of clarity regarding the indications for vitamin B_{12} treatment for cognitive dysfunction, the determination of vitamin B_{12} (or methylmaleonate or homocysteine) remains a part of the basic laboratory investigations. Other tests can also be of importance and are taken whenever indicated (e.g. serological tests for syphilis and HIV).

Lumbar puncture and examination of cerebrospinal fluid

General practitioners seldom perform lumbar puncture in Europe and North America. However, this examination has a low incidence of complications and does not require hospitalization. Investigation of the cerebrospinal fluid provides information on possible blood–brain barrier damage and inflammatory or infectious processes. A new diagnostic marker is tau-protein in cerebrospinal fluid, which is increased in 80 to 90 per cent of patients with Alzheimer's disease, vascular dementia, or frontal lobe degeneration (Blennow *et al.*, 1995)[1], but further validation is required before it becomes a routine diagnostic marker.

Anatomical and functional imaging of the brain

The availability of anatomical or functional imaging for the general practitioner is highly variable between countries. Computed tomography (CT) of the brain should be performed on the majority of patients with suspected early dementia. A CT scan is performed chiefly to detect treatable conditions (tumour, subdural haematoma, cysts, hydrocephalus). In other cases the CT scan may be important in the differential diagnosis. Blood flow measurement, usually with single photon emission tomography (SPECT) can be performed at some hospitals, but the technique is not established as part of the routine dementia investigation.

Electroencephalography (EEG)

EEG can sometimes be of value in early dementia cases where CT can be normal and the clinical picture difficult to evaluate. Most dementias, apart from some frontal lobe dementias, usually present with an abnormal EEG. EEG should always be performed when epileptic manifestations are suspected, and can be useful in confirming the diagnosis of Cruetzfeld–Jakob disease. Chapter 6 reviews radiological and neurophysiological investigations in more detail.

Functional evaluation

An evaluation of the patient in his or her home environment is helpful in determining the care resources needed, either by the individual with dementia or their caregiver, and to assess the need for institutionalization. An occupational therapist often performs these evaluations, as outlined in Chapter 10.

---

[1] Determination of tau-protein in cerebrospinal fluid is a routine analysis available at Department of Clinical Chemistry, Mölndal Hospital, S-141 83 Mölndal, Sweden Fax +46 31 862426.

Neuropsychological evaluation

It is sometimes difficult to detect cognitive impairment in very early dementia cases. A neuropsychological evaluation is essential for establishing the presence of early or mild decline in such cases (in particular because this allows for the estimation of premorbid function by standardized techniques), in determining specific areas of brain dysfunction, and in ruling out depression (see Chapter 7). However, neuropsychological assessment is not available in primary care settings in all countries, and often requires referral on to clinical psychology services.

Evaluation and planning of future care

In the case of confirmed dementia, the specific disease or type of dementia should be considered together with possible pharmacological treatment of the dementia or associated somatic or psychological symptoms. It is of great importance that relatives and other caregivers receive all necessary information, if possible in writing, about the results of the investigations which have been undertaken. This information enables the caregiver to assist the person with dementia, and may also decrease feelings of guilt in the family who feel they are not doing enough for their relative. In the long run, adequate information to relatives and caregivers together with instructions about contacting their general practitioner, can decrease the need for hospitalization. It is important to clarify who is responsible for which aspects of the management of the patient, so that relatives or professional care givers know whom to contact when needed.

In summary, investigation of dementia in primary care should achieve all the objectives presented in Table 20.1. However, if the general practitioner prefers to limit investigations to the exclusion of secondary dementia (e.g. depressive pseudodementia and associated somatic conditions) the patient should be referred to a specialist for diagnostic evaluation regarding type of dementia and possible treatment.

Who takes care of individuals with dementia living in nursing or care homes?

The general practitioner is often responsible for the medical care of people with dementia living in nursing or care homes. However, sometimes the general practitioner has very limited time allocated for this work and is most often involved in the management of acute medical conditions only. There are of course local variations in how these obligations are managed by the general practitioner. In cases where there is inadequate primary care support in the home or nursing home, admission to hospital emergency services is often the result. It is clearly preferable, in most cases, for the general practitioner to manage the care of individuals with dementia in the community environment. When an ideal primary care system is available, there is time for adequate evaluation of the patient's condition and documentation, including evaluation of the effect of medications. Efficient co-operation between well educated and competent staff in nursing homes and the attending general practitioner is required if patients with dementia are to be offered quality care and unnecessary admissions to hospital avoided.

The management of patients with dementia in different kinds of nursing homes can follow the principles shown in Fig. 20.2. Regular visits by the general practitioner enables detection of problems in the early stages, even before they become acute. Nursing home residents with dementia most often suffer from moderate or advanced disease, where communication is usually difficult. Rapid worsening of the physical condition should be followed by an appropriate physical evaluation, often including laboratory tests.

A common problem for the general practitioner is the appearance of agitation in different forms (physical violence, escape attempts, repeated screaming). In these situations, a systematic approach according to Fig. 20.2 is of great importance. Understimulation, too little physical exercise, and even poorly trained staff at the home can be underlying causes of agitation. Sleep disturbances are often caused by too much sleep during the day time. The other major cause of agitation is the occurrence of intercurrent illness, sometimes accompanied by an acute confusional/delirious state. The basic management principal for the general practitioner in handling these is to exclude social and somatic causes of symptoms of agitation. Only when this has been done, should psychoactive medications be used to reduce the symptoms. An important practical consequence of this is the use of a 'family medicine approach' with an investigation of the patient in his home situation, including a careful history taken by talking both to staff and relatives.

What organization of the primary health care system is needed in order to care for individuals with dementia during the disease process?

Care of persons with dementia requires both time and commitment. Medical competence is important, as is availability, although in practice the general practitioner may be busy with patients in his or her clinic when an acute evaluation of a patient with dementia in their own home is needed. Therefore, in many communities, dementia care 'teams' have been developed. One or several nurses together with an occupational therapist have the ability to visit the patient in his home, and when necessary they will be assisted by a general

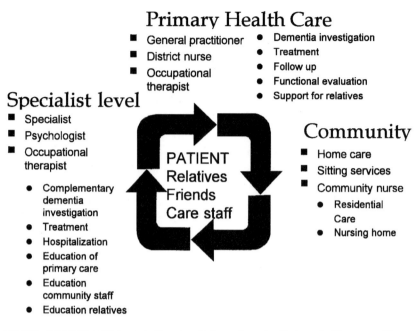

Fig. 20.3 Organization of the community and medical care of people with dementia. The person with dementia and their family should be the focus of attention. Primary care can increase its availability by organizing 'dementia teams' which can take care of many of the problems that occur during the disease process. If the general practitioner manages neither the dementia investigation nor the handling of the problems that arise during the disease process, she/he should refer either to a specialist or to another general practitioner with a special interest in dementia.

practitioner who is on call for the whole community. One model for the organization of the medical care of individuals with dementia living in the community is shown in Fig. 20.3. Chapter 11 describes such an approach.

In many cases the community, the primary care system, and hospital care have written contracts or agreements where each area of responsibility has been clearly indicated. These 'care programmes for dementia' have improved the quality of the medical and community care of people with dementia. Especially in a future with more limited financial resources and an increasing number of people with dementia, efficient organization in the community for the care of dementia will be needed more than ever.

References

Key references recommended by the authors are marked with an *.

Blennow K. *et al.* (1995). Tau protein in cerebrospinal fluid: a biochemical diagnostic marker for Alzheimer's disease? *Molecular and Chemical Neuropathology*, **26**, 231–245.

*Folstein M.F., Folstein S.E., McHugh P.R. (1975). 'Mini-mental state' A practical method for grading the cognitive state of patients for the clinician. *Journal of Psychiatric Research*, **12**, 189–198.

*Glasser M., Stearns J.A., De Kemp E., Van Hout J., Hott D. (1994). Dementia and Depression symptomatology as assessed through screening tests of older patients in an outpatient clinic. *Family Practice Research Journal*, **14**, 261–272.

*Iliffe S., Mitchley S., Gould M., Haines A. (1994). Evaluation of the use of brief screening instruments for dementia, depression and problem drinking among elderly people in general practice. *British Journal of General Practice*, **44**, 503–507.

*Lepeleire J.A., Heyrman J., Baro F., Buntinx F., Lasuy C. (1994). How do general practitioners diagnose dementia? *Family Practice*, **11**, 148–151.

*Pond C.D., Mant A., Kehoe L., Hewitt H., Brodaty H. (1994). General practitioner diagnosis of depression and dementia in the elderly: can academic detailing make a difference? *Family Practice*, **2**, 141–147.

Appendix: A survey of the Memory Disorder Teams represented by the contributors

R. S. Bucks, L. M. T. Byrne, G. K. Wilcock and K. Rockwood

Introduction

A structured questionnaire was sent to all the centres represented by the authors of this book, in all, 28; 12 in North America, nine in the United Kingdom, six in the rest of Europe, and one in Australasia. The questionnaire asked about the running of the memory disorders clinics or teams operated by those centres. Survey responses were coded and analysed using SPSS for Windows and the charts were created in MS-Excel. The results are reported question by question from the survey.

Results

Nineteen (68%) questionnaires were returned; nine from North America (75%), six from the United Kingdom (66%), three from the rest of Europe (50%), and one from Australasia. Most of those who did not fill in questionnaires responded by saying that they did not run memory clinics, nor operated within the context of a multidisciplinary memory disorders or dementia team.

The team

Who is the lead clinician?

Three teams did not specify who their lead clinician was. One team was jointly lead by a geriatrician and a psychiatrist (see Fig. A.1).

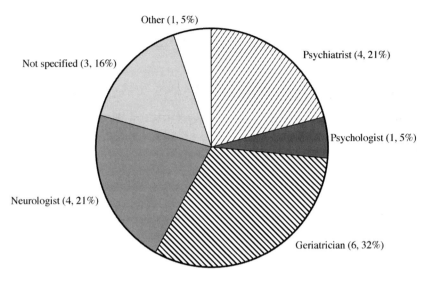

Other (1, 5%)

Not specified (3, 16%)

Psychiatrist (4, 21%)

Psychologist (1, 5%)

Neurologist (4, 21%)

Geriatrician (6, 32%)

Fig. A.1 Specialty of lead clinician (N=19).

Which specialties are represented in the team?

Table A.1 shows the number of staff from each specialty within the clinics/ teams. As can be seen, few teams are staffed by occupational therapists or speech and language therapists. Few teams are staffed by neurologists, although when they are the neurologist is typically the lead clinician (refer to Fig. A.1). Most teams have at least one geriatrician/ physician, psychologist, psychiatrist, and nurse.

Does the Team have an administrator?

Sixteen (84%) of the teams have an administrator. Two teams (11%), employ an individual solely as an administrator. In the other teams, the administrator is another member of staff who has taken on the role in addition

Table A.1 Staff in clinics/ teams (n (%))

Number of staff from each specialty	0	1	2	3 or more
Geriatricians/ physicians	5 (26)	3 (16)	2 (11)	9 (47)
Neurologists	11 (58)	5 (26)	3 (16)	0
Psychologists	4 (21)	9 (47)	3 (16)	3 (16)
Psychiatrists	7 (37)	4 (21)	4 (21)	4 (21)
Occupational therapists	12 (63)	4 (21)	1 (5)	2 (11)
Speech and language therapists	13 (68)	5 (26)	1 (5)	0
Nurses	2 (11)	7 (37)	5 (26)	5 (26)

to their other work; either a researcher (in two, 10% of cases), a member of administrative or clerical staff (seven, 37%) or a nurse (three, 16%). Five of the teams (26%) did not specify who their administrator was.

> Does the team use a database?—If 'yes', who manages the database? What kind of database? (Dbase, mainframe etc.)

Eighteen (95%) of the teams use a database for storing information. This database is managed by a specialist database manager in four (21%) teams. In other teams, the database is managed by other staff. Four of the teams (21%) did not specify who runs their database. The databases used are mainly PC based (11 teams; 61%), including SPSS and MS-Access. Two (11%) of the databases used are mainframe/local network databases.

> Does the team use volunteers?—If 'yes' in what capacity?

Only six (32%) of the teams use volunteers. Volunteers offer assistance with patient relations, administration, and research.

> Additional comments (other team members etc.)

Other staff employed include geneticists and additional research staff. Two teams reported the involvement of trainees and Senior House Officers in addition to the usual staff.

The clinic

> How many clinics are held per week?

There is a wide range in the number of clinical sessions each team runs per week; from one per fortnight to 15 per week (mode 1). Four (21%) reported only one session per week. Four of the teams (21%) found that this question was not applicable to them as they did not run a 'clinic' in this sense (see Fig. A.2).

> How long does the first visit/appointment usually take?

The duration of the first visit ranged from 45 minutes to 2 days with breaks, although it was over 1 day in only one of the teams. In twelve of the teams (63%) the typical first visit length is 1 to 2 hours. Disregarding the team which sees patients over 2 days, the longest first visit duration is 4.5 hours, the mean being 2 hours (SD 0.9).

> Whom do the patients see and how long are the appointments?

At the first visit, in 15 (79%) of the teams, each patient is seen by one to three staff members, with the other teams using more than three staff members. In all but one of the teams the patients see a physician at the first visit (95%). In the two teams where a physician is not necessarily seen at the initial visit, the patient sees either a psychologist or a psychiatrist in one and

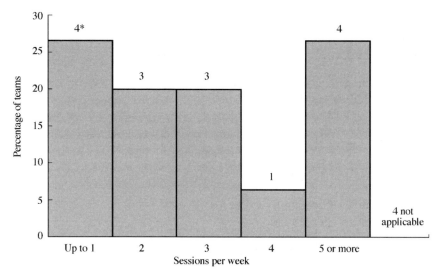

Fig. A.2 Number of clinical sessions per week. * Indicates number of teams.

either a psychologist or a nurse in the other. In ten of the teams (53%) there is always some psychological input at the first visit. In ten teams (53%), patients are seen at their first visit by a nurse.

How many subsequent visits do the patients have? At what intervals are they?

All but one of the teams offer at least one follow-up visit. Generally, the number of subsequent visits offered depends on the patient. Seven (37%) of the teams gave a precise number of subsequent visits and these range between one and five. Others gave a range of possible visits offered. These ranges are all between none and six. Seven (37%) of the teams see each patient again within 4 weeks of the initial visit. Eight (42%) of the teams continue to follow up patients for over a year after their initial visit.

Which imaging techniques do you use? Please delete as applicable—None / CT / SPECT / PET / MRI / Ultrasound / Other (please specify)

Figure A.3 shows the percentage of teams using certain imaging techniques. One of the teams reported using no imaging techniques. The most popular combination of scans, used by six (32%) of the teams, was CT, SPECT, and MRI, with five (26%) of the teams using CT and MRI alone. Only two (11%) of the teams routinely use all of the different types of scans.

Which electrophysiological scans do you use? Please delete as applicable. None / EEG / ECG / Other (please specify)

Thirteen (68%) of the teams use electrophysiological tests. Nine (48%) use both EEG and ECG and four (21%) use EEG alone. None of the teams use ECG and not EEG.

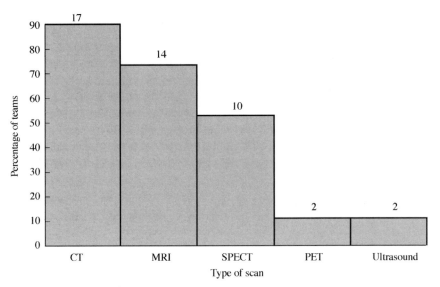

Fig. A.3 Percentage use of imaging techniques.

> Which laboratory tests do you routinely use? Please delete as applicable—None / Full Blood Count / Plasma Viscosity / Red Cell Folate / Serum Folate / Calcium group / Vitamin B$_{12}$ / TFTs / Random glucose / VDRL / U and E / LFTs / Cholesterol / gamma GT / Red cell transketolase / TPP effect / Blood alcohol / Glycated haemoglobin / MSU / Other (please specify)
>
> Who usually carries out these tests? (please specify)

All of the teams perform at least two laboratory tests. Ten (53%) of the teams carry out between two and ten tests. When only two tests are used, these are mid-stream urine and a full blood count. The tests used are summarized in Table A.2. No teams reported using any laboratory tests not included in the list. In two (10%) of the clinics, the primary care physician is asked to carry out the laboratory tests. The remaining 17 (89%) specified that the tests are carried out at a secondary health-care level.

> Which diagnostic criteria do you use? (e.g. NINCDS-ADRDA, NINDS-AIREN, DSM-IV)

Fifteen (79%) of the teams report using diagnostic criteria for the diagnosis of dementia. Twelve (63%) of the teams employ the DSM-IV criteria for the diagnosis of dementia. One team employs the ICD-10 criteria and one team employs the Wash-U criteria. One team reported using both DSM-IV and ICD-10 criteria. Fourteen (74%) of the teams employ the NINCDS-ARDA criteria for diagnosis of Alzheimer's disease and six (32%) use the NINDS-AIREN criteria for the diagnosis of vascular dementia. Only two (10%) of the teams report using the consensus criteria for the diagnosis of Lewy body dementia.

Table A.2 Percentage of memory disorders teams carrying out laboratory tests

Test	Number of teams using test	%
Full blood count	17	94
Vitamin B$_{12}$	17	94
Venereal disease reference laboratory	14	77
Calcium	13	72
Thyroid function test	13	72
Random glucose	12	66
Liver function test	12	66
Serum folate	11	61
Red cell folate	8	44
Urea and electrolytes	8	44
Cholesterol	7	39
Plasma viscosity	6	33
Gamma GT	5	27
Glycated haemoglobin	4	22
Mid-stream urine	4	22
Tpp effect	2	11
Red cell transketolase	1	6
Blood alcohol (EOH)	1	6

Which cognitive / screening test(s) do you use? (e.g. MMSE, Brief Cognitive Rating Scale)

Fifteen (79%) of the teams use the MMSE. Three (16%) of the teams use the CAMCOG and the MMSE together. There was enormous variation in the numbers of other psychological assessment tools used. These are listed in Table A.3.

Six (32%) of the teams use a depression scale. The most popular is the Geriatric Depression Scale. Other scales specified were the Cornell and the Pichot.

Do you use a formal staging protocol (please specify)?

Twelve (63%) of the teams employ a staging protocol; six (32%) use the CDR and two (10%) use the FAST. Other staging protocols employed are the Reisberg Global Deterioration Scale (GDS) and the Brief Cognitive Rating Scale (BCRS).

How do you assess risk factors (formal questionnaire e.g. Hachinski, clinical history etc.)?

Eight of the teams (42%) assess vascular risk factors through both the Hachinski questionnaire and clinical history. Five (26%) teams assess using

Table A.3 Summary of neuropsychological and other tests used

Test	Number of clinics (%)
Estimation of premorbid IQ	
National Adult Reading Test (NART)	3 (16)
Cognitive scales	
Mini Mental State Examination (MMSE)	15 (79)
Modified MMSE	2 (11)
KEW	1 (5)
Cambridge Cognitive Examination (CAMCOG)	4 (21)
Weschsler Adult Intelligence Scale—Revised (WAIS-R) - various subtests	4 (21)
Consortium for the Establishment of a Registry for Alzheimer's Disease (CERAD) Battery	1 (5)
Middlesex Elderly Assessment of Mental State (MEAMS) - subtests of, especially visual recognition	1 (5)
Severe Impairment Battery	1 (5)
Wide Range Achievement Test L-Revised (subtests, especially arithmetic)	1 (5)
Memory scales	
Rivermead Behavioural Memory Test (RBMT)	1 (5)
Adult Memory and Information Processing Battery (AMIPB) -various subtests, especially story recall	1 (5)
Weschsler Memory Scale—Revised (subtests of)	4 (21)
Benton Visual Retention Test	3 (16)
Doors and People Test	1 (5)
Anomalous Sentence Repetition Test	1 (5)
Fuld Object-Memory Evaluation	1 (5)
Rey-Osterrieth Complex Figure Test	1 (5)
DAFS Grocery Recall Task	1 (5)
Buschke Cued Recall	1 (5)
Luria Nebraska Neuropsychological Battery (LNNB) - memory for designs subtest	1 (5)
Verbal learning	
Hopkins Verbal Learning Test (HVLT)	1 (5)
Rey Auditory Verbal Learning Test (RAVLT)	1 (5)
Weschsler Adult Learning Test	1 (5)
Executive function and problem solving	
Benton Verbal Fluency (FAS)	5 (26)
Category Test	1 (5)
Weigl's Colour Form Sorting Test	1 (5)
Trail Making Test	5 (26)
Wisconsin Card Sorting Test	1 (5)
Raven's Progressive Matrices (inc. Coloured)	1 (5)
Stroop Colour and Word Test	1 (5)
Harbor-UCLA Frontal Battery	1 (5)
Language and semantic function	
Graded Naming Test	1 (5)

Table A.3 Continued

Test	Number of clinics (%)
Frenchay Aphasia Screening Test (FAST)	2 (11)
Famous Names	1 (5)
Boston Naming Test (BNT)	2 (11)
Boston Diagnostic Aphasia Examination	1 (5)
Repetition, story retelling, reading, and comprehension test	1 (5)
Generative Naming	2 (11)
Token Test	1 (5)
Speed, visuoperceptual skills, and praxis	
Visual Object Space Perception Battery (VOSP)	1 (5)
Hooper Visual Organization Test	1 (5)
Kendrick Digit Copying Test (KDCT)	1 (5)
Clock Drawing Test	4 (21)
Finger Tapping Test	1 (5)
Depression and anxiety scales	
Geriatric Depression Scale	2 (11)
Cornell Depression Scale in Dementia	3 (16)
Pichot Depression Scale	1 (5)
Multidimensional and staging scales	
Clinical Dementia Rating scale (CDR)	6 (32)
Functional Rating Scale (FRS)	1 (5)
Blessed Dementia Rating Scale (inc. short version)	3 (16)
IQCODE	1 (5)
Gottfries Braane Steens (GBS)	1 (5)
Functional Assessment Staging (FAST)	1 (5)
Global Deterioration Scale (GDS)	1 (5)
Brief Cognitive Rating Scale (BCRS)	1 (5)
Other scales	
Cognitive Abilities Screening Instrument (CASI)	1 (5)
Clinicians Assessment (CIBIC)	1 (5)
Cognitive Failures	1 (5)
Benton Handedness Questionnaire	1 (5)
Cognitive Efficiency Profile (PEC)	1 (5)
Frontal Behavioural Inventory (FBI)	1 (5)
Caregiver Stress Inventory	1 (5)

clinical history alone. Six (32%) teams do not report any formal method of assessing vascular risk factors.

> How do you assess comorbid illness (formal questionnaire e.g. Cumulative Illness Rating Scale, clinical history etc.)?

Two of the teams did not report their method of assessing comorbid illness. Eleven of the teams (58%) reported using clinical history alone, whilst three (16%) use both clinical history and formal questionnaire and three (16%)

employ only a formal questionnaire. The only formal questionnaire named (by two teams), was the Cumulative Illness Rating Scale.

Does the clinic/team have links with other specialist services (please elaborate)?

Sixteen (84%) of the teams specified that they maintain links with other services. Eleven (58%) of the teams have links with other hospital medical services. These services are; genetics, psychiatry, neurosurgery, neuro-physiology, rheumatology, and internal medicine. Four (21%) of the teams reported links with neuroimaging and neuroradiology. Three (16%) reported links with care services and three (16%) links with research centres and projects. Two (10%) reported links with psychological services.

The patients

What is the waiting time for an appointment (weeks/months)?

The waiting time for a first appointment ranges from 1.5 weeks to 2.5 months (mode 4 weeks). Some of the teams reported that this question was not applicable to them as they did not run a clinic in this sense and some did not specify a typical waiting time (see Table A.4). One of the teams reported two different referral times depending on whether the referral was an acute or a standard referral.

Approximately how many patients are seen per year, including follow-ups?
Approximately how many of these are new patients?

The total numbers of patients seen in the past year in the teams, summarized in Fig. A.4, ranges from 50 to 1203. The number of *new* patients seen by the teams, summarized in Fig. A.5, ranges from 25 to 655. Those teams with the greatest number of patients do not necessarily have the most new patients. This is possibly due to some teams following patients over a longer period of time and therefore their clinical sessions incorporating more current patients and less new patients.

What type of referrals do you take?

Only one of the teams (5%) specified that they do not take general practitioner referrals. This team takes only referrals from secondary health

Table A.4 Estimated typical waiting time for first appointment (N = 13)

Weeks	Number of teams (%)
1–4	8 (42)
5–8	3 (16)
9–12	2 (11)

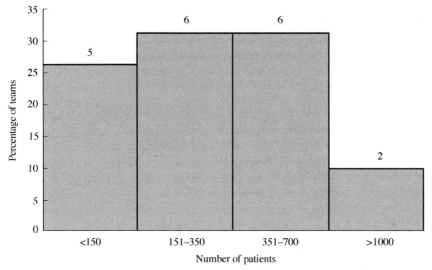

Fig. A.4 Total number of patients seen in the last year (N = 19).

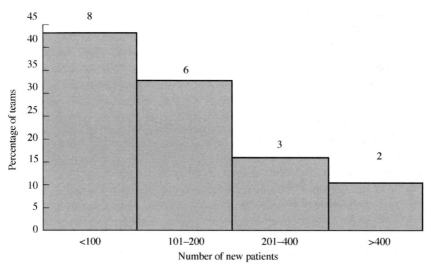

Fig. A.5 Number of new patients seen in the last year (N = 19).

care—neuropsychology and psychogeriatrics. Only five (26%) of the teams specified that they would take self referrals.

Is there a minimum age for patients? (Please state)

Fifteen (79%) of the teams reported no minimum age for patients. The other four teams employ a minimum age of between 40 and 50 years.

Who usually attends with the patient?

All of the teams reported that patients typically attend the clinic with someone, usually carers, relatives (spouses or children), or friends.

To whom do you tell the diagnosis (please elaborate)?

Patients are always told something about their condition by all teams. Teams vary in what they tell the patient, depending on how much the patient wants to know and seems able to understand. If it was considered clinically appropriate, the patient may not be told their diagnosis. In sharing the diagnosis some clinicians rely on the use of euphemisms such as memory loss, whilst others give a specific disease diagnosis.

Funding

What are your sources of funding? Please delete as applicable The State / Health insurance / Research grants / Pharmaceutical industry / Charitable donation / Other (please specify).

Table A.5 shows the sources of funding for the teams, with the most common sources towards the left of the table. Health insurance, although not a source of funding in the United Kingdom or Australia, funds some teams in North America and the rest of Europe. The Australian teams is funded solely from research.

Table A.5 Sources of funding, N = 19, (n (%))

	n	Research	Pharmaceutical industry	State	Charitable donation	Health insurance
North America	9	7 (78)	6 (66)	4 (44)	4 (44)	6 (66)
United Kingdom	6	6 (66)	3 (50)	3 (50)	3 (50)	
Other European	3	1 (33)		2 (66)	1 (33)	1 (33)
Australia	1	1 (100)				
TOTAL	19	13 (68)	9 (47)	9 (47)	8 (42)	7 (37)

Note: the sources of funding are not mutually exclusive since most teams are funded from more than one source.

Conclusion

As can be seen, there is considerable variation in the types of service offered by the teams, although the majority have some common features. This reflects a healthy diversity and is an indicator of the fact that there is no blueprint for a memory disorders team. This diversity may reflect the different starting point of the teams as well as the differing specialties of the lead clinicians. There may also be some variation caused by the differing longevity of the teams, and by the culture of the continent in which the team is based. The diversity may simply reflect the different needs of the community the team serves.

Acknowledgements

Many thanks to the teams taking part in the survey (listed alphabetically):

Alzheimer's Disease Research Centre
Alzheimer Centre
12200 Fairhill Road
Cleveland, OH 44106
UNITED STATES OF AMERICA

Bristol Memory Disorders Clinic
Blackberry Hill Hospital
Manor Road
Fishponds
Bristol, BS16 2EW
UNITED KINGDOM

Challenging Behaviours in Dementia Project
Health Aging Research Unit
Hornsby / Ku-Ring Gai Hospital
Palmerston Road
Hornsby
NSW 2077
AUSTRALIA

Clinic for Alzheimer Disease and Related Disorders
Vancouver Hospital and Health Sciences Centre
2211 Westbrook Mall
Vancouver, BC, V6T 123
CANADA

Dementia Team
Department of Geriatric Medicine
University Hospital
S-58185
Linkoping
SWEDEN

Department of Clinical Neuroscience and Family Medicine
Division of Geriatric Medicine at Geriatric Clinic
Hudinge University Hospital
S-141 86
Huddinge
SWEDEN

Hammersmith Hospital Memory Clinic
Psychological Medicine Department
Hammersmith Hospital
Do Cane Road
London, W12 0HS
UNITED KINGDOM

Harbor-UCLA Medical Centre
1000 West Carson Street
Building F-9
Torrance, CA 90509
UNITED STATES OF AMERICA

Hôpital de jai d'Évaluation Gérontologique
Groupe Hospitalier Broca-La Rochefoucauld
54–56 Rue Pasca;
75013, Paris
FRANCE

The Leicester Memory Clinic
Psychiatry for the Elderly
Leicester General Hospital
Leicester, LE5 4PW
UNITED KINGDOM

McGill Centre for Studies in Aging
Douglas Hospital
6825 LaSalle Boulevard
Verdun
Quebec, H4H 1R3
CANADA

Memory Disability Clinic
Queen Elizabeth II Health Sciences Centre
PO Box 9000
Halifax, Nova Scotia, B3K 6A3
CANADA

Neuropsychiatry and Memory Group
Osler 320
The Johns Hopkins Hospital
Baltimore, MD 21287–5371
UNITED STATES OF AMERICA

Northern Memory Clinic
Newcastle General Hospital
Westgate Road
Newcastle-Upon-Tyne, NE4 6BE
UNITED KINGDOM

Older Adult Health Centre
Washington University
Division of Geriatrics
4488 Forest Park
St Louis, Mo 63108
UNITED STATES OF AMERICA

Pacific Neuroscience Institute
Memory Disorders Clinic
109–1026 Johnson Street
Victoria, BC V8V 3N7
CANADA

The Research Institute for the Care of the Elderly
St Martin's Hospital
Bath, BA2 5RP
UNITED KINGDOM

South Manchester Memory Clinic
University Department of Old Age Psychiatry
Withington Hospital
Nell Lane
West Didsbury
Manchester, M20 8LR
UNITED KINGDOM

Wien Centre for Alzheimer's Disease and Memory Disorders
Mount Sinai Medical Centre
4300 Alton Road
Miami Beach
Florida 33140
UNITED STATES OF AMERICA

Bibliography

American Psychiatric Association (1994). *Diagnostic and Statistical Manual of Mental Disorders* (4th edn). American Psychiatric Association, Washington, DC.

Alexopoulos, G.S., Abrams, R.C., Young, R.C. and Shamoian, C.A. (1988). Cornell scale for depression in dementia. *Biological Psychiatry* **23**: 271–284.

Baddeley, A., Emslie, H. and Nimmo Smith, I. (1994). *Doors and people.* Thames Valley Test Company, Bury St. Edmunds.

Battersby, W.S., Bender, M.B., Pollack, M. and Kahn, R.L. (1956). Unilateral 'spatial agnosia' ('inattention') in patients with cerebral lesions. *Brain* **79**: 68–93.

Benton, A.L. (1973). Test de praxie constructive tri-dimensionnelle: Forme alternative pour la clinique et la recherche. *Revue de psychologie appliquée* **23**: 1–5.

Benton, A.L. and Hamisher, K. deS. (1989). *Multilingual aphasia examination.* AJA Associates, Iowa City.

Blessed, G., Tomlinson, B.E. and Roth, M. (1968). The association between quantitative measures of dementia and of senile changes in the cerebral grey matter of elderly subjects. *British Journal of Psychiatry* **114**: 797–811.

Brandt, J. (1991). The Hopkins Verbal Learning Test: Development of a new memory test with six equivalent forms. *Clinical Neuropsychologist* **5**: 125–142.

Conwell, Y., Forbes, N.T., Cox, C. and Caine, E.D. (1993). Validation of a measure of physical illness burden at autopsy: The Cumulative Illness Rating Scale. *Journal of the American Geriatric Society* **41**: 38–41.

Coughlan, A.K. and Hollows, S.E. (1985). *The Adult Memory and Information Processing Battery (AMIPB).* Psychology Department, St. James's University Hospital, Leeds.

De Renzi, E. and Vignolo, L.A. (1962). The token test: A sensitive test to detect disturbances in aphasics. *Brain* **85**: 665–678.

Enderby, P., Wood, V. and Wade, D. (1987). *Frenchay Aphasia Screening Test (FAST) test manual.* NFER-NELSON, Windsor, England.

Folstein, M.F., Folstein, S.E. and McHugh, P.R. (1975). Mini-Mental State; a practical method of grading the cognitive state of patients for the clinician. *Journal of Psychiatric Research* **12**: 189–198.

Fuld, P.A. (1981). *Fuld Object-Memory Evaluation.* Stoelting Instrument Company, Chicago, IL

Golden, C.J. (1978). *The Stroop Color and Word Test.* Psychological Assessment Resources, Odessa, FL.

Golden, C.J., Purisch, A.D., and Hammeke, T.A. (1985). *Luria-Nebraska*

Neuropsychological Battery: Forms I and II. Western Psychological Services, Los Angeles.

Golding, E. (1989). *The Middlesex Elderly Assessment of Mental State.* Thames Valley Test Company, Bury St. Edmunds.

Goldstein, K. and Scheerer, M. (1941). Abstract and concrete behaviour: An experimental study with specific tests. *Psychological Monographs* **53**: 1–150.

Goodglass, H. and Kaplan, E. (1983). *The Boston Diagnostic Aphasia Examination.* Lea and Febiger, Philadelphia, distributed by Psychological Assessment Resources, Odessa, FL.

Grewal, B.S. and Harward, L.R.C. (1984). Validation of a new Weigl scoring system in neurological diagnosis. *Medical Science* **12**: 602–603.

Hachinski, V.C., Iliff, L.D., Ziihka, E., Du Boulay, G.H., McAllister, V.L., Marshall, J., Russell, R.W.R. and Syman, L. (1975). Cerebral blood flow in dementia. *Archives of Neurology* **32**: 632–637.

Halstead, W.C. (1947) *Brain and intelligence.* University of Chicago Press: Chicago.

Heaton, R.K. (1991). *Wisconsin Card Sorting Test.* Psychological Assessment Resources, Odessa, FL.

Hooper, H.E. (1983). *Hooper Visual Organisation Test (VOT).* Western Psychological Services, Los Angeles.

Huppert, F.A., Brayne, C., Gill, C., Paykel, E.S., and Beardsall, L. (1995). CAMCOG—A concise neuropsychological test to assist dementia diagnosis: Socio-demographic determinants in an elderly population sample. *British Journal of Clinical Psychoogy* **34**: 529–542.

Jastak, J.F. and Wilkinson, G.S. (1984). *Wide Range Acheivement Test— revised.* Jastak Assessment Systems, Wilmington, DE.

Kaplan, E.F., Goodglass, H., and Weintraub, S. (1983). *The Boston Naming Test* (2nd edn). Lea and Febiger, Philadelphia.

Kendrick, D.C. (1985). *Kendrick Cognitive Tests for the Elderly.* NFER-NELSON, Windsor.

Maj, M., D'Elia, L., Satz, P., Jansen, R., Zandig, M., Uchiyama, C., Statace, F., Galderisi, S., Chevinsky, A. (1993). *Archives of Clinical Neuropsychology*, **8**, 123–35.

McDonald, C. (1969). Clinical heterogeneity in senile dementia. *British Journal of Psychiatry* **115**: 267–271.

McKeith, I.G., Galesko, D., Kosalle, K., Perry, E.K., Dickson, D.W., Hansen, L.A., *et al.* (1996). Consensus guidelines for the clinical and pathological diagnosis of dementia with Lewy bodies (DLB): report of the consortium on DLB international workshop. *Neurology*, **47**, 1113–24.

McKenna, P. and Warrington, E. (1983). *Graded Naming Test: Manual.* NFER-NELSON, Windsor.

McKhann, G., Drachman, D., Folstein, M.F., Katzman, R., Price, D. and

Stadlan, E.M. (1984). Clinical diagnosis of Alzheimer's disease: Report of the NINCDS-ADRDA Work Group under the auspices of Department of Health and Human Services Task Force on Alzheimer's Disease. *Neurology* **34**: 939–944.

Morris, J.C. (1993). The Clinical Dementia Rating (CDR)—Current version and scoring rules. *Neurology* **43**: 2412–2414.

Morris, J.C., Heyman, A., Mohs, R.C., Hughes, J.P., van Belle, G., Fillenbaum, G., Mellits, E.D., and Clark, C. (1989). The Consortium to Establish a Registry for Alzheimer's Disease (CERAD). Part 1. Clinical and neuropsychological assessment of Alzheimer's disease. *Neurology* **39**:1159–1165.

Nelson, H.E., and Willison, J. (1991). *The National Adult Reading Test (NART): Test Manual including new data supplement.* NFER-Nelson, Windsor, Berks, UK.

Pichot, P. and Brun, J.P. (1984). Short Self-Assessment Questionnaire on the depressive, asthenic and anxious dimensions *Annales Medico-Psycho - logiques* **142**: 862–865.

Price, JL. (1997). Diagnostic criteria for Alzheimer's disease. *Neurobiology of Aging* **18**: S67–S70.

Raven, J.C. (1965). *Guide to the standard progressive matrices.* H.K. Lewis, London.

Reisberg, B. (1988) Functional Assessment Staging (FAST) *Psycho - pharmacology* **24**: 653–655.

Reisberg, B., Ferris, S.H., DeLeon, M.J. and Crook, T. (1982). The Global Deterioration Scale for assessment of primary degenerative dementia. *American Journal of Psychiatry* **139**: 1136–1139.

Reisberg, B., Schneck, M.K., Ferris, S.H., *et al.* (1983). The Brief Cognitive Rating Scale (BCRS). Findings in primary degenerative dementia (PDD). *Psychopharmacology Bulletin* **19**: 734–739.

Rey, A. (1941). L'examen psychologique dans les cas d'encephalopathie traumatique. *Archives de psychologie* **28**: 286–340 (translated by Cormin, J. and Bylsma, F.W., 1993, *Clinical Neuropsychologist* **7**: 9–15).

Rey, A. (1964). *L'examen clinique en psychologie.* Presses Universitaires de France: Paris.

Roman, G.C., Tatemichi, T.K., Erkinjuntti, T., Cummings, J.L., Masdeu, J.C., Garcia, J.H., Amaducci, L., Orgogozo, J.M., Brun, A., Hofman, A., *et al.* (1993). Vascular dementia: diagnostic criteria for research studies. Report of the NINDS-AIREN International Workshop. *Neurology* **43**: 250–260.

Saxton, J.A., McGonigle-Gibson, K.L. and Swihart, A.A. (1988). An assessment device for the severely demented patient. *Journal of Clinical and Experimental Neuropsychology* **10**: 62 (abstract).

Shua-Haim, J., Koppuzha, G., and Gross, J. (1996). A simple scoring system for clock drawing in patients with Alzheimer's disease. *Journal of the American Geriatrics Society* **44**: 335.

Teng, E.L. and Chang Chui, H. (1987) The modified Mini-Mental State (3MS) Examination. *Journal of ClinicalPsychiatry* **48**: 314–318.

Towk, D., Wilcock, G.K., and Sumon, D.J. (1987). The KEW test—a study of reliability and validity. *Journal of Clinical and Experimental Geontology*, **9**, 245–56.

Warrington, E.K. and James, M. (1991). *Visual Object and Space Perception battery (VOSP)*. Thames Valley Test Company, Bury St. Edmunds.

Wechsler, D. (1981). *WAIS-R Manual*. The Psychological Corporation, New York.

Wechsler, D. (1987). *Wechsler Memory Scale—Revised*. The Psychological Corporation, San Antonio, TX.

Wilson, B.A., Cockburn, J. and Baddeley, A. (1995). *The Rivermead Behavioural Memory Test (RBMT)*. Thames Valley Test Company, Bury St. Edmunds.

World Health Organisation (1992). *The ICD-10 classification of mental and behavioural disorders*. WHO, Geneva.

Yesavage, J.A., Brink, T.L., Rose, T.L., Lum, O., Huang, V.S., *et al*. (1983). Development and validation of a geriatric depression screening scale: A preliminary report. *Journal of Psychiatric Research* **17**: 37–39.

Index

Note: References in **bold** indicate chapters